Contemporary Management and Controversies of Sarcoma

Editor

CHANDRAJIT P. RAUT

SURGICAL ONCOLOGY CLINICS OF NORTH AMERICA

www.surgonc.theclinics.com

Consulting Editor
NICHOLAS J. PETRELLI

October 2016 • Volume 25 • Number 4

ELSEVIER

1600 John F. Kennedy Boulevard ● Suite 1800 ● Philadelphia, Pennsylvania, 19103-2899

http://www.theclinics.com

SURGICAL ONCOLOGY CLINICS OF NORTH AMERICA Volume 25, Number 4
October 2016 ISSN 1055-3207, ISBN-13: 978-0-323-46339-3

Editor: John Vassallo (j.vassallo@elsevier.com)
Developmental Editor: Meredith Clinton

Surgical Oncology Clinics of North America (ISSN 1055-3207) is published quarterly by Elsevier Inc., 360 Park Avenue South, New York, NY 10010-1710. Months of publication are January, April, July, and October. Business and Editorial Offices: 1600 John F. Kennedy Blvd., Ste. 1800, Philadelphia, PA 19103-2899. Customer Service Office: 3251 Riverport Lane, Maryland Heights, MO 63043. Periodicals postage paid at New York, NY and additional mailing offices. Subscription prices are $290.00 per year (US individuals), $471.00 (US institutions) $100.00 (US student/resident), $330.00 (Canadian individuals), $596.00 (Canadian institutions), $205.00 (Canadian student/resident), $410.00 (foreign individuals), $596.00 (foreign institutions), and $205.00 (foreign student/resident). Foreign air speed delivery is included in all *Clinics* subscription prices. All prices are subject to change without notice. **POSTMASTER**: Send address changes to *Surgical Oncology Clinics of North America,* Elsevier Health Science Division, Subscription Customer Service, 3251 Riverport Lane, Maryland Heights, MO 63043. **Customer Service: 1-800-654-2452 (US and Canada). 314-447-8871 (outside US and Canada). Fax: 314-447-8029. E-mail: journalscustomerservice-usa@elsevier.com (for print support); journalsonline support-usa@elsevier.com (for online support).**

Reprints. For copies of 100 or more, of articles in this publication, please contact the Commercial Reprints Department, Elsevier Inc., 360 Park Avenue South, New York, New York 10010-1710. Tel. 212-633-3874; Fax: 212-633-3820; E-mail: reprints@elsevier.com.

Surgical Oncology Clinics of North America is covered in *MEDLINE/PubMed (Index Medicus)* and *EMBASE/ Excerpta Medica, Current Contents/Clinical Medicine, and ISI/BIOMED.*

Contributors

CONSULTING EDITOR

NICHOLAS J. PETRELLI, MD, FACS
Bank of America Endowed Medical Director, Helen F. Graham Cancer Center & Research Institute, Christiana Care Health Systems, Newark, Delaware; Professor of Surgery, Thomas Jefferson University, Philadelphia, Pennsylvania

EDITOR

CHANDRAJIT P. RAUT, MD, MSc
Associate Surgeon, Division of Surgical Oncology, Department of Surgery, Brigham and Women's Hospital, Surgery Director, Center for Sarcoma and Bone Oncology, Dana-Farber Cancer Institute, Associate Professor of Surgery, Harvard Medical School, Boston, Massachusetts

AUTHORS

MATTHEW G. CABLE, MD
Huntsman Cancer Institute, University of Utah, Salt Lake City, Utah

ROBERT J. CANTER, MD, MAS
Associate Professor of Surgery, Division of Surgical Oncology, Department of Surgery, University of California Davis Comprehensive Cancer Center, Davis School of Medicine, University of California, Sacramento, California

CHARLES N. CATTON, MD, FRCPC
Professor, Department of Radiation Oncology, University of Toronto; Radiation Medicine Program, Princess Margaret Cancer Centre, Toronto, Ontario, Canada

CHIARA COLOMBO, MD
Sarcoma Service, Department of Surgery, Fondazione IRCCS Istituto Nazionale dei Tumori, Milan, Italy

YOLONDA L. COLSON, MD, PhD
Professor of Surgery, Division of Thoracic Surgery, Department of Surgery, Brigham and Women's Hospital, Harvard Medical School, Boston, Massachusetts

AIMEE M. CRAGO, MD, PhD, FACS
Assistant Attending Surgeon, Sarcoma Disease Management Team; Gastric and Mixed Tumor Service, Department of Surgery, Memorial Sloan Kettering Cancer Center; Department of Surgery, Weill Cornell Medical College, New York, New York

BRIAN G. CZITO, MD
Gary Hock and Lynn Proctor Associate Professor, Department of Radiation Oncology, Duke University Medical Center, Durham, North Carolina

MARK A. DICKSON, MD
Assistant Attending, Sarcoma Disease Management Team; Sarcoma Oncology Service, Department of Medicine, Memorial Sloan Kettering Cancer Center; Department of Medicine, Weill Cornell Medical College, New York, New York

CHRISTOPHER S. DIGESU, MD
Clinical Research Fellow, Division of Thoracic Surgery, Department of Surgery, Brigham and Women's Hospital, Harvard Medical School, Boston, Massachusetts

LEONA A. DOYLE, MD
Department of Pathology, Brigham and Women's Hospital, Harvard Medical School, Boston, Massachusetts

SARAH M. DRY, MD
Professor, Department of Pathology & Laboratory Medicine, University of California, Los Angeles, Los Angeles, California

FRITZ C. EILBER, MD
Associate Professor of Surgery; Associate Professor of Molecular and Medical Pharmacology, Division of Surgical Oncology, University of California, Los Angeles, Los Angeles, California

MARCO FIORE, MD
Sarcoma Service, Department of Surgery, Fondazione IRCCS Istituto Nazionale dei Tumori, Milan, Italy

REBECCA A. GLADDY, MD, PhD, FACS, FRCSC
Assistant Professor, Department of Surgery, Mount Sinai Hospital, University of Toronto; Department of Surgical Oncology, Princess Margaret Cancer Centre, Toronto, Ontario, Canada

ALESSANDRO GRONCHI, MD
Sarcoma Service, Department of Surgery, Fondazione IRCCS Istituto Nazionale dei Tumori, Milan, Italy

ABHA GUPTA, MD, MSc, FRCPC
Associate Professor, Division of Pediatric Hematology/Oncology, Department of Pediatrics, The Hospital For Sick Children, University of Toronto; Department of Medical Oncology, Princess Margaret Cancer Centre, Toronto, Ontario, Canada

DAPHNE HOMPES, MD, PhD
Department of Surgical Oncology, University Hospitals Gasthuisberg Leuven, Leuven, Belgium

JYOTHI P. JAGANNATHAN, MD
Department of Imaging, Dana-Farber Cancer Institute; Department of Radiology, Brigham and Women's Hospital, Harvard Medical School, Boston, Massachusetts

AARON W. JAMES, MD
Department of Pathology, Johns Hopkins University, Baltimore, Maryland

VICKIE Y. JO, MD
Department of Pathology, Brigham and Women's Hospital, Harvard Medical School, Boston, Massachusetts

DAVID G. KIRSCH, MD, PhD
Barbara Levine University Professor, Departments of Radiation Oncology and Pharmacology & Cancer Biology, Duke University Medical Center, Durham, North Carolina

NICOLE A. LARRIER, MD, MSc
Assistant Professor, Department of Radiation Oncology, Duke University Medical Center, Durham, North Carolina

ALEXANDER J. LAZAR, MD, PhD
Department of Pathology, University of Texas MD Anderson Cancer Center, Houston, Texas

ANDREA MACNEILL, MD, FRCSC
Sarcoma Service, Department of Surgery, Fondazione IRCCS Istituto Nazionale dei Tumori, Milan, Italy; Department of Surgery, University of Toronto, Toronto, Ontario, Canada

JOHN T. MULLEN, MD
Division of Surgical Oncology, Massachusetts General Hospital, Associate Professor of Surgery, Harvard Medical School, Boston, Massachusetts

NIKHIL H. RAMAIYA, MD
Department of Imaging, Dana-Farber Cancer Institute; Department of Radiology, Brigham and Women's Hospital, Harvard Medical School, Boston, Massachusetts

R. LOR RANDALL, MD, FACS
Huntsman Cancer Institute, University of Utah, Salt Lake City, Utah

CHRISTINA L. ROLAND, MD
Department of Surgical Oncology, University of Texas MD Anderson Cancer Center, Houston, Texas

PIOTR RUTKOWSKI, MD, PhD
Department of Soft Tissue, Bone Sarcoma and Melanoma, Maria Sklodowska-Curie Memorial Cancer Center, Institute of Oncology, Warsaw, Poland

ELIZABETH SHURELL, MD
Department of Surgery, Memorial Sloan Kettering Cancer Center, New York, New York

ARUN SINGH, MD
Assistant Professor, Sarcoma Service, Division of Hematology/Oncology, University of California, Los Angeles, Santa Monica, California

KATHERINE THORNTON, MD
Center for Sarcoma and Bone Oncology, Dana-Farber Cancer Institute, Boston, Massachusetts

SREE HARSHA TIRUMANI, MD
Department of Imaging, Dana-Farber Cancer Institute; Department of Radiology, Brigham and Women's Hospital, Harvard Medical School, Boston, Massachusetts

KEILA E. TORRES, MD, PhD
Department of Surgical Oncology, University of Texas MD Anderson Cancer Center, Houston, Texas

ARA A. VAPORCIYAN, MD
Professor of Surgery, Division of Surgery, Department of Thoracic and Cardiovascular Surgery, University of Texas MD Anderson Cancer Center, Houston, Texas

WEI-LIEN WANG, MD
Department of Pathology, University of Texas MD Anderson Cancer Center, Houston, Texas

ORY WIESEL, MD
Clinical Fellow, Division of Thoracic Surgery, Department of Surgery, Brigham and Women's Hospital, Harvard Medical School, Boston, Massachusetts

Contents

The 4th edition of the World Health Organization (WHO) *Classification of Tumours of Soft Tissue and Bone* was published in February 2013. The 2013 WHO volume provides an updated classification scheme and reproducible diagnostic criteria, which are based on recent clinicopathologic studies and genetic and molecular data that facilitated refined definition of established tumor types, recognition of novel entities, and the development of novel diagnostic markers. This article reviews updates and changes in the classification of bone and soft tissue tumors from the 2002 volume.

Soft tissue sarcomas (STS) are heterogeneous malignant tumors that have nonspecific imaging features. A combination of clinical, demographic, and imaging characteristics can aid in the diagnosis. Imaging provides important information regarding the tumor extent, pretreatment planning, and surveillance of patients with STS. In this article, we illustrate the pertinent imaging characteristics of the commonly occurring STS and some uncommon sarcomas with unique imaging characteristics.

Soft tissue sarcomas comprise tumors originating from mesenchymal or connective tissue. Histologic grade is integral to prognosis. Because sarcoma management is multimodal, histologic subtype should inform optimum treatment. Appropriate biopsy and communication between surgeon and pathologist can help ensure a correct diagnosis. Treatment often involves surgical excision with wide margins and adjuvant radiotherapy. There is no consensus on what constitutes an adequate margin for histologic subtypes. An appreciation of how histology corresponds with tumor biology and surgical anatomic constraints is needed for management of this disease. Even with the surgical goal of wide resection being obtained, many patients do not outlive their disease.

After diagnosis of retroperitoneal sarcoma (RPS), detailed imaging and multidisciplinary discussion should guide treatment including surgical resection and in select cases, neoadjuvant therapy. Local recurrence is common in RPS and is associated with grade, histologic subtype, completeness of resection, and size. As guidelines to standardize RPS patient management emerge, expert pathologic assessment and management in centers of excellence are benchmarks of quality of care. The efficacy of current chemotherapy is limited and there is a critical need to understand the molecular basis of sarcoma so that new drug therapies are developed. Multicenter clinical trials are needed to limit opinion and controversy in this complex and challenging disease.

Breast sarcomas are a diverse group of neoplasms arising from the non-epithelial and mesenchymal tissues of the breast. Their behaviors vary from the more indolent tumors like cystosarcoma phyllodes to the extremely aggressive angiosarcoma. They should be approached in a similar fashion to their soft tissue sarcoma counterparts in other locations and managed by multidisciplinary sarcoma specialists with attention to wide-margin surgical excision. The use of adjuvant chemotherapy is controversial and should be discussed on a case-by-case basis and preferably given in the context of a clinical trial.

For decades, surgical resection of pulmonary metastases has been performed; despite limited randomized data, surgery is increasingly accepted as an integral part in the management of metastatic disease. Long-term results indicate resection is potentially curative with significantly improved survival following complete resection. Recurrence, however, is not uncommon with many patients undergoing repeat resection. With advancing surgical technique and adjuvant therapies, patients with high or recurrent tumor burden are increasingly afforded disease control and potential cure. In this review, the prognostic characteristics of pulmonary metastases from sarcoma, preoperative evaluation, operative technique, long-term outcomes, and management of complex patients are highlighted.

Radical surgery is the mainstay of therapy for primary resectable, localized gastrointestinal stromal tumors (GIST). Nevertheless, approximately 40% to 50% of patients with potentially curative resections develop recurrent or metastatic disease. The introduction of imatinib mesylate has revolutionized the therapy of advanced (inoperable and/or metastatic) GIST and has become the standard of care in treatment of patients with advanced GIST. This article discusses the proper selection of candidates for adjuvant and neoadjuvant treatment in locally advanced GIST, exploring the available evidence behind the combination of preoperative imatinib and surgery.

There are 3 biologic groups of liposarcoma: well-differentiated and dedifferentiated liposarcoma, myxoid/round cell liposarcoma, and pleomorphic liposarcoma. In all 3 groups, complete surgical resection is central in treatment aimed at cure and is based on grade. Radiation can reduce risk of local recurrence in high-grade lesions or minimize surgical morbidity in the myxoid/round cell liposarcoma group. The groups differ in chemosensitivity, so adjuvant chemotherapy is selectively used in histologies with metastatic potential but not in the resistant subtype dedifferentiated liposarcoma. Improved understanding of the genetic aberrations that lead to liposarcoma initiation is allowing for the rapid development of targeted therapies for liposarcoma.

Myxofibrosarcoma is a unique subtype of soft tissue sarcoma with a locally infiltrative behavior. High-quality MRI imaging is critical for preoperative planning. Wide surgical resection with a 2 cm soft tissue margin is the mainstay of treatment and can require complex vascular and plastic surgery reconstruction. Local recurrence is common, and a subset of patients with higher-grade lesions will develop distant metastases. Radiation may be beneficial in reducing local recurrence.

Malignant peripheral nerve sheath tumor (MPNST) is the sixth most common type of soft tissue sarcoma. Most MPNSTs arise in association with a peripheral nerve or preexisting neurofibroma. Neurofibromatosis type is the most important risk factor for MPNST. Tumor size and fludeoxyglucose F 18 avidity are among the most helpful parameters to distinguish MPNST from a benign peripheral nerve sheath tumor. The histopathologic diagnosis is predominantly a diagnosis of light microscopy. Immunohistochemical stains are most helpful to distinguish high-grade MPNST from its histologic mimics. Current surgical management of high-grade MPNST is similar to that of other high-grade soft tissue sarcomas.

Desmoid-type fibromatosis is a rare nonmetastasizing neoplasm with variable behavior. Recent discoveries into the biology of this disease hold promise for identifying prognostic and predictive features and novel therapeutic targets. Surgery has been the historical standard of care but carries considerable drawbacks in terms of high local recurrence rates and poor functional outcomes. Improved understanding of the natural history of desmoid-type fibromatosis has resulted in a paradigm shift toward nonoperative management. Effective medical treatment options include nonsteroidal anti-inflammatory drugs, hormone therapy, cytotoxic chemotherapy, and targeted agents. A treatment algorithm has been proposed with the objective of optimizing treatment.

Dermatofibrosarcoma protuberans (DFSP) is a rare dermal soft tissue sarcoma characterized by a typically indolent clinical course. The greatest clinical challenge in management of DFSP is achieving local control. There is vigorous debate in the literature as to the optimal surgical approach to these tumors. The choice between wide local excision and Mohs micrographic surgery for DFSP should be governed by the attainment of three goals: (1) to completely excise the tumor with negative margins, tantamount to cure; (2) to preserve function, optimize cosmesis, and minimize morbidity of resection; and (3) to minimize cost and inconvenience to the patient and the health care system at large.

Soft tissue sarcomas are rare mesenchymal cancers that pose a treatment challenge. Although small superficial soft tissue sarcomas can be managed by surgery alone, adjuvant radiotherapy, in addition to limb-sparing surgery, substantially increases local control of extremity sarcomas. Compared with postoperative radiotherapy, preoperative radiotherapy doubles the risk of a wound complication, but decreases the risk for late effects, which are generally irreversible. For retroperitoneal sarcomas, intraoperative radiotherapy can be used to safely escalate the radiation dose to the tumor bed. Patients with newly diagnosed sarcoma should be evaluated before surgery by a multidisciplinary team that includes a radiation oncologist.

Since preoperative chemotherapy has been clearly shown to improve outcomes for patients with Ewing sarcoma, rhabdomyosarcoma, and osteosarcoma, practitioners have attempted to extend the use of adjuvant/neoadjuvant chemotherapy to other types of adult soft tissue sarcoma. Given the high risk of distant recurrence and disease-specific death for patients with soft tissue sarcoma tumors larger than 10 cm, these patients should be considered candidates for neoadjuvant chemotherapy as well as investigational therapies. Yet, potential toxicity from cytotoxic chemotherapy is substantial, and there remains little consensus and wide variation regarding the indications for use of chemotherapy in the adjuvant/neoadjuvant setting.

SURGICAL ONCOLOGY CLINICS OF NORTH AMERICA

FORTHCOMING ISSUES

January 2017
Anal Canal Cancers
Cathy Eng, *Editor*

April 2017
Advances in Esophageal and Gastric Cancer
David Ilson, *Editor*

July 2017
Radiation Oncology
Adam Raben, *Editor*

RECENT ISSUES

July 2016
Lung Cancer
Mark J. Krasna, *Editor*

April 2016
Pancreatic Neoplasms
Nipun B. Merchant, *Editor*

January 2016
Endocrine Tumors
Douglas L. Fraker, *Editor*

RELATED INTEREST

Surgical Clinics of North America, October 2016 (Vol. 96, Issue 5)
New Trends in the Treatment of Sarcoma
Jeffrey M. Farma and Andrea S. Porpiglia, *Editors*
Available at: http://www.surgical.theclinics.com/

Foreword

Sarcomas 2016

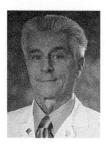

Nicholas J. Petrelli, MD, FACS
Consulting Editor

This issue of the *Surgical Oncology Clinics of North America* discusses the topic of sarcomas. The guest editor is Chandrajit P. Raut, MD, MSc. Dr Raut is Associate Professor of Surgery at the Harvard Medical School and Director of Surgical Oncology at the Dana Farber Cancer Institute in Boston, Massachusetts. Dr Raut completed his general surgery residency at the Massachusetts General Hospital, and this was followed by a fellowship in surgical oncology at the University of Texas MD Anderson Cancer Center.

The last issue of the *Surgical Oncology Clinics of North America* that dealt with soft tissue sarcomas was in April of 2002, where the guest editor was John M. Kane, MD from the Roswell Park Cancer Institute in Buffalo, New York. In that issue, Dr Raut had contributed an article devoted to limb salvage and the role of amputation for extremity soft tissue sarcomas. Dr Raut's experience with sarcomas makes him well qualified to be the guest editor of this issue of *Surgical Oncology Clinics of North America*.

Dr Raut has assembled an outstanding group of physicians to discuss this topic. When it comes to treating patients with the diagnosis of sarcoma, there is no question that it is imperative that the patient be approached by a multidisciplinary team. Dr Raut has brought together experts in the field of radiology, surgical oncology, pathology, radiation oncology, and medical oncology to discuss this important topic. For example, there is an excellent article discussing refinements in sarcoma classification by Drs Vickie Y. Jo and Leona A. Doyle from the Department of Pathology at the Brigham and Women's Hospital in Boston. The article on imaging in soft tissue sarcomas by Dr Jyothi P. Jagannathan and associates from the Dana Farber Cancer Institute describes the challenge of differentiating benign and malignant soft tissue tumors as well as the various histologic subtypes of sarcoma on imaging.

Last, the article on "Retroperitoneal Sarcomas: Fact, Opinion, and Controversy" by Rebecca Gladdy and associates has an extensive discussion on the diagnostic challenges of retroperitoneal sarcomas and their management. Outcomes and recurrence are also described in detail in a section in this article.

Surg Oncol Clin N Am 25 (2016) xiii–xiv
http://dx.doi.org/10.1016/j.soc.2016.05.015
1055-3207/16/$ – see front matter © 2016 Published by Elsevier Inc.

surgonc.theclinics.com

I would like to thank Dr Chandrajit Raut for this excellent issue of the *Surgical Oncology Clinics of North America* and his colleagues for taking the time to complete outstanding articles on this subject.

Nicholas J. Petrelli, MD, FACS
Helen F. Graham Cancer Center
& Research Institute
Christiana Care Health Systems
4701 Ogletown-Stanton Road, Suite 1233
Newark, DE 19713, USA

E-mail address:
npetrelli@christianacare.org

Preface

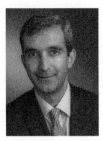

Chandrajit P. Raut, MD, MSc
Editor

Sarcomas are among the oldest malignancies known, identified in mummies from ancient Egypt and even further back in dinosaur fossils. Despite being recognized for such a long time, their rarity complicates effective management, as many clinicians may only encounter patients with sarcomas a handful of times during their career.

Historically, much of what has been reported about soft tissue sarcomas has been categorized by site of origin. However, it has become increasingly apparent over the last several decades that histology-specific management should be central to the approach to sarcoma care, and that is reflected in the organization of this special issue devoted to sarcomas. Herein, we have compiled a series of articles relevant to clinical practice. They focus on some of the most controversial, contemporary topics in sarcoma care.

The first two articles focus on histologic and radiographic features of sarcomas, respectively. The first reflects changes within and since the 2013 World Health Organization Classification. Most sarcomas are now classified according to differentiation as determined by morphologic, immunohistochemical, and genetic characteristics. Importantly, terms such as hemangiopericytoma and malignant fibrous histiocytoma (MFH) are now eliminated.

The second article dovetails nicely with the first. Organized to reflect current classification, this article details how radiographic findings coupled with pattern of spread and other findings can help winnow the differential diagnosis of the potential histologies, but cannot in the absence of a diagnostic biopsy confirm an exact diagnosis.

SITE-SPECIFIC SARCOMA MANAGEMENT

The next four articles describe site-specific sarcomas, emphasizing the importance of histology for each site. The article on extremity soft tissue sarcomas covers general management principles and highlights the lack of consensus on what constitutes an adequate margin, which can be histology specific.

Surg Oncol Clin N Am 25 (2016) xv–xvii
http://dx.doi.org/10.1016/j.soc.2016.07.011
1055-3207/16/© 2016 Published by Elsevier Inc.

surgonc.theclinics.com

The article on retroperitoneal sarcoma sorts through fact, opinion, and controversy, including the recent discussions about extended resections. Patterns of failure for retroperitoneal sarcomas are different than for sarcomas at other body sites and are further compounded by histology-specific behavior.

The next article on breast sarcomas covers a variety of different histologies arising in the breast, spanning the spectrum from the often indolent phyllodes to the aggressive angiosarcoma, including, most commonly, radiation-associated angiosarcoma.

Finally, the article on pulmonary metastases highlights the fact that although pulmonary metastasectomies are performed commonly, they are not guided by phase III trials but rather by retrospective historical data. Nevertheless, data suggest that long disease-free intervals and margin-negative resections have prognostic value.

HISTOLOGY-SPECIFIC MANAGEMENT

The emphasis of this issue then shifts to specific sarcoma histologies. This section starts with a comprehensive article on gastrointestinal stromal tumors, now recognized as the most common sarcoma subtype.

The article on liposarcomas stresses the key differences between what are now recognized as a heterogeneous group of four distinct diseases with different molecular events, different presentations, and different responses to systemic therapy.

The article on myxofibrosarcoma details the unique behavior of this subtype with a high predilection for tenacious, repeated local recurrence. It can be challenging to distinguish myxofibrosarcomas from unclassified pleomorphic sarcomas, both of which used to fall into the now abandoned MFH classification.

The article on malignant peripheral nerve sheath tumors describes its association with type 1 neurofibromatosis and the important role of PET scans in guiding treatment planning.

Desmoid tumors, the subject of the next article, are technically benign clonal proliferations without a propensity for metastasis. There has been a significant shift over the last decade away from aggressive multimodal management to initial watchful waiting when appropriate.

The final article in this section focuses on dermatofibrosarcoma protuberans and the roles of wide local excision and Moh micrographic surgery, another controversial topic.

NEOADJUVANT AND ADJUVANT THERAPY

The last two articles focus on radiation therapy and chemotherapy. The former focuses on radiation's role as a local therapy whose efficacy should be assessed by its impact on local control, not tumor shrinkage. However, there can be significant consequences to radiation therapy, in either the preoperative (wound complications) or postoperative setting (fibrosis, edema, and joint stiffness).

The last article addresses the controversy over the role of adjuvant and neoadjuvant chemotherapy for primary sarcomas, with experts passionate on both sides. Once again, histology-specific data are discussed.

I hope that this collection of articles provides an informative framework for clinical care. I would like to thank the authors for thoughtfully crafting their detailed and balanced articles, all submitted well in advance of the publishing deadline. This issue would not have been possible without Meredith Clinton, Developmental Editor, who has kept me on track—thank you for your guidance. And finally, I would like to thank Dr Nicholas Petrelli for the opportunity to work on this issue.

Chandrajit P. Raut, MD, MSc
Division of Surgical Oncology
Department of Surgery
Brigham and Women's Hospital
Center for Sarcoma and Bone Oncology
Dana-Farber Cancer Institute
Harvard Medical School
75 Francis Street
Boston, MA 02115, USA

E-mail address:
craut@bwh.harvard.edu

Refinements in Sarcoma Classification in the Current 2013 World Health Organization *Classification of Tumours of Soft Tissue and Bone*

Vickie Y. Jo, MD*, Leona A. Doyle, MD

KEYWORDS

- Sarcoma • Soft tissue • Bone • Tumor • Classification • Histology
- World Health Organization

KEY POINTS

- The 2013 World Health Organization *Classification of Tumours of Soft Tissue and Bone* provides updated and reproducible diagnostic criteria based on morphologic, immunohistochemical, and genetic/molecular data.
- Most soft tissue and bone tumors can be classified according to differentiation as determined by morphologic, immunohistochemical, and genetic features.
- The numerous advances in the genetic/molecular features of soft tissue and bone tumors has facilitated more accurate classification and the development of useful diagnostic tools.

INTRODUCTION

The fourth edition of the World Health Organization (WHO) *Classification of Tumours of Soft Tissue and Bone*[1] was published in 2013, and represents an updated consensus text assembled by an expert working group. The WHO classification propagates reproducible diagnostic criteria and is organized by tumor type as determined by morphologic, immunohistochemical, and genetic features. The classification of soft tissue and bone tumors has evolved considerably in the 11 years since the third volume,[2] primarily because of genetic insights that have led to the development of useful diagnostic markers, reclassification of certain entities, and recognition of novel distinct

Disclosures: The authors have nothing to disclose.
Department of Pathology, Brigham and Women's Hospital, Harvard Medical School, 75 Francis Street, Boston, MA 02115, USA
* Corresponding author.
E-mail address: vjo@partners.org

Surg Oncol Clin N Am 25 (2016) 621–643
http://dx.doi.org/10.1016/j.soc.2016.05.001
1055-3207/16/$ – see front matter © 2016 Elsevier Inc. All rights reserved.

tumor types. For soft tissue and bone neoplasms, this consensus work is important given the diagnostic challenges caused by the rarity of sarcomas, diversity of tumor types, and rapid rate of immunohistochemical and genetic/molecular advances. The WHO classification stratifies soft tissue and bone tumors into 4 categories based on clinical behavior: (1) benign; (2) intermediate, locally aggressive; (3) intermediate, rarely metastasizing; and (4) malignant (ie, sarcoma). Accurate pathologic diagnosis is critical for appropriate prognostication and management, and requires correlation with clinical and radiologic data. This article reviews updates in the 2013 WHO classification (as well as new findings since its publication), outlining changes from the 2002 volume; although the focus of this article is sarcoma classification, selected benign tumors are also reviewed.

TUMORS OF SOFT TISSUE
Adipocytic Tumors

No major changes in the category of adipocytic tumors were effected, with the exception of the removal of the terms round cell liposarcoma and mixed-type liposarcoma. Myxoid liposarcoma is graded based on cellularity using a 3-tier system (low, intermediate, and high); transition between different grades is often seen within a tumor. Histologic grade is prognostic and high-grade tumors show greater risk for recurrence, metastasis, and tumor-related death, thus tumors are classified according to the highest grade present. Although some high-grade myxoid liposarcomas show a predominance of round cell morphology (hence previously classified as round cell liposarcoma), the hypercellular high-grade areas more commonly show a spindle cell morphology. All myxoid liposarcomas, regardless of grade, harbor FUS-DDIT3 gene fusion,[3] or rarely an alternate EWSR1-DDIT3 fusion.[4]

Most tumors previously classified as mixed-type liposarcoma are now considered to represent unusual examples of dedifferentiated liposarcoma, based on currently available immunohistochemical and molecular studies that confirm the presence of amplification of chromosome 12q13-15. Amplification of 12q13-15 (via supernumerary ring or giant marker chromosomes) results in overexpression of the encoded gene products, MDM2 and CDK4. Since 2002, MDM2 and CDK4 immunohistochemistry and/or fluorescence in situ hybridization for MDM2 gene amplification have come into widespread use for the diagnosis of atypical lipomatous tumor (ALT)/well-differentiated liposarcoma (WDLPS) and dedifferentiated liposarcoma (DDLPS).[5] In addition to enabling accurate reclassification of mixed-type liposarcoma, these immunohistochemical and molecular studies also facilitate the diagnosis of retroperitoneal lipoma and exclude the more likely possibility of WDLPS at this anatomic site; the former follows a benign clinical course,[6,7] unlike WDLPS, which requires surgical resection given its risk for recurrence and dedifferentiation.

Note that although the 2013 WHO classification lists the term ALT as the section heading, it is pointed out that the retention of WDLPS in practice is still appropriate for tumors in sites at which complete resection is often not feasible, such as the mediastinum and retroperitoneum, and there is associated significant morbidity by locally aggressive growth, recurrence, and extensive surgical resections that often requires removal of multiple organs.

DDLPS, previously defined as a nonlipogenic sarcoma, is now known to occasionally show homologous lipoblastic differentiation by having morphologic features indistinguishable from pleomorphic liposarcoma.[8] Since publication of the 2013 WHO classification, a subset of such lipogenic DDLPS have been reported to show low nuclear grade.[9] It has also recently been suggested that the histologic grade of DDLPS is prognostically significant, with one study showing 5-year survival rates of 93%, 57%, and 21% associated with grade 1, 2, and 3, respectively, of retroperitoneal liposarcoma graded according to the French National Federation of the Centers for the Fight Against Cancer grading system, as well as worse survival for tumors with heterologous myogenic and rhabdomyoblastic differentiation.[10]

In addition, the benign tumor chondroid lipoma is now known to harbor the recurrent translocation t(11;16) (q13;p13), resulting in *C11orf95-MKL2* fusion,[11] which was confirmed in a larger study of 8 cases after the 2013 publication.[12]

Fibroblastic/Myofibroblastic Tumors

The pathobiology of many neoplasms in this category has been updated to reflect significant genetic and molecular discoveries. Two entities are no longer included here: myofibroma/myofibromatosis (now described under pericytic tumors) and giant cell angiofibroma, which is now listed as a synonym for extrapleural solitary fibrous tumor (SFT).

The 2013 WHO classification includes giant cell fibroblastoma and dermatofibrosarcoma protuberans (DFSP), which were formerly classified in the WHO skin tumor volume. Both giant cell fibroblastoma and DFSP are characterized by the translocation t(17;22) (q21;q13) (resulting in *PDGFB-COL1A1* fusion),[13,14] and occasionally occur together as hybrid tumors. Giant cell fibroblastoma shows frequent local recurrence but has no metastatic potential; DFSP also shows locally aggressive behavior and can metastasize if it undergoes fibrosarcomatous transformation.

Nodular fasciitis was long considered to be a reactive process, because of self-limited presentation of rapid growth with spontaneous regression over the course of months. On histology, some cases may be worrisome for sarcoma, especially if biopsied during the active growth phase when abundant mitotic activity is present. Nodular fasciitis is now understood to represent a transient neoplasia with the discovery of a recurrent *MYH9-USP6* gene fusion resulting from translocation t(17p;22q) (p13;q13.1).[15]

Mammary-type myofibroblastoma, cellular angiofibroma, and the adipocytic tumor spindle cell lipoma/pleomorphic lipoma (all benign tumors), have long been appreciated to share morphologic features and are now known to share the genetic features of consistent 13q and 16q rearrangements or deletions.[16–18] Aberrations involving the 13q14 locus include the region encoding the tumor suppressor gene *Retinoblastoma* (Rb); after publication of the 2013 WHO classification it has been reported that immunohistochemical detection of loss of Rb expression secondary to 13q14 rearrangement is characteristic of mammary-type myofibroblastoma, cellular angiofibroma, and spindle cell lipoma/pleomorphic lipoma.[19,20] In addition, a subset of cellular angiofibroma is now known to show severe cytologic atypia or sarcomatous transformation; despite the worrisome histologic features, such tumors do not show increased recurrence risk compared with conventional cellular angiofibroma.[21]

For extrapleural SFT, the prior synonym hemangiopericytoma has now been omitted. Since publication of the WHO volume, there have been several significant advances in the understanding of SFT. SFTs are characterized by the *NAB2-STAT6* fusion oncogene resulting from inversion of 2 genes located on chromosome 12q13[22,23]; this intrachromosomal fusion cannot be detected by conventional cytogenetic methods. *NAB2-STAT6* fusion results in overexpression of STAT6, immunohistochemistry for which is highly sensitive and specific for SFT.[24,25]

Myxoinflammatory fibroblastic sarcoma is now known to harbor the translocation t(1;10) (p22–31;q24–25); this is also a feature of the newly described entity hemosiderotic fibrolipomatous tumor (classified under tumors or uncertain differentiation).

Myxoinflammatory fibroblastic sarcoma may recur but rarely metastasizes, hence the introduction of the synonym atypical myxoinflammatory fibroblastic tumor. Tumors with hybrid features of both myxoinflammatory fibroblastic sarcoma and hemosiderotic fibrolipomatous tumor are now recognized.[26,27]

Low-grade fibromyxoid sarcoma (LGFMS) is characterized by the translocation t(7;16) (q33;p11) resulting in the FUS-CREB3L2 fusion gene.[28] Some cases have alternate fusions with EWSR1 in lieu of FUS and in such instances CREB3L1 (encoded on 11p11) is the fusion partner; this occurs more frequently in tumors with hybrid LGFMS and sclerosing epithelioid fibrosarcoma (SEF) or in pure SEF.[29–32] MUC4 is a newly described immunohistochemical marker that was shown to have high sensitivity and specificity for LGFMS and SEF[30,33] after overexpression in LGFMS was identified by gene expression studies.[34] LGFMS shows low recurrence and metastatic rates within the first 5 years, but rates increase (up to 50%) over the course of decades after initial diagnosis. In contrast, SEF shows high rates of recurrence, and metastases occur in up to 80% of patients.

Recognition of distinct morphologic variants of existing tumor types has also been facilitated by the increased understanding of defining immunohistochemical and genetic features. One such example is the epithelioid variant of inflammatory myofibroblastic tumor (IMT), which has a characteristic ALK-RANBP2 gene fusion that results in a characteristic nuclear membrane staining pattern for ALK immunohistochemistry, because RANBP2 localizes ALK to the nuclear membrane.[35] This epithelioid variant is important to recognize because it shows far more aggressive biological behavior than conventional IMT, and is considered by some investigators to be better designated as epithelioid inflammatory myofibroblastoma sarcoma because of its high rate of metastasis and death from disease.

So-Called Fibrohistiocytic Tumors

The most significant change in this category is the abandonment of the outdated (and largely meaningless) term malignant fibrous histiocytoma (MFH). Most tumors previously classified as MFH can now be classified as specific sarcoma types with currently available immunohistochemical and genetic/molecular tests. Some sarcomas remain unclassified or undifferentiated, and are discussed in the newly introduced section on undifferentiated/unclassified sarcomas (discussed later in this article).

No other major changes were made in this section. Both localized and diffuse types of tenosynovial giant cell tumors are now known to harbor translocations involving the CSF1 gene (encoded on chromosome 1p13), most frequently with COL6A3 (encoded on chromosome 2q37).[36–38]

Smooth Muscle Tumors

The only change in this tumor group is the removal of angioleiomyoma, which is now classified under pericytic (perivascular) tumors (discussed later).

Pericytic (Perivascular) Tumors

Several classification changes were made in this section. This category now includes angioleiomyoma, a benign tumor characterized by perivascular concentric arrangement of smooth muscle cells. Myopericytomas now include myofibromas (previously classified as a fibroblastic/myofibroblastic tumor) based on the morphologic continuum between these two tumors.

The 2013 WHO classification revised recommendations for the designation of glomus tumors as malignant and of uncertain malignant potential. Malignant glomus tumors applies to tumors having marked nuclear atypia and any mitotic activity, or if atypical mitotic figures are present. Tumor size greater than 2.0 cm and deep location are no longer criteria for malignancy, and tumors with these features (and without nuclear atypia) are now considered to be glomus tumors of uncertain malignant potential. Glomus tumors may be associated with type 1 neurofibromatosis,[39,40] and *BRAF* (V600E) and *KRAS* (G12A) mutations occur in some sporadic cases.[41] Since publication of the 2013 WHO classification, *NOTCH* mutations (of either *NOTCH2* or *NOTCH3*) have also been described in glomus tumors.[42]

Skeletal Muscle Tumors

The major change in this section is that spindle cell/sclerosing rhabdomyosarcoma (RMS) is now considered a distinct entity constituting a morphologic continuum; both spindle and sclerosing subtypes were previously considered to be variants of embryonal RMS (**Fig. 1**). Clinicopathologic and genetic differences have been recognized in spindle cell/sclerosing RMS. In pediatric patients, spindle cell RMS most frequently arises in paratesticular sites, and is associated with a more favorable outcome compared with other RMS subtypes. In contrast, spindle cell RMS in adults more frequently arise in the head and neck, and are associated with a significantly worse outcome than in children, with up to 50% risk for recurrence and metastasis.[43] Although many spindle cell/sclerosing RMSs harbor recurrent *NCOA2* and *VGLL2* rearrangements in congenital/infantile tumors,[44,45] a separate subset in children and adults has recurrent *MyoD1* mutations.[46,47]

Vascular Tumors

The 2013 WHO classification includes updates in the molecular genetics of several entities, as well as the introduction of the newly recognized tumor, pseudomyogenic hemangioendothelioma.

Pseudomyogenic (epithelioid sarcomalike) hemangioendothelioma is a recently recognized entity with distinct clinicopathologic and genetic features.[48–50] Tumors most frequently arise in the limbs of young adult men, and have a distinctive clinical presentation as multifocal discontiguous nodules involving multiple tissue planes (dermal, subcutaneous, subfascial, intramuscular, and intraosseous) (**Fig. 2A**). Pseudomyogenic hemangioendothelioma has the microscopic appearance of uniform

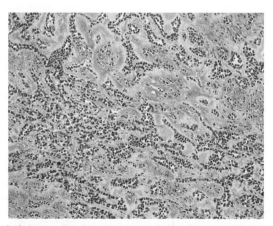

Fig. 1. Sclerosing rhabdomyosarcoma is composed of small to medium-sized cells with variable amounts of eosinophilic cytoplasm, embedded in a densely sclerotic stroma, and often producing a pseudovascular appearance (H&E, 200×).

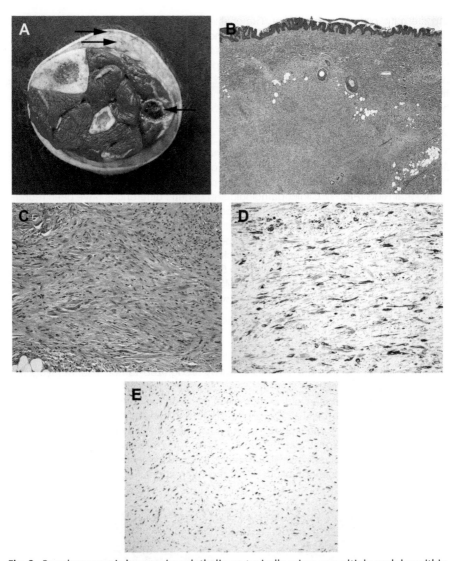

Fig. 2. Pseudomyogenic hemangioendothelioma typically arises as multiple nodules within different tissue planes; in this case nodules can be seen in skin, subcutaneous tissue, and soleus muscle (*A, arrows*). Skin lesions have a vaguely circumscribed nodular appearance but infiltrative edges (H&E, 40×) (*B*). The tumor cells grow in fascicles and are typically spindled with mild cytologic atypia and pleomorphism; the eosinophilic cytoplasm imparts a myoid appearance to the cells (H&E, 200×) (*C*). The characteristic immunoprofile is expression of cytokeratin AE1/AE3 (200×) (*D*) and endothelial markers such as ERG, which shows nuclear reactivity in tumor cells (400×) (*E*).

plump myoid-appearing spindle cells distributed singly or in sheets and loose fascicles (**Fig. 2**B, C), with the characteristic immunophenotype of positivity for cytokeratin AE1/AE3 (**Fig. 2**D) and expression of vascular markers ERG (**Fig. 2**E) and CD31; CD34 and desmin are negative. This tumor is characterized by the translocation t(7:19) (q22;q13), which results in a *SERPINE-FOSB* fusion gene.[50] Despite the worrisome and dramatic clinical presentation as well as frequent local recurrences or regional development of new nodules, most cases seem to follow a fairly indolent course and distant metastasis is infrequent, although rare cases showing an aggressive clinical course and pulmonary metastases have been reported.[51,52] Conservative management via local control by surgical resection or curettage of bone lesions is currently the mainstay of treatment.

It is now known that epithelioid hemangioendothelioma (EHE) is characterized by the recurrent translocation t(1;3) (p36;q23–25), which results in the *WWTR1-CAMTA1* fusion gene.[53,54] It was further elucidated via breakpoint analysis that multifocal EHE likely represents monoclonal metastases rather than synchronous primary tumors.[55] Since the 2013 WHO publication, CAMTA1 expression by immunohistochemistry has been shown to be a useful diagnostic marker for EHE.[56] Another recent study found recurrent *YAP1-TFE3* fusion genes in a distinct subset of epithelioid EHE that occurs most frequently in young adults and morphologically shows abundant eosinophilic cytoplasm and well-formed vascular channels.[57] EHE shows overall indolent clinical behavior but up to 30% of tumors eventually metastasize. A risk stratification scheme for EHE has been proposed based on 1 large study that reported that tumors larger than 3.0 cm and having more than 3 mitoses per 50 high-power fields (HPF) were associated with 59% 5-year survival, in contrast with 100% 5-year disease-specific survival in patients with tumors lacking these features.[58]

Some insights have been gained into the genetics of angiosarcomas in the past decade. Most secondary angiosarcomas associated with radiation treatment or pre-existing lymphedema are associated with *MYC* gene amplification, and *FLT4* coamplification is identified in 25% of cases[59–61]; *MYC* amplification can be shown by corresponding MYC protein expression using immunohistochemistry, and this is particularly helpful in distinguishing radiation-associated angiosarcoma from atypical postradiation vascular proliferation, which does not show *MYC* amplification or overexpression. However, *MYC* amplification is also present in a subset of primary angiosarcoma[62] and therefore these methods cannot be used to determine whether a given angiosarcoma is radiation associated or not. *KDR* mutations are also present in up to 10% of primary and secondary angiosarcomas.[63,64] *CIC* gene rearrangements have recently been reported in a subset of angiosarcomas, predominantly in young patients.[64] Although angiosarcomas have a wide morphologic spectrum, the histologic grade is not predictive of biological behavior.[65]

Chondro-Osseous Tumors

There were no major changes in this category.

Gastrointestinal Stromal Tumors

The 2013 WHO classification now includes gastrointestinal stromal tumors (GISTs), which had previously been part of the WHO volume on gastrointestinal tumors. The National Comprehensive Cancer Network (NCCN) guidelines for risk stratification are now widely used in reporting GISTs. The guidelines were first established in 2006 and then modified in 2010,[66] and are based on anatomic site, tumor size, and mitotic count, features determined to be highly predictive of malignant behavior in several large retrospective studies.[67,68]

GIST classification now reflects numerous advances in genetic characterization and subsequent phenotypic correlations. Most GISTs harbor oncogenic mutations in the tyrosine kinase receptor gene *KIT*, and a smaller subset have *PDGFRA* mutations; both result in constitutive activation of the type III receptor tyrosine kinase family. Most of these conventional GISTs have a spindle or mixed spindle and epithelioid morphology; epithelioid-predominant morphology is often associated with *PDGFRA* mutation or succinate dehydrogenase (SDH) deficiency. SDH-deficient GISTs are a newly recognized category of GIST and were first recognized among pediatric GISTs (and therefore initially known as pediatric-type GIST), having the distinct features of wild-type *KIT* and *PDGFRA* mutational status, exclusive location in the stomach with a typical multinodular growth pattern within the gastric wall (**Fig. 3**A), epithelioid morphology (**Fig. 3**B), and frequent lymph node metastases.[69] SDH deficiency results from dysfunction of the mitochondrial SDH complex of the Krebs cycle, secondary to inactivation of any of the SDH subunit genes (*SDHA*, *SDHB*, *SDHC*, or *SDHD*) by mutation or dysfunction by other mechanisms (such as SDHC promoter hypermethylation), and correlates with loss of expression of SDHB by immunohistochemistry (**Fig. 3**C).[70–72] Immunohistochemical loss of SDHB is caused by mutations or dysfunction in any of the 4 subunits, whereas loss of both SDHB and SDHA is seen only in the presence of *SDHA* mutation.[73–75] The behavior of SDH-deficient tumors cannot be predicted using conventional NCCN risk stratification; despite frequent lymph node metastases (which are exceptionally rare in conventional GIST) the overall clinical behavior is indolent. SDH-deficient GIST is also imatinib resistant, but in most cases shows clinical response to second-generation and third-generation tyrosine kinase inhibitors, such as sunitinib, sorafenib, and dasatinib.[76] Most SDH-deficient GISTs are sporadic, but a subset arise in the setting of Carney triad (GIST, paraganglioma,

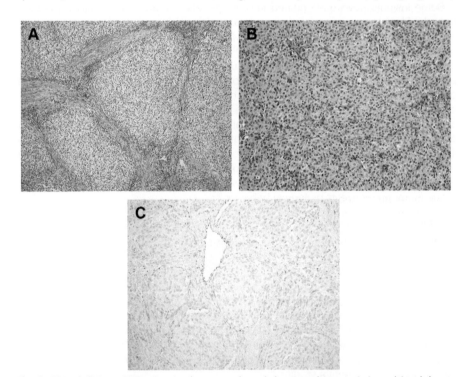

Fig. 3. SDH-deficient GIST arises in the stomach and shows a characteristic multinodular or plexiform architecture (H&E, 40×) (*A*). The tumor cells are usually epithelioid, grow in a nested pattern, and have mild cytologic atypia and abundant palely eosinophilic cytoplasm (H&E, 100×) (*B*). Similar to most GIST, SDH-deficient GIST expresses KIT and DOG1, but is differentiated by loss of cytoplasmic expression of SDHB in tumor cells, which is normally expressed in all cells, including endothelium and inflammatory cells, as shown (100×) (*C*).

pulmonary chondroma) or the autosomal dominant Carney-Stratakis syndrome (characterized by GIST and paraganglioma), which is caused by germline *SDH* mutations.[77,78] Identification of SDH-deficient GIST thus has strong clinical implications with regard to prognostication and therapeutics, and patients should be referred for genetic counseling to assess for possible inherited disorders.

Nerve Sheath Tumors

Nerve sheath tumors are now included in the 2013 WHO volume, although no major changes in the classification of malignant peripheral nerve sheath tumors were introduced. Several new subtypes of benign tumors were added, including hybrid tumors that have features of more than 1 type of conventional nerve sheath tumor. The most common is hybrid schwannoma and perineurioma, which is typically sporadic,[79] whereas hybrid neurofibroma/schwannoma is associated with type 1 neurofibromatosis.[80]

Tumors of Uncertain Differentiation

There were 4 tumor types included for the first time in this category: acral fibromyxoma, atypical fibroxanthoma, hemosiderotic fibrolipomatous tumor (HFLT), and phosphaturic mesenchymal tumor. Many existing entities have been further characterized by immunohistochemical and molecular advances.

Acral fibromyxoma (or digital fibromyxoma) is a benign tumor that arises in subungual/periungual sites on the hands or feet.[81,82] Atypical fibroxanthoma (AFX) is a benign dermal tumor that, when strictly defined by complete confinement to the dermis, has no risk for recurrence of metastasis. AFX often has microscopic features of a pleomorphic sarcoma caused by the presence of marked cytologic atypia and pleomorphism, and thus requires complete excision for thorough evaluation of the lesion base in order to exclude the presence of invasion of tumor into subcutaneous tissue, in which case the diagnosis of pleomorphic dermal sarcoma is applied.

HFLT is a locally aggressive tumor that frequently arises on the distal lower extremities of adult women[83,84] and shares the same translocation t(1;10) as myxoinflammatory fibroblastic sarcoma; hybrid tumors of these entities may occur. HFLT is composed of an admixture of adipocytes and bland spindle cells with hemosiderin deposition and lymphocytic inflammation. HFLT has recurrence rates of 30% to 50%, often associated with incomplete excision.

Phosphaturic mesenchymal tumor most commonly affects adults and arises over a wide anatomic distribution. It is associated with a distinct clinical picture of tumor-associated osteomalacia and phosphaturia secondary to overexpression of FGF23, which is also at increased levels in serum and inhibits renal tubule phosphate reabsorption.[85,86] *FN1-FGFR1* fusion gene has recently been identified as a recurrent finding that drives the formation of these tumors.[87] Tumors are composed of bland spindle and stellate cells with admixed thin-walled slitlike vessels and so-called grungy stromal calcifications. Most tumors follow a benign clinical course with recurrence secondary to incomplete excision; malignant examples that metastasize are rare. Osteomalacia resolves after resection.

Since the 2002 WHO publication, myoepithelial tumors of soft tissues have been further characterized. Tumors are now known to affect patients over a wide age range and can arise at all anatomic sites (including visceral locations). Mixed tumors are related to their salivary gland counterparts, and show ductal differentiation and similarly harbor *PLAG1* gene rearrangement.[88-91] Myoepithelioma is composed of benign myoepithelial cells; malignant tumors (myoepithelial carcinoma) are defined by the presence of cytologic atypia and are often associated with high mitotic rate and necrosis. Mixed tumors and myoepithelioma are benign tumors; however; myoepithelial carcinoma follows an aggressive clinical course.[92,93] A subset of myoepitheliomas and myoepithelial carcinomas are associated with *EWSR1* rearrangement,[94–100] and a small subset have alternate *FUS* rearrangement.[100] SMARCB1/INI1 protein expression is lost in a subset of myoepitheliomas and myoepithelial carcinomas, likely secondary to functional loss of material on chromosome 22q.

Recurrent rearrangements of *PHF1* (on chromosome 6p21) have been identified in ossifying fibromyxoid tumor (OFMT), including atypical and malignant examples.[101,102] Criteria for atypical and malignant OFMT remain to be well defined, but some investigators suggest that high nuclear grade, hypercellularity, mitotic activity greater than 2 mitoses per 50 HPF, and atypical ossification within tumor nodules are features of malignancy.

Criteria for malignancy in PEComa also remain to be clearly defined and validated, but the features of mitotic activity, necrosis, marked atypia, pleomorphism, large tumor size, and infiltrative growth seem predictive of malignant behavior.[103,104] Sclerosing PEComa is a recently recognized variant that occurs most frequently at retroperitoneal sites in adult women and is typically benign.[105] Although most PEComas show both myoid and melanocytic differentiation, a subset is negative for melanocytic markers (HMB-45, Mart-1, and MiTF) and instead harbor *TFE3* gene fusions and show nuclear expression for TFE3 by immunohistochemistry.[103,106]

Undifferentiated/Unclassified Sarcomas

This newly introduced section encompasses unclassified tumors that have no distinct histologic, immunohistochemical, or genetic features, which comprise 20% to 25% of all soft tissue sarcomas.[107] Tumors in this category are subclassified according to the predominant morphologic patterns of round cell, spindled, epithelioid, or pleomorphic. Many pleomorphic tumors are high grade and associated with poor prognosis, and would have been classified as MFH in the past. Distinct genetic subsets of round cell sarcomas have been increasingly recognized, including round cell sarcomas having *EWSR1* translocations involving non-*ETS* fusion partners,[108,109] *CIC-DUX4* fusion,[110–113] and *BCOR-CCNB3* fusion.[114–117] Many of these tumors may have been classified as atypical Ewing sarcoma in the past given the variable staining pattern for CD99 within these molecularly distinct groups (**Fig. 4**). *CIC-DUX4* sarcoma

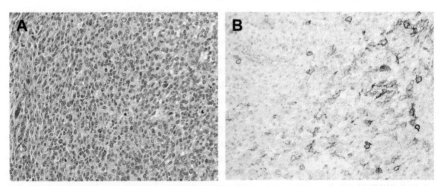

Fig. 4. Round cell sarcoma with *CIC-DUX4* fusion gene. In contrast with Ewing sarcoma, the tumor cells have amphophilic cytoplasm, greater cytologic pleomorphism, and often show areas with spindle cell morphology (H&E, 400×) (*A*). In addition, CD99 staining is often multifocal or patchy in distribution (200×) (*B*), unlike the diffuse pattern seen in Ewing sarcoma.

shows nuclear WT1 immunoreactivity,[118] and immunohistochemistry for CCNB3 is a useful marker for sarcomas with *BCOR-CCNB3* fusion.[119] Tumors with *BCOR-CCNB3* gene fusion are more common in bone than in soft tissue and usually occur in young adult male patients, whereas those with *CIC-DUX4* fusion most often arise in soft tissue and show a slight male predominance. These tumors have generally been treated similarly to Ewing sarcoma, but to date data have shown limited or poor responses to Ewing sarcoma treatment regimens.

TUMORS OF BONE
Chondrogenic Tumors

The 2013 WHO classification effected a significant change in the grading and classification for chondrosarcoma, which now separates grade 1 chondrosarcoma from grade 2 and grade 3 tumors. The most important prognostic predictor for recurrence and metastasis of chondrosarcoma is the histologic grade, which is assigned on a 3-tier system based on nuclear size, hyperchromasia, cellularity, and mitotic count; some tumors show coexistence of various histologic grades and the highest grade present should be reported. The terminology atypical cartilaginous tumor was introduced as a synonym for grade 1 chondrosarcoma (analogous to ALT). This new terminology was introduced to reflect the clinical behavior of grade 1 tumors, which have an excellent prognosis, showing predominantly locally aggressive behavior but essentially no risk of metastasis, with a 5-year survival of 83% to 99%.[120–122] A worse prognosis is associated with grade 2 and 3 chondrosarcomas, which are associated with metastatic rates of 10% and 71%, respectively.[120] Grade 2 chondrosarcoma is associated with a 5-year-survival from 62% to 93% and 10-year survival from 58% to 86%; reported 5-year and 10-year survival rates for grade 3 chondrosarcomas are 0% to 77% and 0% to 55%, respectively.[120,122] En bloc resection is recommended for grade 2 and 3 chondrosarcomas. The advised treatment of atypical cartilaginous tumor/grade 1 chondrosarcoma is curettage or excision; tumors that recur often show higher grade and should be treated accordingly. Chondrosarcoma was also further separated into 3 main groups: primary central chondrosarcoma (arising intraosseously without a precursor lesion), secondary central chondrosarcoma (intraosseous and arising in association with a preexisting enchondroma), and peripheral chondrosarcoma (arising in association with osteochondroma).

Knowledge of the genetics of chondrosarcoma has also been expanded; *IDH1* and *IDH2* mutations are present in both primary and secondary central chondrosarcoma (70%–80%), most periosteal chondrosarcoma, and dedifferentiated chondrosarcoma (50%), as well as in enchondroma and periosteal chondroma (including those associated with endochondromatosis syndromes, Maffucci disease and Ollier syndrome).[123–125]

Osteochondromyxoma was introduced in the 2013 WHO classification. This rare benign tumor occurs in ~ 1% of patients with Carney complex, and commonly arises in the tibia and craniofacial bones.[126] Tumors are composed of a hypocellular proliferation of bland cells in a myxoid stroma with osteoid and chondroid production; some clinicians consider this to represent the osseous counterpart of Carney complex–type myxomas. Osteochondromyxomas show locally aggressive growth and may recur with incomplete excision, but no cases with metastasis have been reported.

Chondroblastoma was classified as a benign tumor in 2002, but the 2013 volume designates it as a tumor of intermediate biological potential (locally aggressive, rarely metastasizing).

Additional genetic data were updated for existing entities, including the identification of recurrent translocation t(1;17) (q32;q21) in bizarre parosteal osteochondromatous proliferation,[127,128] frequent chromosome 6 aberrations in chondromyxoid fibroma[129] and synovial chondromatosis,[130] and recurrent *HEY1-NCOA2* fusion gene in mesenchymal chondrosarcoma.[131]

Osteogenic Tumors

No major classification changes were effected for osteogenic tumors. The section for conventional osteosarcoma now includes secondary osteosarcoma, and although histologic subtypes are outlined for conventional osteosarcoma (eg, osteoblastic, fibroblastic, chondroblastic), the subtype has no therapeutic or prognostic significance.

Amplification of 12q13-15 (which encodes *MDM2* and *CDK4*) is a well-established aberration in low-grade central osteosarcoma[132] and parosteal osteosarcoma.[133] MDM2 and CDK4 immunostains are useful diagnostic markers for both entities,[134,135] and may be particularly useful for recognizing dedifferentiated low-grade central osteosarcomas. Low-grade central osteosarcoma is composed of bland spindle cells and bony trabeculae (and may resemble fibrous dysplasia), whereas dedifferentiated tumors appear as high-grade osteosarcomas. The prognosis of low-grade central osteosarcoma is excellent, with 5-year survival rates greater than 90%, but recurrence and dedifferentiation is reported in 15% of patients. Parosteal osteosarcoma is low grade and has a 5-year survival rate of 91%; tumors are composed of mildly atypical spindle cells and collagenous stroma, and 25% of tumors have a cartilaginous cap and may mimic the benign tumor osteochondroma.

Fibrogenic Tumors

Fibrosarcoma of bone is retained as a tumor type, but is a diagnosis of exclusion. Fibrosarcoma of bone is defined in the 2013 WHO classification as an intermediate-grade to high-grade spindle cell sarcoma lacking significant pleomorphism, and showing no demonstrable line of differentiation other than fibroblastic. Diagnosis requires thorough histologic examination of a tumor, and cannot be made on biopsies. Historically, fibrosarcoma encompassed many different tumor types with a fascicular or herringbone growth pattern; however, modern ancillary studies have allowed more specific classification of most such cases. Tumors showing no line of differentiation but having pleomorphism and significant cytologic atypia are best classified as undifferentiated high-grade pleomorphic sarcoma (discussed later), because these tumors show more aggressive biological behavior.

Desmoplastic fibroma of bone is now designated as a tumor of intermediate biological potential (locally aggressive), from its 2002 classification as a benign tumor. Recurrence rates are 17% with complete resection and up to 72% with incomplete resection.[136]

Fibrohistiocytic Tumors

MFH has been removed as a tumor type in bone; similar to soft tissue counterparts, this previously served as a so-called wastebasket term for many tumors that can now be more specifically classified.

Ewing Sarcoma

Peripheral neuroectodermal tumor (PNET) has been removed as a synonym for Ewing sarcoma, because true PNET of the central nervous system and female genital tract is a pathologically and genetically distinct neoplasm. As described for undifferentiated/ unclassified tumors in soft tissue tumor classification, there has been increasing recognition of distinct genetic subsets of undifferentiated round cell sarcomas in bone (eg, sarcomas with *EWSR1* translocations involving non-*ETS* fusion partners,[108,109] *CIC-DUX4* fusion,[110–113] and *BCOR-CCNB3* fusion[114–117]).

Osteoclastic Giant Cell–Rich Tumors

Previously grouped together, giant cell tumor of bone and giant cell lesion of the small bones are now separated despite sharing morphologic appearances. Giant cell lesion of the small bones is common in younger patients during the first and second decades, and arises most frequently in small tubular bones; tumors are treated by curettage, and despite recurrence rates up to 50% after initial treatment they are virtually always cured after a second procedure. Giant cell tumor of bone is a locally aggressive neoplasm, typically arising in young adults (most often in women with mature skeletons after closure of epiphyseal growth plates); most tumors arise in the epiphysis of long bones. These tumors show significant rates of local recurrence; metastasis of histologically benign giant cell tumors and malignant transformation into a high-grade sarcoma are rare occurrences.

Notochordal Tumors

Benign notochordal cell tumor (also known as giant notochordal rest or notochordal hamartoma) was added to this section. Benign notochordal cell tumors often arise in the skull base, vertebral bodies, and sacrococcygeal bones, and are typically detected incidentally. Some investigators consider these tumors to resemble persistent notochord, whereas others hypothesize that these are neoplasms that develop after birth and have potential to progress to chordoma.[137]

Vascular Tumors

There was only 1 major change to this section: the addition of epithelioid hemangioma. Epithelioid hemangioma is distinguished from hemangioma because of its locally aggressive behavior, with recurrence rates up to 10%.[99] Clinical management requires complete resection, sometimes followed by radiation therapy.

Hematopoietic Neoplasms and Myogenic, Lipogenic, and Epithelial Tumors

There were no major changes in classification of these tumors; diagnostic criteria for these tumors occurring in intraosseous sites are the same as for their conventional counterparts.

Tumors of Undefined Neoplastic Nature

This newly introduced section includes many lesions classified as miscellaneous lesions in the 2002 volume. Most existing entities have been further characterized by genetics means. It has been well established that most cases of primary aneurysmal bone cysts (ABC) are characterized by recurrent rearrangements of the *USP6* gene (encoded on chromosome 17p13), most commonly fused with *CDH11* encoded on 16q22.[138] However, secondary ABC lacks *USP6* gene rearrangements. *BRAF* (V600E) mutations have been identified in both Langerhans cell histiocytosis[139] and Erdheim-Chester disease.[140]

Fibrous dysplasia, chondromesenchymal hamartoma, and osteofibrous dysplasia are now categorized as benign tumors; all were previously designated in 2002 as having unspecified/borderline/uncertain behavior.

Undifferentiated High-Grade Pleomorphic Sarcoma

This terminology replaced MFH and applies to high-grade pleomorphic malignances that lack any specific line of differentiation. This diagnosis is one exclusion, and thorough sampling and histologic evaluation are necessary; most cases previously classified as MFH show focal histologic features suggestive of a line of differentiation (eg, malignant osteoid production for osteosarcoma) or can be further classified by immunohistochemical of molecular/genetic means.[141,142] Tumors show aggressive behavior with frequent metastases (up to 50%), and treatment requires neoadjuvant chemotherapy and complete resection. Similar to conventional osteosarcoma, the extent of tumor necrosis in response to neoadjuvant therapy is an important prognostic factor.[143]

SUMMARY

This article outlines the major updates in the 2013 WHO *Classification of Tumours of Soft Tissue and Bone*, many of which are based on detailed clinicopathologic and immunohistochemical studies and significant discoveries in the molecular pathogenesis of both benign and malignant mesenchymal tumors. These advances have facilitated more accurate classification of tumor types, recognition of novel variants and entities, the development of useful diagnostic immunohistochemical and molecular tests, and uniform diagnostic criteria.

REFERENCES

1. Fletcher C, Bridge J, Hogendoorn P, et al, editors. WHO classification of tumours of soft tissue and bone. Pathology and genetics of tumours of soft tissue and bone. Lyon (France): IARC Press; 2013.
2. Fletcher C, Unni K, Mertens F, editors. WHO classification of tumours of soft tissue and bone. 3rd edition. Lyon (France): IARC Press; 2002.
3. Crozat A, Aman P, Mandahl N, et al. Fusion of CHOP to a novel RNA-binding protein in human myxoid liposarcoma. Nature 1993;363:640–4.
4. Panagopoulos I, Hoglund M, Mertens F, et al. Fusion of the EWS and CHOP genes in myxoid liposarcoma. Oncogene 1996;12:489–94.
5. Binh MB, Sastre-Garau X, Guillou L, et al. MDM2 and CDK4 immunostainings are useful adjuncts in diagnosing well-differentiated and dedifferentiated liposarcoma subtypes: a comparative analysis of 559 soft tissue neoplasms with genetic data. Am J Surg Pathol 2005;29:1340–7.
6. Ida CM, Wang X, Erickson-Johnson MR, et al. Primary retroperitoneal lipoma: a soft tissue pathology heresy? Report of a case with classic histologic, cytogenetics, and molecular genetic features. Am J Surg Pathol 2008;32:951–4.
7. Macarenco RS, Erickson-Johnson M, Wang X, et al. Retroperitoneal lipomatous tumors without cytologic atypia: are they lipomas? A clinicopathologic and molecular study of 19 cases. Am J Surg Pathol 2009;33:1470–6.
8. Marino-Enriquez A, Fletcher CD, Dal Cin P, et al. Dedifferentiated liposarcoma with "homologous" lipoblastic (pleomorphic liposarcoma-like) differentiation: clinicopathologic and molecular analysis of a series suggesting revised diagnostic criteria. Am J Surg Pathol 2010;34:1122–31.
9. Liau JY, Lee JC, Wu CT, et al. Dedifferentiated liposarcoma with homologous lipoblastic differentiation: expanding the spectrum to include low-grade tumours. Histopathology 2013;62:702–10.
10. Gronchi A, Collini P, Miceli R, et al. Myogenic differentiation and histologic grading are major prognostic determinants in retroperitoneal liposarcoma. Am J Surg Pathol 2015;39:383–93.

11. Huang D, Sumegi J, Dal Cin P, et al. C11orf95-MKL2 is the resulting fusion onco-gene of t(11;16)(q13;p13) in chondroid lipoma. Genes Chromosomes Cancer 2010;49:810–8.

12. Flucke U, Tops BB, de Saint Aubain Somerhausen N, et al. Presence of C11orf95-MKL2 fusion is a consistent finding in chondroid lipomas: a study of eight cases. Histopathology 2013;62:925–30.

13. Pedeutour F, Simon MP, Minoletti F, et al. Translocation, t(17;22)(q22;q13), in dermatofibrosarcoma protuberans: a new tumor-associated chromosome rear-rangement. Cytogenet Cell Genet 1996;72:171–4.

14. Patel KU, Szabo SS, Hernandez VS, et al. Dermatofibrosarcoma protuberans COL1A1-PDGFB fusion is identified in virtually all dermatofibrosarcoma protu-berans cases when investigated by newly developed multiplex reverse tran-scription polymerase chain reaction and fluorescence in situ hybridization assays. Hum Pathol 2008;39:184–93.

15. Erickson-Johnson MR, Chou MM, Evers BR, et al. Nodular fasciitis: a novel model of transient neoplasia induced by MYH9-USP6 gene fusion. Lab Invest 2011;91:1427–33.

16. Pauwels P, Sciot R, Croiset F, et al. Myofibroblastoma of the breast: genetic link with spindle cell lipoma. J Pathol 2000;191:282–5.

17. Maggiani F, Debiec-Rychter M, Vanbockrijck M, et al. Cellular angiofibroma: another mesenchymal tumour with 13q14 involvement, suggesting a link with spindle cell lipoma and (extra)-mammary myofibroblastoma. Histopathology 2007;51:410–2.

18. Flucke U, van Krieken JH, Mentzel T. Cellular angiofibroma: analysis of 25 cases emphasizing its relationship to spindle cell lipoma and mammary-type myofibro-blastoma. Mod Pathol 2011;24:82–9.

19. Chen BJ, Marino-Enriquez A, Fletcher CD, et al. Loss of retinoblastoma protein expression in spindle cell/pleomorphic lipomas and cytogenetically related tu-mors: an immunohistochemical study with diagnostic implications. Am J Surg Pathol 2012;36:1119–28.

20. Howitt BE, Fletcher CD. Mammary-type myofibroblastoma: clinicopathologic characterization in a series of 143 cases. Am J Surg Pathol 2016;40(3):361–7.

21. Chen E, Fletcher CD. Cellular angiofibroma with atypia or sarcomatous transfor-mation: clinicopathologic analysis of 13 cases. Am J Surg Pathol 2010;34:707–14.

22. Mohajeri A, Tayebwa J, Collin A, et al. Comprehensive genetic analysis identifies a pathognomonic NAB2/STAT6 fusion gene, nonrandom secondary genomic im-balances, and a characteristic gene expression profile in solitary fibrous tumor. Genes Chromosomes Cancer 2013;52:873–86.

23. Robinson DR, Wu YM, Kalyana-Sundaram S, et al. Identification of recurrent NAB2-STAT6 gene fusions in solitary fibrous tumor by integrative sequencing. Nat Genet 2013;45:180–5.

24. Schweizer L, Koelsche C, Sahm F, et al. Meningeal hemangiopericytoma and solitary fibrous tumors carry the NAB2-STAT6 fusion and can be diagnosed by nuclear expression of STAT6 protein. Acta Neuropathol 2013;125:651–8.

25. Doyle LA, Vivero M, Fletcher CD, et al. Nuclear expression of STAT6 distin-guishes solitary fibrous tumor from histologic mimics. Mod Pathol 2014;27:390–5.

26. Elco CP, Marino-Enriquez A, Abraham JA, et al. Hybrid myxoinflammatory fibroblastic sarcoma/hemosiderotic fibrolipomatous tumor: report of a case

providing further evidence for a pathogenetic link. Am J Surg Pathol 2010;34: 1723–7.

27. Antonescu CR, Zhang L, Nielsen GP, et al. Consistent t(1;10) with rearrangements of TGFBR3 and MGEA5 in both myxoinflammatory fibroblastic sarcoma and hemosiderotic fibrolipomatous tumor. Genes Chromosomes Cancer 2011; 50:757–64.

28. Panagopoulos I, Storlazzi CT, Fletcher CD, et al. The chimeric FUS/CREB3I2 gene is specific for low-grade fibromyxoid sarcoma. Genes Chromosomes Cancer 2004;40:218–28.

29. Guillou L, Benhattar J, Gengler C, et al. Translocation-positive low-grade fibromyxoid sarcoma: clinicopathologic and molecular analysis of a series expanding the morphologic spectrum and suggesting potential relationship to sclerosing epithelioid fibrosarcoma: a study from the French Sarcoma Group. Am J Surg Pathol 2007;31:1387–402.

30. Doyle LA, Wang WL, Dal Cin P, et al. MUC4 is a sensitive and extremely useful marker for sclerosing epithelioid fibrosarcoma: association with FUS gene rearrangement. Am J Surg Pathol 2012;36:1444–51.

31. Lau PP, Lui PC, Lau GT, et al. EWSR1-CREB3L1 gene fusion: a novel alternative molecular aberration of low-grade fibromyxoid sarcoma. Am J Surg Pathol 2013; 37:734–8.

32. Arbajian E, Puls F, Magnusson L, et al. Recurrent EWSR1-CREB3L1 gene fusions in sclerosing epithelioid fibrosarcoma. Am J Surg Pathol 2014;38:801–8.

33. Doyle LA, Moller E, Dal Cin P, et al. MUC4 is a highly sensitive and specific marker for low-grade fibromyxoid sarcoma. Am J Surg Pathol 2011;35:733–41.

34. Moller E, Hornick JL, Magnusson L, et al. FUS-CREB3L2/L1-positive sarcomas show a specific gene expression profile with upregulation of CD24 and FOXL1. Clin Cancer Res 2011;17:2646–56.

35. Marino-Enriquez A, Wang WL, Roy A, et al. Epithelioid inflammatory myofibroblastic sarcoma: an aggressive intra-abdominal variant of inflammatory myofibroblastic tumor with nuclear membrane or perinuclear ALK. Am J Surg Pathol 2011;35:135–44.

36. West RB, Rubin BP, Miller MA, et al. A landscape effect in tenosynovial giant-cell tumor from activation of CSF1 expression by a translocation in a minority of tumor cells. Proc Natl Acad Sci U S A 2006;103:690–5.

37. Cupp JS, Miller MA, Montgomery KD, et al. Translocation and expression of CSF1 in pigmented villonodular synovitis, tenosynovial giant cell tumor, rheumatoid arthritis and other reactive synovitides. Am J Surg Pathol 2007;31:970–6.

38. Moller E, Mandahl N, Mertens F, et al. Molecular identification of COL6A3-CSF1 fusion transcripts in tenosynovial giant cell tumors. Genes Chromosomes Cancer 2008;47:21–5.

39. Brems H, Park C, Maertens O, et al. Glomus tumors in neurofibromatosis type 1: genetic, functional, and clinical evidence of a novel association. Cancer Res 2009;69:7393–401.

40. Stewart DR, Pemov A, Van Loo P, et al. Mitotic recombination of chromosome arm 17q as a cause of loss of heterozygosity of NF1 in neurofibromatosis type 1-associated glomus tumors. Genes Chromosomes Cancer 2012;51:429–37.

41. Chakrapani A, Warrick A, Nelson D, et al. BRAF and KRAS mutations in sporadic glomus tumors. Am J Dermatopathol 2012;34:533–5.

42. Mosquera JM, Sboner A, Zhang L, et al. Novel MIR143-NOTCH fusions in benign and malignant glomus tumors. Genes Chromosomes Cancer 2013;52: 1075–87.

43. Nascimento AF, Fletcher CD. Spindle cell rhabdomyosarcoma in adults. Am J Surg Pathol 2005;29:1106–13.

44. Mosquera JM, Sboner A, Zhang L, et al. Recurrent NCOA2 gene rearrangements in congenital/infantile spindle cell rhabdomyosarcoma. Genes Chromosomes Cancer 2013;52:538–50.

45. Alaggio R, Zhang L, Sung YS, et al. A molecular study of pediatric spindle and sclerosing rhabdomyosarcoma: identification of novel and recurrent VGLL2-related fusions in infantile cases. Am J Surg Pathol 2016;40:224–35.

46. Szuhai K, de Jong D, Leung WY, et al. Transactivating mutation of the MYOD1 gene is a frequent event in adult spindle cell rhabdomyosarcoma. J Pathol 2014;232:300–7.

47. Agaram NP, Chen CL, Zhang L, et al. Recurrent MYOD1 mutations in pediatric and adult sclerosing and spindle cell rhabdomyosarcomas: evidence for a common pathogenesis. Genes Chromosomes Cancer 2014;53:779–87.

48. Billings SD, Folpe AL, Weiss SW. Epithelioid sarcoma-like hemangioendothelioma. Am J Surg Pathol 2003;27:48–57.

49. Hornick JL, Fletcher CD. Pseudomyogenic hemangioendothelioma: a distinctive, often multicentric tumor with indolent behavior. Am J Surg Pathol 2011; 35:190–201.

50. Walther C, Tayebwa J, Lilljebjorn H, et al. A novel SERPINE1-FOSB fusion gene results in transcriptional up-regulation of FOSB in pseudomyogenic haemangioendothelioma. J Pathol 2014;232:534–40.

51. Sheng W, Pan Y, Wang J. Pseudomyogenic hemangioendothelioma: report of an additional case with aggressive clinical course. Am J Dermatopathol 2013;35: 597–600.

52. Shah AR, Fernando M, Musson R, et al. An aggressive case of pseudomyogenic haemangioendothelioma of bone with pathological fracture and rapidly progressive pulmonary metastatic disease: case report and review of the literature. Skeletal Radiol 2015;44:1381–6.

53. Errani C, Zhang L, Sung YS, et al. A novel WWTR1-CAMTA1 gene fusion is a consistent abnormality in epithelioid hemangioendothelioma of different anatomic sites. Genes Chromosomes Cancer 2011;50:644–53.

54. Tanas MR, Sboner A, Oliveira AM, et al. Identification of a disease-defining gene fusion in epithelioid hemangioendothelioma. Sci Transl Med 2011;3:98ra82.

55. Errani C, Sung YS, Zhang L, et al. Monoclonality of multifocal epithelioid hemangioendothelioma of the liver by analysis of WWTR1-CAMTA1 breakpoints. Cancer Genet 2012;205:12–7.

56. Doyle LA, Fletcher CD, Hornick JL. Nuclear expression of CAMTA1 distinguishes epithelioid hemangioendothelioma from histologic mimics. Am J Surg Pathol 2016;40:94–102.

57. Antonescu CR, Le Loarer F, Mosquera JM, et al. Novel YAP1-TFE3 fusion defines a distinct subset of epithelioid hemangioendothelioma. Genes Chromosomes Cancer 2013;52:775–84.

58. Deyrup AT, Tighiouart M, Montag AG, et al. Epithelioid hemangioendothelioma of soft tissue: a proposal for risk stratification based on 49 cases. Am J Surg Pathol 2008;32:924–7.

59. Manner J, Radlwimmer B, Hohenberger P, et al. MYC high level gene amplification is a distinctive feature of angiosarcomas after irradiation or chronic lymphedema. Am J Pathol 2010;176:34–9.

60. Guo T, Zhang L, Chang NE, et al. Consistent MYC and FLT4 gene amplification in radiation-induced angiosarcoma but not in other radiation-associated atypical vascular lesions. Genes Chromosomes Cancer 2011;50:25–33.

61. Mentzel T, Schildhaus HU, Palmedo G, et al. Postradiation cutaneous angiosarcoma after treatment of breast carcinoma is characterized by MYC amplification in contrast to atypical vascular lesions after radiotherapy and control cases: clinicopathological, immunohistochemical and molecular analysis of 66 cases. Mod Pathol 2012;25:75–85.

62. Italiano A, Thomas R, Breen M, et al. The miR-17-92 cluster and its target THBS1 are differentially expressed in angiosarcomas dependent on MYC amplification. Genes Chromosomes Cancer 2012;51:569–78.

63. Antonescu CR, Yoshida A, Guo T, et al. KDR activating mutations in human angiosarcomas are sensitive to specific kinase inhibitors. Cancer Res 2009;69:7175–9.

64. Huang SC, Zhang L, Sung YS, et al. Recurrent CIC gene abnormalities in angiosarcomas: a molecular study of 120 cases with concurrent investigation of PLCG1, KDR, MYC, and FLT4 gene alterations. Am J Surg Pathol 2016;40(5):645–55.

65. Nascimento AF, Raut CP, Fletcher CD. Primary angiosarcoma of the breast: clinicopathologic analysis of 49 cases, suggesting that grade is not prognostic. Am J Surg Pathol 2008;32:1896–904.

66. Demetri GD, von Mehren M, Antonescu CR, et al. NCCN task force report: update on the management of patients with gastrointestinal stromal tumors. J Natl Compr Canc Netw 2010;8(Suppl 2):S1–41 [quiz: S42–4].

67. Miettinen M, Sobin LH, Lasota J. Gastrointestinal stromal tumors of the stomach: a clinicopathologic, immunohistochemical, and molecular genetic study of 1765 cases with long-term follow-up. Am J Surg Pathol 2005;29:52–68.

68. Miettinen M, Makhlouf H, Sobin LH, et al. Gastrointestinal stromal tumors of the jejunum and ileum: a clinicopathologic, immunohistochemical, and molecular genetic study of 906 cases before imatinib with long-term follow-up. Am J Surg Pathol 2006;30:477–89.

69. Rege TA, Wagner AJ, Corless CL, et al. "Pediatric-type" gastrointestinal stromal tumors in adults: distinctive histology predicts genotype and clinical behavior. Am J Surg Pathol 2011;35:495–504.

70. Gill AJ, Chou A, Vilain RE, et al. "Pediatric-type" gastrointestinal stromal tumors are SDHB negative ("type 2") GISTs. Am J Surg Pathol 2011;35:1245–7 [author reply: 1247–8].

71. Doyle LA, Nelson D, Heinrich MC, et al. Loss of succinate dehydrogenase subunit B (SDHB) expression is limited to a distinctive subset of gastric wild-type gastrointestinal stromal tumours: a comprehensive genotype-phenotype correlation study. Histopathology 2012;61:801–9.

72. Killian JK, Miettinen M, Walker RL, et al. Recurrent epimutation of SDHC in gastrointestinal stromal tumors. Sci Transl Med 2014;6:268ra177.

73. Wagner AJ, Remillard SP, Zhang YX, et al. Loss of expression of SDHA predicts SDHA mutations in gastrointestinal stromal tumors. Mod Pathol 2013;26:289–94.

74. Dwight T, Benn DE, Clarkson A, et al. Loss of SDHA expression identifies SDHA mutations in succinate dehydrogenase-deficient gastrointestinal stromal tumors. Am J Surg Pathol 2013;37:226–33.

75. Oudijk L, Gaal J, Korpershoek E, et al. SDHA mutations in adult and pediatric wild-type gastrointestinal stromal tumors. Mod Pathol 2013;26:456–63.

76. Agaram NP, Laquaglia MP, Ustun B, et al. Molecular characterization of pediatric gastrointestinal stromal tumors. Clin Cancer Res 2008;14:3204–15.
77. Pasini B, McWhinney SR, Bei T, et al. Clinical and molecular genetics of patients with the Carney-Stratakis syndrome and germline mutations of the genes coding for the succinate dehydrogenase subunits SDHB, SDHC, and SDHD. Eur J Hum Genet 2008;16:79–88.
78. Janeway KA, Kim SY, Lodish M, et al. Defects in succinate dehydrogenase in gastrointestinal stromal tumors lacking KIT and PDGFRA mutations. Proc Natl Acad Sci U S A 2011;108:314–8.
79. Hornick JL, Bundock EA, Fletcher CD. Hybrid schwannoma/perineurioma: clinicopathologic analysis of 42 distinctive benign nerve sheath tumors. Am J Surg Pathol 2009;33:1554–61.
80. Harder A, Wesemann M, Hagel C, et al. Hybrid neurofibroma/schwannoma is overrepresented among schwannomatosis and neurofibromatosis patients. Am J Surg Pathol 2012;36:702–9.
81. Fetsch JF, Laskin WB, Miettinen M. Superficial acral fibromyxoma: a clinicopathologic and immunohistochemical analysis of 37 cases of a distinctive soft tissue tumor with a predilection for the fingers and toes. Hum Pathol 2001;32:704–14.
82. Hollmann TJ, Bovee JV, Fletcher CD. Digital fibromyxoma (superficial acral fibromyxoma): a detailed characterization of 124 cases. Am J Surg Pathol 2012;36:789–98.
83. Marshall-Taylor C, Fanburg-Smith JC. Hemosiderotic fibrohistiocytic lipomatous lesion: ten cases of a previously undescribed fatty lesion of the foot/ankle. Mod Pathol 2000;13:1192–9.
84. Browne TJ, Fletcher CD. Haemosiderotic fibrolipomatous tumour (so-called haemosiderotic fibrohistiocytic lipomatous tumour): analysis of 13 new cases in support of a distinct entity. Histopathology 2006;48:453–61.
85. Folpe AL, Fanburg-Smith JC, Billings SD, et al. Most osteomalacia-associated mesenchymal tumors are a single histopathologic entity: an analysis of 32 cases and a comprehensive review of the literature. Am J Surg Pathol 2004;28:1–30.
86. Bahrami A, Weiss SW, Montgomery E, et al. RT-PCR analysis for FGF23 using paraffin sections in the diagnosis of phosphaturic mesenchymal tumors with and without known tumor induced osteomalacia. Am J Surg Pathol 2009;33:1348–54.
87. Lee JC, Jeng YM, Su SY, et al. Identification of a novel FN1-FGFR1 genetic fusion as a frequent event in phosphaturic mesenchymal tumour. J Pathol 2015;235:539–45.
88. Matsuyama A, Hisaoka M, Hashimoto H. PLAG1 expression in cutaneous mixed tumors: an immunohistochemical and molecular genetic study. Virchows Arch 2011;459:539–45.
89. Bahrami A, Dalton JD, Krane JF, et al. A subset of cutaneous and soft tissue mixed tumors are genetically linked to their salivary gland counterpart. Genes Chromosomes Cancer 2012;51:140–8.
90. Matsuyama A, Hisaoka M, Hashimoto H. PLAG1 expression in mesenchymal tumors: an immunohistochemical study with special emphasis on the pathogenetical distinction between soft tissue myoepithelioma and pleomorphic adenoma of the salivary gland. Pathol Int 2012;62:1–7.
91. Antonescu CR, Zhang L, Shao SY, et al. Frequent PLAG1 gene rearrangements in skin and soft tissue myoepithelioma with ductal differentiation. Genes Chromosomes Cancer 2013;52:675–82.

92. Hornick JL, Fletcher CD. Myoepithelial tumors of soft tissue: a clinicopathologic and immunohistochemical study of 101 cases with evaluation of prognostic parameters. Am J Surg Pathol 2003;27:1183–96.

93. Gleason BC, Fletcher CD. Myoepithelial carcinoma of soft tissue in children: an aggressive neoplasm analyzed in a series of 29 cases. Am J Surg Pathol 2007; 31:1813–24.

94. Flucke U, Palmedo G, Blankenhorn N, et al. EWSR1 gene rearrangement occurs in a subset of cutaneous myoepithelial tumors: a study of 18 cases. Mod Pathol 2011;24:1444–50.

95. Brandal P, Panagopoulos I, Bjerkehagen B, et al. Detection of a t(1;22)(q23;q12) translocation leading to an EWSR1-PBX1 fusion gene in a myoepithelioma. Genes Chromosomes Cancer 2008;47:558–64.

96. Brandal P, Panagopoulos I, Bjerkehagen B, et al. t(19;22)(q13;q12) Translocation leading to the novel fusion gene EWSR1-ZNF444 in soft tissue myoepithelial carcinoma. Genes Chromosomes Cancer 2009;48:1051–6.

97. Antonescu CR, Zhang L, Chang NE, et al. EWSR1-POU5F1 fusion in soft tissue myoepithelial tumors. A molecular analysis of sixty-six cases, including soft tissue, bone, and visceral lesions, showing common involvement of the EWSR1 gene. Genes Chromosomes Cancer 2010;49:1114–24.

98. Jo VY, Antonescu CR, Zhang L, et al. Cutaneous syncytial myoepithelioma: clinicopathologic characterization in a series of 38 cases. Am J Surg Pathol 2013; 37:710–8.

99. Agaram NP, Chen HW, Zhang L, et al. EWSR1-PBX3: a novel gene fusion in myoepithelial tumors. Genes Chromosomes Cancer 2015;54:63–71.

100. Huang SC, Chen HW, Zhang L, et al. Novel FUS-KLF17 and EWSR1-KLF17 fusions in myoepithelial tumors. Genes Chromosomes Cancer 2015;54(5):267–75.

101. Gebre-Medhin S, Nord KH, Moller E, et al. Recurrent rearrangement of the PHF1 gene in ossifying fibromyxoid tumors. Am J Pathol 2012;181:1069–77.

102. Graham RP, Weiss SW, Sukov WR, et al. PHF1 rearrangements in ossifying fibromyxoid tumors of soft parts: a fluorescence in situ hybridization study of 41 cases with emphasis on the malignant variant. Am J Surg Pathol 2013;37: 1751–5.

103. Folpe AL, Mentzel T, Lehr HA, et al. Perivascular epithelioid cell neoplasms of soft tissue and gynecologic origin: a clinicopathologic study of 26 cases and review of the literature. Am J Surg Pathol 2005;29:1558–75.

104. Doyle LA, Hornick JL, Fletcher CD. PEComa of the gastrointestinal tract: clinicopathologic study of 35 cases with evaluation of prognostic parameters. Am J Surg Pathol 2013;37:1769–82.

105. Hornick JL, Fletcher CD. Sclerosing PEComa: clinicopathologic analysis of a distinctive variant with a predilection for the retroperitoneum. Am J Surg Pathol 2008;32:493–501.

106. Argani P, Aulmann S, Illei PB, et al. A distinctive subset of PEComas harbors TFE3 gene fusions. Am J Surg Pathol 2010;34:1395–406.

107. Fletcher CD, Gustafson P, Rydholm A, et al. Clinicopathologic re-evaluation of 100 malignant fibrous histiocytomas: prognostic relevance of subclassification. J Clin Oncol 2001;19:3045–50.

108. Wang L, Bhargava R, Zheng T, et al. Undifferentiated small round cell sarcomas with rare EWS gene fusions: identification of a novel EWS-SP3 fusion and of additional cases with the EWS-ETV1 and EWS-FEV fusions. J Mol Diagn 2007; 9:498–509.

109. Deng FM, Galvan K, de la Roza G, et al. Molecular characterization of an EWSR1-POU5F1 fusion associated with a t(6;22) in an undifferentiated soft tissue sarcoma. Cancer Genet 2011;204:423–9.

110. Kawamura-Saito M, Yamazaki Y, Kaneko K, et al. Fusion between CIC and DUX4 up-regulates PEA3 family genes in Ewing-like sarcomas with t(4;19)(q35;q13) translocation. Hum Mol Genet 2006;15:2125–37.

111. Graham C, Chilton-MacNeill S, Zielenska M, et al. The CIC-DUX4 fusion transcript is present in a subgroup of pediatric primitive round cell sarcomas. Hum Pathol 2012;43:180–9.

112. Italiano A, Sung YS, Zhang L, et al. High prevalence of CIC fusion with double-homeobox (DUX4) transcription factors in EWSR1-negative undifferentiated small blue round cell sarcomas. Genes Chromosomes Cancer 2012;51:207–18.

113. Choi EY, Thomas DG, McHugh JB, et al. Undifferentiated small round cell sarcoma with t(4;19)(q35;q13.1) CIC-DUX4 fusion: a novel highly aggressive soft tissue tumor with distinctive histopathology. Am J Surg Pathol 2013;37:1379–86.

114. Pierron G, Tirode F, Lucchesi C, et al. A new subtype of bone sarcoma defined by BCOR-CCNB3 gene fusion. Nat Genet 2012;44:461–6.

115. Cohen-Gogo S, Cellier C, Coindre JM, et al. Ewing-like sarcomas with BCOR-CCNB3 fusion transcript: a clinical, radiological and pathological retrospective study from the Societe Francaise des Cancers de L'Enfant. Pediatr Blood Cancer 2014;61:2191–8.

116. Puls F, Niblett A, Marland G, et al. BCOR-CCNB3 (Ewing-like) sarcoma: a clinicopathologic analysis of 10 cases, in comparison with conventional Ewing sarcoma. Am J Surg Pathol 2014;38:1307–18.

117. Peters TL, Kumar V, Polikepahad S, et al. BCOR-CCNB3 fusions are frequent in undifferentiated sarcomas of male children. Mod Pathol 2015;28:575–86.

118. Specht K, Sung YS, Zhang L, et al. Distinct transcriptional signature and immunoprofile of CIC-DUX4 fusion-positive round cell tumors compared to EWSR1-rearranged Ewing sarcomas: further evidence toward distinct pathologic entities. Genes Chromosomes Cancer 2014;53:622–33.

119. Shibayama T, Okamoto T, Nakashima Y, et al. Screening of BCOR-CCNB3 sarcoma using immunohistochemistry for CCNB3: a clinicopathological report of three pediatric cases. Pathol Int 2015;65:410–4.

120. Evans HL, Ayala AG, Romsdahl MM. Prognostic factors in chondrosarcoma of bone: a clinicopathologic analysis with emphasis on histologic grading. Cancer 1977;40:818–31.

121. Gelderblom H, Hogendoorn PC, Dijkstra SD, et al. The clinical approach towards chondrosarcoma. Oncologist 2008;13:320–9.

122. Nota SP, Braun Y, Schwab JH, et al. The identification of prognostic factors and survival statistics of conventional central chondrosarcoma. Sarcoma 2015;2015:623746.

123. Pansuriya TC, van Eijk R, d'Adamo P, et al. Somatic mosaic IDH1 and IDH2 mutations are associated with enchondroma and spindle cell hemangioma in Ollier disease and Maffucci syndrome. Nat Genet 2011;43:1256–61.

124. Amary MF, Bacsi K, Maggiani F, et al. IDH1 and IDH2 mutations are frequent events in central chondrosarcoma and central and periosteal chondromas but not in other mesenchymal tumours. J Pathol 2011;224:334–43.

125. Damato S, Alorjani M, Bonar F, et al. IDH1 mutations are not found in cartilaginous tumours other than central and periosteal chondrosarcomas and enchondromas. Histopathology 2012;60:363–5.

126. Carney JA, Boccon-Gibod L, Jarka DE, et al. Osteochondromyxoma of bone: a congenital tumor associated with lentigines and other unusual disorders. Am J Surg Pathol 2001;25:164–76.

127. Zambrano E, Nose V, Perez-Atayde AR, et al. Distinct chromosomal rearrangements in subungual (Dupuytren) exostosis and bizarre parosteal osteochondromatous proliferation (Nora lesion). Am J Surg Pathol 2004;28:1033–9.

128. Nilsson M, Domanski HA, Mertens F, et al. Molecular cytogenetic characterization of recurrent translocation breakpoints in bizarre parosteal osteochondromatous proliferation (Nora's lesion). Hum Pathol 2004;35:1063–9.

129. Romeo S, Duim RA, Bridge JA, et al. Heterogeneous and complex rearrangements of chromosome arm 6q in chondromyxoid fibroma: delineation of breakpoints and analysis of candidate target genes. Am J Pathol 2010;177: 1365–76.

130. Buddingh EP, Krallman P, Neff JR, et al. Chromosome 6 abnormalities are recurrent in synovial chondromatosis. Cancer Genet Cytogenet 2003;140:18–22.

131. Panagopoulos I, Gorunova L, Bjerkehagen B, et al. Chromosome aberrations and HEY1-NCOA2 fusion gene in a mesenchymal chondrosarcoma. Oncol Rep 2014;32(1):40–4.

132. Tarkkanen M, Bohling T, Gamberi G, et al. Comparative genomic hybridization of low-grade central osteosarcoma. Mod Pathol 1998;11:421–6.

133. Mejia-Guerrero S, Quejada M, Gokgoz N, et al. Characterization of the 12q15 MDM2 and 12q13-14 CDK4 amplicons and clinical correlations in osteosarcoma. Genes Chromosomes Cancer 2010;49:518–25.

134. Dujardin F, Binh MB, Bouvier C, et al. MDM2 and CDK4 immunohistochemistry is a valuable tool in the differential diagnosis of low-grade osteosarcomas and other primary fibro-osseous lesions of the bone. Mod Pathol 2011;24:624–37.

135. Yoshida A, Ushiku T, Motoi T, et al. Immunohistochemical analysis of MDM2 and CDK4 distinguishes low-grade osteosarcoma from benign mimics. Mod Pathol 2010;23:1279–88.

136. Bohm P, Krober S, Greschniok A, et al. Desmoplastic fibroma of the bone. A report of two patients, review of the literature, and therapeutic implications. Cancer 1996;78:1011–23.

137. Yamaguchi T, Suzuki S, Ishiiwa H, et al. Benign notochordal cell tumors: a comparative histological study of benign notochordal cell tumors, classic chordomas, and notochordal vestiges of fetal intervertebral discs. Am J Surg Pathol 2004;28:756–61.

138. Oliveira AM, Perez-Atayde AR, Inwards CY, et al. USP6 and CDH11 oncogenes identify the neoplastic cell in primary aneurysmal bone cysts and are absent in so-called secondary aneurysmal bone cysts. Am J Pathol 2004;165:1773–80.

139. Badalian-Very G, Vergilio JA, Degar BA, et al. Recurrent BRAF mutations in Langerhans cell histiocytosis. Blood 2010;116:1919–23.

140. Haroche J, Charlotte F, Arnaud L, et al. High prevalence of BRAF V600E mutations in Erdheim-Chester disease but not in other non-Langerhans cell histiocytoses. Blood 2012;120:2700–3.

141. Mertens F, Romeo S, Bovee JV, et al. Reclassification and subtyping of so-called malignant fibrous histiocytoma of bone: comparison with cytogenetic features. Clin Sarcoma Res 2011;1:10.

142. Romeo S, Bovee JV, Kroon HM, et al. Malignant fibrous histiocytoma and fibrosarcoma of bone: a re-assessment in the light of currently employed

morphological, immunohistochemical and molecular approaches. Virchows Arch 2012;461:561–70.

143. Jeon DG, Song WS, Kong CB, et al. MFH of bone and osteosarcoma show similar survival and chemosensitivity. Clin Orthop Relat Res 2011;469:584–90.

Imaging in Soft Tissue Sarcomas: Current Updates

Jyothi P. Jagannathan, MD[a,b,*], Sree Harsha Tirumani, MD[a,b],
Nikhil H. Ramaiya, MD[a,b]

KEYWORDS

- Soft tissue sarcomas • CT • MRI • Liposarcoma • Leiomyosarcoma

KEY POINTS

- Differentiation of benign and malignant soft tissue tumors as well as differentiating various histologic subtypes of sarcoma on imaging alone is challenging.
- Patient demographics, pertinent clinical data, location of the mass, multiplicity of lesions, growth pattern, and specific imaging findings may help to narrow down the differential.
- Tissue sampling remains the gold standard for definitive diagnosis; the optimal biopsy site and route depends on imaging findings and is determined with the surgical/orthopedic oncologist.
- Certain soft tissue sarcomas have characteristic imaging features: fat in adipocytic sarcomas, high T2 signal intensity in myxoid tumors, low T2 signal intensity in tumors with fibrosis and flow voids in highly vascular tumors.

INTRODUCTION

Soft tissue sarcomas (STS) are rare, accounting for only 1% of malignant tumors, with an estimated incidence of 2.7 per 100,000. However, it is a heterogeneous group with more than 50 subtypes exhibiting varying clinical behavior from indolent to highly aggressive. Although the majority arise in the extremities, the retroperitoneum, trunk, and head and neck are also common locations.[1–3]

Patient age is an important discriminating factor in the differential diagnosis of STS. The most common STS in adults are gastrointestinal stromal tumors (GIST), followed by unclassified pleomorphic sarcoma, liposarcoma (LPS), and leiomyosarcoma (LMS), and myxofibrosarcoma (MFS), whereas in the pediatric population, rhabdomyosarcomas (RMS) constitutes the most common STS. Certain histologic subtypes

The authors have nothing to disclose.
^a Department of Imaging, Dana-Farber Cancer Institute, Harvard Medical School, 450 Brookline Avenue, Boston, MA 02215, USA; ^b Department of Radiology, Brigham and Women's Hospital, Harvard Medical School, 75 Francis Street, Boston, MA 02115, USA
* Corresponding author. Department of Imaging, Dana-Farber Cancer Institute, Harvard Medical School, 450 Brookline Avenue, Boston, MA 02215.
E-mail address: jjagannathan@partners.org

Surg Oncol Clin N Am 25 (2016) 645–675
http://dx.doi.org/10.1016/j.soc.2016.05.002
1055-3207/16/$ – see front matter © 2016 Elsevier Inc. All rights reserved.

surgonc.theclinics.com

like synovial sarcoma, alveolar soft part sarcoma (ASPS) and Ewing sarcoma tend to occur predominantly in young adults. Imaging plays an important role in the diagnostic workup of STS, including tissue characterization, guiding biopsy, staging, and pretreatment planning of STS. Although most STS have nonspecific imaging features, certain STS can have a characteristic imaging appearance, which can help in their diagnosis. Furthermore, certain histologic subtypes have a unique metastatic pattern, like nodal metastases in synovial sarcoma and brain metastases in ASPS, which can aid in their primary diagnosis as well as posttreatment surveillance.

A comprehensive review of the imaging findings of all STS is beyond the scope of this paper. In this paper, we illustrate pertinent imaging characteristics of commonly occurring STS and some uncommon sarcomas with unique imaging characteristics, and provide an overview of role of imaging in intraabdominal sarcomas and extremity STS (ESTS).

SPECIFIC HISTOLOGIC SUBTYPES BASED ON THE WORLD HEALTH ORGANIZATION CLASSIFICATION
Adipocytic Tumors: Liposarcomas

The major changes in the recent 2013 World Health Organization (WHO) classification has been the removal of the terms 'round cell LPS' and 'mixed-type LPS' and introduction of new subtype "LPS, not otherwise specified."[1] Round cell LPS are currently thought to represent high-grade myxoid LPS, and mixed-type LPS are considered variant of dedifferentiated LPS based on molecular testing.[1,4]

Atypical lipomatous tumor/well-differentiated liposarcoma

ALT and well-differentiated LPS are intermediate (locally aggressive) neoplasms that do not metastasize. ALT and well-differentiated LPS have a predilection for the extremities, retroperitoneum, and paratesticular and the inguinal regions[5] (**Fig. 1**). Although imaging findings of lipoma and ALT/well-differentiated LPS overlap, owing to the predominant fat component, features that favor ALT/well-differentiated LPS over lipoma include age greater than 60 years, lesion size greater than 10 cm, lower

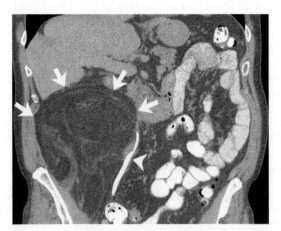

Fig. 1. A 76-year-old man with retroperitoneal well-differentiated liposarcoma. Coronal contrast enhanced computed tomography of the abdomen reveals a large multicompartmental intraabdominal mass (*arrows*) with predominantly fat attenuation compressing and displacing the ureter medially (*arrowhead*). The thick internal septations and mass effect differentiate the mass form the normal intraabdominal fat. Surgical resection included right nephrectomy.

extremity location, presence of thickened septa (>2 mm), globular/nodular enhancing foci, and greater portion of nonfatty (solid or amorphous) areas[5–7] (**Fig. 2**). The sclerosing variant of well-differentiated LPS seen most commonly in the retroperitoneum, has a predominant nonfatty component, simulating dedifferentiated LPS or other aggressive neoplasms.[8]

Dedifferentiated liposarcoma

Dedifferentiated LPS are aggressive sarcomas seen in up to 15% of well-differentiated LPS of the retroperitoneum, and rarely in the extremities and mediastinum. Dedifferentiation can occur in primary tumors or within the recurrences and metastases. Both well-differentiated and dedifferentiated LPS are characterized on pathology by 12q13 to 15 amplification and MDM2 and CDK4 positivity.[4] Dedifferentiated areas most frequently resemble undifferentiated high-grade pleomorphic sarcoma in 90% of cases, but may exhibit heterologous differentiation (eg, myogenic, osteo/chondrosarcomatous). On imaging, dedifferentiated component is identified by focal nodular nonlipomatous region greater than 1 cm, often showing enhancement[9] (**Fig. 3**). Calcifications/ossification may be present. The proportion of lipomatous component decreases with increasing grade of tumor, and measurement of this component maybe more significant than the entire tumor size when evaluating rate of growth and response to treatment.[7,10] Distant metastases from dedifferentiated LPS occur in 15% to 20% of cases, most commonly to the liver and lungs.[11,12]

Myxoid liposarcoma

Myxoid LPS is another subtype of LPS, often occurring in the extremities of young to middle-aged adults, usually in the deep soft tissues of the thigh. On imaging, myxoid LPS are usually seen as well-circumscribed, multilobulated (often septated), deep subcutaneous or intramuscular masses.[9,13] On MRI, the myxoid content leads to characteristically low signal intensity (SI) on T1-weighted imaging and very high SI on T2-weighted imaging, with marked heterogeneous enhancement (**Fig. 4**).[13,14]

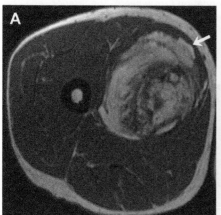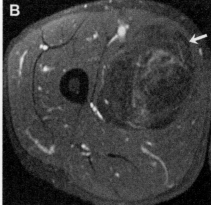

Fig. 2. A 57-year-old male with atypical lipomatous tumor. Axial T1 turbo spin echo (A) and fat-suppressed postgadolinium (B) T1-weighted MRI demonstrates a heterogeneous mass (arrows in A and B) in the medial thigh. The mass has predominantly T1 hyperintense signal areas, which are suppressed on fat-suppressed sequence consistent with macroscopic fat. There are, however, linear T1 hypointense enhancing areas in the mass, which is atypical for simple lipoma and raising the possibility of liposarcoma. Histopathology confirmed atypical lipomatous tumor with spindle cell histology.

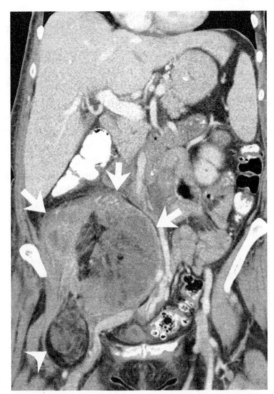

Fig. 3. A 69-year-old woman with retroperitoneal dedifferentiated liposarcoma. Coronal contrast-enhanced computed tomography of the abdomen reveals a large heterogeneous predominantly soft tissue containing retroperitoneal mass (*arrows*) extending into the right inguinal region with variable areas of fat attenuation (*arrowhead*). The inferior vena cava and the right iliac vessels are displaced by the mass.

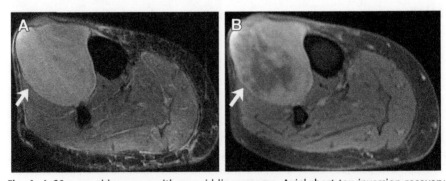

Fig. 4. A 66- year-old woman with myxoid liposarcoma. Axial short-tau inversion recovery (*A*) and fat-suppressed postgadolinium (*B*) T1-weighted MRIs demonstrates a well-circumscribed markedly T2 hyperintense lobulated intramuscular mass in the anterior compartment of the leg, which shows marked heterogeneous enhancement after contrast administration (*arrow*). There is no significant surrounding edema.

Macroscopic fat is usually less than 10% of the tumor volume, although quite variable. Myxoid LPS is graded using a 3-tier system as low, intermediate, or high grade, based on the degree of cellularity. On imaging, large tumor size (>10 cm), deep location, lack of lobulations, and greater than 5% of nonfatty, nonmyxoid contrast enhancing component was associated with higher grader tumors.[15,16] Myxoid LPS has an unusual pattern of metastases to extrapulmonary sites, often to other fat-containing areas, such as the paraspinal regions, intermuscular fat pad, bone, retroperitoneum, and the opposite extremity.[17] Osseous metastases, although frequent and readily apparent on MRI, are exceedingly hard to detect on computed tomography (CT) and PET-CT, because lesions cause minimal disruption of the bony trabeculae and may not be avid owing to the myxoid matrix. Several investigators, including ourselves, have found whole body MRI to be a promising tool for screening for osseous and soft tissue metastases in patients with myxoid LPS, and should be strongly considered, especially in high-grade tumors[18,19] **(Fig. 5)**.

Pleomorphic liposarcoma
Pleomorphic LPS is the least common subtype of LPS, often seen in deep soft tissues of the extremities of elderly patients.[9] The tumors are often high grade with high rates

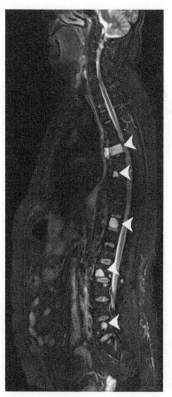

Fig. 5. A 55-year-old man with myxoid liposarcoma and presumed solitary thoracic vertebral body metastasis. Whole body MRI was subsequently performed. Sagittal whole-body short-tau inversion recovery MRI demonstrates multifocal T2 hyperintense osseous disease (*arrowheads*) throughout the spine and the pelvic bones (images not shown).

of local recurrence and metastases. The imaging appearance resembles other aggressive sarcomas because they contain little or no fat.

FIBROBLASTIC/MYOFIBROBLASTIC TUMORS
Dermatofibrosarcoma Protuberans

Dermatofibrosarcoma protuberans was included in STS for the first time in the 2013 WHO classification (previously was categorized under tumors of the skin).[1] Dermatofibrosarcoma protuberans is a rare soft tissue tumor, comprising 6% of STS. Tumors are characterized by t(17; 22) translocation, resulting in the activation of platelet-derived growth factor receptor.[4] Although the majority of the tumors are intermediate in grade and rarely metastasizing, fibrosarcomatous transformation to higher grade with metastatic potential may occur in up to 20% of cases.[20] Dermatofibrosarcoma protuberans affects men more often than women, and most commonly occurs in the third to fifth decades of life. The trunk is most commonly involved (50%), followed by proximal extremities (35%–40%) and the head and neck (14%) (**Fig. 6**). Surgery with wide local excision is the treatment of choice.[21] However, owing to infiltrative margins, local recurrence is common, ad is seen in up to 20% of cases. Although imaging is not performed routinely owing to its superficial location, it is helpful for preoperative planning especially in deep and infiltrative tumors.[22] MRI demonstrates a lobular or nodular enhancing intermediate SI lesion involving the subcutaneous fat and the skin, often causing a focal protuberance[2,23] (**Fig. 7**). Myxoid lesions may be extremely T2 hyperintense. Satellite nodules and plaque like lesions with ill-defined

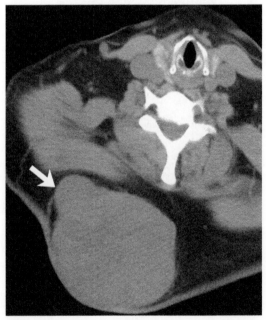

Fig. 6. A 54-year-old male with dermatofibrosarcoma protuberans. Axial noncontrast computed tomography image of the chest shows an ovoid, lobulated, homogeneous, low-density, subcutaneous mass in the posterior chest wall without invasion of the underlying muscles (*arrow*).

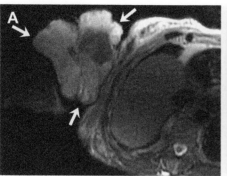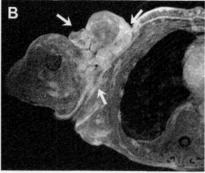

Fig. 7. An 80-year-old woman with high-grade fibrosarcomatous variant of dermatofibrosarcoma protuberans. Axial T2 (*A*) and postcontrast (*B*) T1-weighted MRIs of the chest reveal a large lobulated heterogeneous high signal intensity mass with heterogeneous enhancement protruding from the skin of the right anterior chest wall (*arrows*), with infiltrative margins.

infiltrative margins are also reported.[23,24] Hemorrhage and necrosis is uncommon, except in fibrosarcomatous transformation.[23,25]

Myxofibrosarcoma

Previously known as the myxoid variant of malignant fibrous histiocytoma, MFS is recognized currently as a distinct entity.[1,26] MFS is among the most sarcoma in elderly patients (median age, 65 years), occurring mainly in the extremities (75%), followed by trunk (12%) and retroperitoneum/mediastinum (8%).[2] Masses may be subcutaneous (50%–70%) or intramuscular in location. Histologically, MFS is characterized by multinodular growth pattern with variable degrees of fibrous tissue, cellularity, and pleomorphism on a background of myxoid stroma (usually >5% of tumor). Treatment includes preoperative chemoradiation followed by wide en bloc resection. Local recurrence is seen in 50% to 60% of patients, and is independent of the histologic grade. Low-grade tumors can demonstrate histologic progression and evolve into high-grade lesions after local recurrence.[27,28] Metastases can occur anywhere, but most commonly to the lungs.[29]

The MRI findings are nonspecific, with heterogeneity on all pulse sequences reflecting variable amounts of myxoid stroma (low T1 SI, very high T2 SI, usually markedly enhancing), fibrous tissue, often seen as septa (low SI on T2 with minimal enhancement), cellular (intermediate on T1-weighted imaging, intermediate to high SI on T2-weighted imaging, and moderately enhancing), hemorrhage (high SI on T1 fat-suppressed sequences, fluid levels, nonenhancing), and necrosis (low SI on T1-weighted imaging, high SI on T2-weighted imaging, and nonenhancing)[2,30] **(Fig. 8)**. T2 hypointense pseudocapsule may be present in some cases. The main differential diagnosis includes other myxoid neoplasms (eg, myxoid LPS) and other pleomorphic soft tissue tumors (eg, unclassified pleomorphic sarcoma).[14,30] A characteristic feature of MFS is the presence of unencapsulated margin and a centrifugal infiltrative growth pattern along the fascial planes and intermuscular septa, resulting in positive surgical margins despite wide resection, and a high rate of local recurrence (50%–60%).[31] This growth pattern is often manifest on MRI as the "tail sign," a T2-hyperintense enhancing curvilinear projection (tail) extending from the primary tumor mass into the adjacent soft tissues. The "tail sign" was found to be moderately

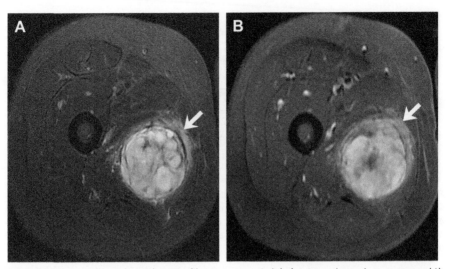

Fig. 8. A 77-year old male with myxofibrosarcoma. Axial short-tau inversion recovery (A) and postgadolinium fat-suppressed (B) T1-weighted MRIs of the thigh reveal a heterogeneous extremely T2 high signal intensity intramuscular mass (*arrows*) with heterogeneous enhancement. There is a T2 hypointense pseudocapsule and T2 hyperintense enhancing peritumoral edema.

specific and sensitive for the diagnosis of MFS compared with other myxoid neoplasms[31,32] and was also found to be associated with worse local recurrence-free survival.[33] Recognition of the infiltrative pattern of tumor spread on preoperative MRI is critical for surgical planning and facilitating complete tumor resection. Thick fascial enhancement without a discrete mass may also be a sign of local recurrence after resection.[32]

Smooth Muscle Tumors

LMS is a common mesenchymal tumor of smooth muscle differentiation, accounting for 9% of all STS. The most common sites of involvement are the uterus, retroperitoneum, and large blood vessels, and less commonly the soft tissues and skin.[2,34] LMS is the second most common retroperitoneal tumor after LPS, and is the most common sarcoma of the large blood vessels (**Fig. 9**).[34] There was no difference between the imaging features and metastatic pattern of non–inferior vena cava and inferior vena cava LMS, with tumors of both subtypes appearing as large, heterogeneously enhancing masses, and frequently metastasizing to the lungs, peritoneum, and liver.[35,36] Extremity LMS, most commonly affecting the thigh, may be deep (intramuscular and intermuscular) or superficial (subcutaneous) in location, and very rarely arise from the bones.[37]

On MRI, imaging features of extremity LMS are nonspecific. Lesions are typically isointense to muscle on T1-weighted images and variably hyperintense relative to muscle on T2-weighted images, with moderate heterogeneous contrast enhancement (**Fig. 10**).[2] Histologically, LMS are usually highly cellular, and may account for T2 hypointensity seen in some of the tumors. Large lesions and those in the deep soft tissue locations are usually more heterogeneous secondary to hemorrhage, necrosis, and cystic change, and may exhibit thick peripheral irregular rim enhancement.[34,37]

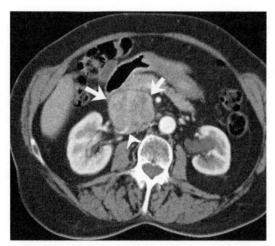

Fig. 9. A 78-year-old man with inferior vena cava (IVC) leiomyosarcoma. Axial contrast-enhanced computed tomography image reveals a large mass (*arrows*) in the retroperitoneum centered in the IVC (*arrowhead*), with intraluminal tumor extension.

Calcification/ossification may be present,[38] and bone involvement is seen in up to 10% of cases.

SKELETAL MUSCLE TUMORS
Rhabdomyosarcomas

RMS arising from striated muscle or its precursor undifferentiated mesenchymal cells is the most common STS in children but also affects adults.[2] Although it can occur anywhere in the body, the most common primary site in adults is the extremities (26% of cases) followed by the genitourinary system (25%), whereas in children the head and neck parameningeal region (25% of cases) is the most common site. Three histologic subtypes of RMS are recognized. The most common embryonal subtype (50%) occurs commonly in children under the age of 10 and affects the head and

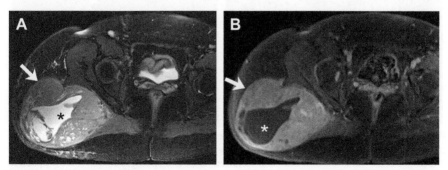

Fig. 10. A 58-year-old woman with right gluteal leiomyosarcoma. Axial short-tau inversion recovery (*A*) and fat-suppressed postgadolinium (*B*) T1-weighted MRIs demonstrate a heterogeneous T2 intermediate signal mass (*arrow*) in the right gluteal region with large central areas of T2 hyperintensity and hypointensity consistent with hemorrhage (*asterisk*). Postcontrast shows moderate homogenous enhancement of the mass.

neck region and genitourinary system. The alveolar subtype (30%) is often seen in the trunk and extremities of adolescents and young adults, 10 to 25 years old, and in the perimaxillary region in adults. The pleomorphic subtype, seen in adults older than 45 years, usually involves the muscles of the thigh and has a poor prognosis.[2]

Embryonal RMS usually presents as heterogeneous, poorly circumscribed mass, with moderately high SI on T2-weighted imaging, with heterogeneous contrast enhancement[39,40] Hemorrhage, necrosis, and calcification are rare. Multiple ring enhancing regions resembling bunch of grapes referred to as "botyroid sign" was noted in some cases.[41] Destruction of the adjacent bone is frequent, seen in approximately 25%, almost exclusively with tumors of the head and neck region.[40,42] Alveolar RMS present as infiltrative heterogenous soft tissue masses with moderately high SI on T2-weighted, and prominent areas of necrosis. Serpentine flow voids and lobulated architecture may also be present. The pleomorphic subtype tends to be markedly hyperintense on T2-weighted imaging with marked heterogeneous enhancement.[40] Lymph node involvement is seen in 33% to 45% of patients with adult RMS,[39] and is most frequent with the alveolar subtype.[43] Lung is the most common site of distant metastases followed by the bones, although any organ may be involved.[39,44]

Vascular Tumors

Angiosarcoma of soft tissue

Soft tissue angiosarcomas are highly aggressive tumors, with high rates of local recurrence and distant metastasis. Angiosarcomas contain both epithelioid and spindle cells, forming rudimentary vascular channels, with frequent infiltration.[1] The majority of soft tissue angiosarcomas are cutaneous tumors, with less than 25% presenting in the deep soft tissues. Risk factors include chronic lymphedema, previous radiation therapy, implanted foreign body, and familial syndromes including type 1 neurofibromatosis and Klippel-Trénaunay-Weber syndrome. MR signal characteristics of angiosarcoma include intermediate SI on T1-weighted images, and high SI on T2-weighted images, with marked, often heterogeneous enhancement (**Fig. 11**).[2] Areas of high signal on T1-weighted imaging suggestive of hemorrhage may be present. Although

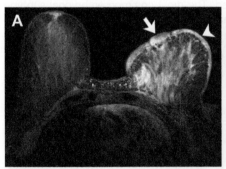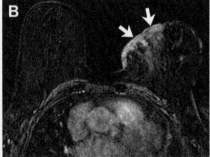

Fig. 11. An 84-year-old woman with radiation-associated angiosarcoma, presenting with violaceous skin lesion and bruising over the left breast 4 years after lumpectomy and radiation for invasive ductal carcinoma. Axial T2-weighted (A) and postgadolinium fat-suppressed T1-weighted (B) MRIs of the breast reveals a heterogenous T2 high signal intensity left medial breast skin thickening, which enhances rapidly after contrast administration (arrows). The diffuse T2 high signal thickening in the skin of the rest of the breast (arrowhead) and within the breast parenchyma do not enhance and represent postradiation edema. The patient underwent neoadjuvant chemotherapy before radical mastectomy and chest wall resection.

flow voids maybe seen in larger deeper tumors, it is characteristically absent with cutaneous lesions. A recent study of MRI findings in 17 women with secondary radiation associated angiosarcoma of the breast demonstrated multifocal T2 hyper or hypointense and rapidly enhancing dermal and intraparenchymal nodules, against a background of T2 hyperintense diffuse skin thickening.[45]

NERVE SHEATH TUMORS

Nerve sheath tumors are included in WHO STS classification for the first time in 2013, previously considered under tumors of the nervous system and skin.[1] Nerve sheath tumors include both benign peripheral nerve sheath tumors, such as neurofibroma and schwannoma, as well as their malignant counterpart, malignant peripheral nerve sheath tumors (MPNST).

MPNST, previously referred to as malignant schwannoma, neurofibrosarcoma, and neurogenic sarcoma, can arise de novo or in preexisting neurofibromas in the setting of neurofibromatosis I. MPNSTs account for 5% to 10% of all STS and usually seen in adult patients 30 to 50 years of age, with males and females affected equally. MPNSTs are associated with neurofibromatosis type 1 in 30% to 70% of cases and that, in that subset, tumors occur a decade earlier with a distinct male predilection (80%).[46] Some MPNSTs have heterologous skeletal muscle (rhabdomyoblastic) differentiation within the tumor, and are classified as malignant triton tumors, demonstrating a more aggressive clinical course and worse prognosis.[47] The most common location is in proximity to large peripheral nerves in the trunk, extremities, head, neck, and retroperitoneum, and most commonly involve the sciatic nerve, brachial plexus, and sacral plexus. Surgical resection is the treatment of choice for MPNSTs. However, local recurrence is seen in 25% to 40%, and distant metastases (commonly to lungs) in 20% to 30%.

Imaging findings of MPNST are nonspecific, with heterogeneous intermediate to high SI on T1-weighted images, and isointense to high SI on T2-weighted images[2,46] (**Fig. 12**). MPNSTs may share some imaging findings with benign neurogenic tumors, such as fusiform appearance with nerve entering/existing the lesion, "split fat" sign,

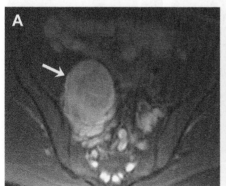
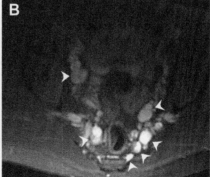

Fig. 12. A 32-year-old man with malignant peripheral nerve sheath tumor in the setting of neurofibromatosis type I. Axial short-tau inversion recovery MRI demonstrates multiple neurofibromas in the pelvis, which are bright on T2-weighted images (*arrowheads, B*). One of the neurogenic tumors in the right pelvic sidewall (*arrow, A*) had significantly enlarged in size when compared with computed tomography scan performed 6 months before (not shown). Biopsy of the mass showed malignant peripheral nerve sheath tumor.

bright rim sign, fascicular sign, and denervation atrophy of the supplied muscles, and differentiation of benign from malignant nerve sheath tumors may be difficult. Imaging features that favor MPNST over benign neurogenic tumors include rapid growth, large size (>5 cm), infiltrative margins, lobulation, heterogeneous high SI on T1, irregular peripheral enhancement with central necrosis, and peritumoral edema.[46,48,49] A study of 45 patients with neurofibromatosis type 1, reported that fluorodeoxyglucose (FDG) PET-CT showed specificity of 72% and a positive predictive value of 71% in detection of MPNSTs.[50] Although imaging findings are similar to other high grade sarcomas, if a lesion has an intermuscular distribution and/or along the course of a large nerve and has a nodular morphology with a fusiform shape, MPNST should be included in the differential diagnosis.[51]

TUMORS OF UNCERTAIN DIFFERENTIATION
Synovial Sarcoma

Synovial sarcoma (SS) is a relatively common sarcoma, mainly affecting young adults, and accounts for 5% to 10% of STS. Pathologically, it is classified as monophasic (composed of only spindle cells), biphasic (composed of both spindle cell and epithelial components) and poorly differentiated. The characteristic t(X;18) translocation is seen in about 95% of tumors.[1] Despite the name, less than 5% of SS originate in a joint or bursa. The most common location are the extremities (80% of cases), especially around the knee and adjacent to tendon sheaths[2] (**Fig. 13**).

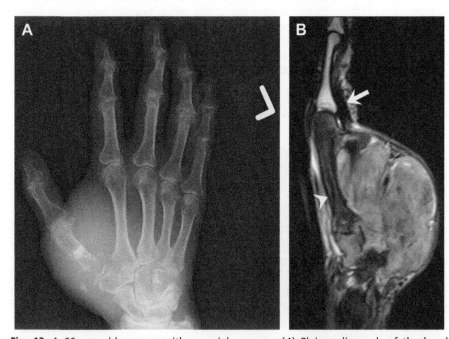

Fig. 13. A 66-year-old woman with synovial sarcoma. (*A*) Plain radiograph of the hand shows a soft tissue mass centered on the thenar eminence of the left hand with destruction of the first metacarpal bone and areas of calcification within. (*B*) Sagittal T2-weighted MRI of the hand reveals a large heterogeneously hyperintense mass with abnormal signal of the first metacarpal bone (*arrowhead*) and invasion of the extensor tendons of the first digit (*arrow*).

On imaging, SS are multilobulated or septated masses with heterogeneous SI on both T1 and T2 W images. Heterogeneity is secondary to areas of cystic change, necrosis, calcification, and hemorrhage within the tumor, and maybe manifest as "triple sign" on T2-weighted imaging (consisting of hypo-, iso-, and hyperintense signal) (**Fig. 14**). "Fluid–fluid levels" secondary to layering hemorrhage and "bowl of grapes" appearance from T2 hyperintense lobulated areas and T2 hypointense septa, may be present in some cases.[52–54] Calcification is seen in up to one third of cases, ranging from fine stippling to marked peripheral calcifications, and is best seen on CT.[53,55,56] Up to 20% show erosion or invasion of adjacent bone (see **Fig. 13**). Smaller tumors may be well-circumscribed and homogeneous and can be mistaken for a benign cystic lesions.[55] SS are commonly high grade tumors, with high incidence of pleuropulmonary metastases, as well as lymph nodal metastases (10%–30%).[54] Although imaging findings are nonspecific, a calcified soft tissue mass in the lower extremity of young adults should prompt the diagnosis of synovial sarcoma.

Alveolar Soft Part Sarcoma

ASPS are extremely rare sarcomas, predominantly affecting the lower extremities (thighs) of children and young adults.[57] ASPS are highly vascular tumors often presenting as pulsating masses with bruits. Histologically, ASPS is composed of large epithelioid cells with abundant cytoplasm arranged in nesting or pseudoalveolar

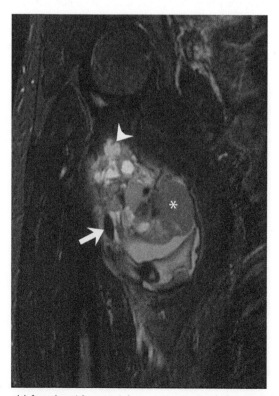

Fig. 14. A 35-year old female with synovial sarcoma. Coronal short-tau inversion recovery MRI reveals a large heterogenous mass in the medial right upper thigh demonstrating triple sign (*arrow, arrowhead,* and *asterisk*).

growth pattern, surrounded by vascularized connective tissue. The tumor cells stain positive for TFE3 in nearly100% of cases, almost exclusively seen in ASPS and in Xp11 translocation-associated pediatric renal cell cancers.[1]

On imaging, ASPS are usually well-circumscribed lobulated masses with moderately high SI on T1-weighted imaging and T2-weighted imaging, and marked heterogeneous contrast enhancement.[2] The tumor often has internal and peripheral, areas of serpentine and linear flow voids from intratumoral vessels[58,59] (**Fig. 15**). Although appearance is similar to other aggressive STS, ASPS should be suggested when children or young adults present with a highly vascular intramuscular mass with flow voids and central scar, especially if concurrent lung metastases are present.[60–62] ASPS has a high propensity for hematogenous metastases, most frequently to the lungs (90%), lymph nodes (60%), bones (50%) and brain (40%).[63,64] Despite high incidence of distant metastases, it a follows a characteristically indolent course with long overall survival.[63,65]

Extraskeletal Ewing Sarcoma

EES belong to the Ewing sarcoma family of tumors comprising of classical skeletal Ewing sarcoma, extraskeletal Ewing sarcoma, primitive neuroectodermal tumor, and Askin tumor.[66] Ewing sarcoma is a malignant small round-blue cell tumor of the bone and soft tissue, arising from neuroectodermal cells, with classical translocation t[11;22], present in approximately 90% of cases.[1] EES can occur anywhere in the body from head to toe, the preferred locations are deep soft tissues of the extremities (**Fig. 16**), retroperitoneum/peritoneum, chest wall and paravertebral regions (most frequent in cervical and sacral spine).[67–69] On imaging, tumors appear as bulky heterogeneous masses with frequent invasion of the adjacent organs. Paravertebral masses

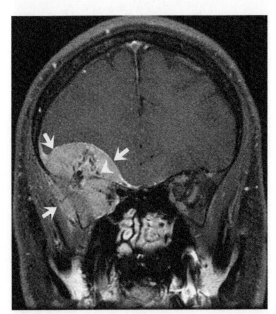

Fig. 15. A 27-year-old with retroocular alveolar soft part sarcoma. Coronal postcontrast fat-suppressed T1-weighted MRI reveals a large retroorbital mass with intracranial extension (*arrows*). The linear hypointense areas in the mass (*arrowhead*) represent flow voids, characteristic of this vascular tumor.

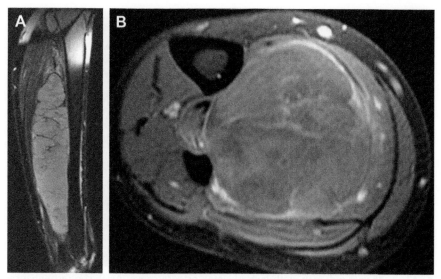

Fig. 16. A 24-year-old man with extraskeletal Ewing sarcoma. Coronal short-tau inversion recovery (*A*) and axial postcontrast fat-suppressed (*B*) T1-weighted MRI reveals a T2 hyperintense lobulated intramuscular mass in the anterior compartment of the leg, with mild diffuse enhancement throughout. The tibia and fibula are intact.

maybe associated with neural foraminal and epidural extension. Tumors are either hypo or isointense to the skeletal muscle on T1-weighted, and heterogenously hyperintense on T2-weighted, with heterogenous enhancement and frequent central necrosis (50%–70%).[66–69] The most common sites of metastases are lung, bones and lymph nodes, although a more recent series of 70 patients with EES in the Asian population reported lymph nodes as the most common site of metastases (71%).[68]

Extraskeletal Osteosarcoma

Extraskeletal osteosarcoma (EO) is an extremely rare, but aggressive, malignant mesenchymal neoplasm histologically indistinguishable from bone osteosarcoma. Tumors are seen in a distinctly older age group, with mean age of 45 to 60 years. The most common site of involvement is the thigh (50% of cases), followed by the upper extremity, retroperitoneum and the trunk. Prior radiation is a documented risk factor and EO is one of the common radiation-associated sarcomas.[1] EO are large, deep-seated soft tissue masses with a variable amount of mineralization. Although EO does not arise from the bone, osseous involvement may be seen. On MRI EO often present as well-circumscribed, inhomogeneous masses on T1-weighted imaging and T2-weighted imaging with pseudocapsule and heterogeneous contrast enhancement. Mineralization is present in up to 50% to 70% of lesions (presenting as signal voids on all sequences), and when present greatly aids diagnosis (**Fig. 17**).[2,70] In contrast to myositis ossificans which shows peripheral and zonal ossification, non-organized mineralization is seen in the center of the lesion. Hemorrhage, necrosis and cystic change are common, and fluid–fluid levels may be seen in aggressive tumors. The overall prognosis is poor, with high rates of local recurrence and metastases occurring in up to 90% of cases.

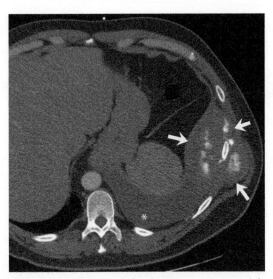

Fig. 17. A 46-year-old man with extraskeletal osteosarcoma. Axial contrast-enhanced computed tomography image of the chest demonstrates a large left chest wall soft tissue mass with internal areas of mineralization (*arrows*). There is associated left pleural effusion (*asterisk*).

Aggressive Angiomyxoma

Aggressive angiomyxoma is a rare locally aggressive mesenchymal tumor most commonly arising from the perineum or lower pelvis, of young women.[2] On imaging, the tumor is large, often greater than 10 cm, and extends from the pelvis into the perineum into the pelvis. Despite its large size, it is frequently asymptomatic as it displaces rather than invades the pelvic viscera. Owing to the myxoid matrix, the tumor is markedly hypoechoic on ultrasonography, hypodense on CT and T2 hyperintense on MRI (**Fig. 18**). Another characteristic finding is "swirling" or "laminated" appearance of swirling T2 hypointense strands, owing to presence of fibrovascular stroma.[71–73]

Desmoplastic Small Round Cell Tumor

Desmoplastic small round cell tumor is a rare, peritoneal malignancy occurring in adolescents and young adults, with a distinct male predilection.[74] It belongs to the family

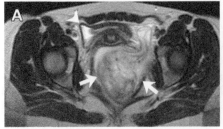
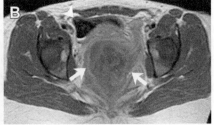

Fig. 18. A 28-year-old woman with aggressive angiomyxoma. Axial T2 (*A*) and contrast-enhanced T1-weighted (*B*) MRIs reveal a T2 hyperintense and T1 hypointense lobulated pelvic mass (*arrows*) displacing the urinary bladder anteriorly (*arrowhead*). There are linear T2-hypointense strands coursing through lesion, giving rise to classic swirling pattern.

of small round blue cell tumors (lymphoma, neuroblastoma, Ewing sarcoma), and is characterized by reciprocal translocation between Ewing sarcoma gene (EWS) and Wilms' tumor gene (WT1) [t(11;22) (q13;p12)].[74] The most common imaging appearance is that of multiple, bulky, heterogeneous peritoneal based masses, without distinct site of origin. The pelvis and paravesical regions are frequently involved, although any serosal surface maybe affected (**Fig. 19**).[74] Ascites is frequent (up to 50%) and lesions may rarely be calcified. It is an aggressive tumor with frequent and early metastatic spread to the peritoneum, liver, lymph nodes, lungs and bones.

Solitary Fibrous Tumor

Solitary fibrous tumors are rare spindle cell neoplasms, affecting middle aged adults with no sex predilection. In the revised 2013 WHO classification, solitary fibrous tumor encompasses tumors that were previously classified hemangiopericytoma, lipomatous hemangiopericytoma and giant cell angiofibroma.[1] Histologic hallmarks of SFTs are CD34 positivity (seen in 80%–100% of tumors) and over expression of STAT6 protein.[4] While the majority of SFTs are benign, up to 20% may demonstrate malignant behavior, and surgical resection in the treatment of choice. The most common site of origin is the pleura. Extrapleural SFTs commonly involves the retroperitoneum, pelvis, proximal extremities, and abdominal wall, although tumors can occur anywhere in the body.[75]

On CT, lesions are well-circumscribed, lobulated masses with avid enhancement and prominent draining vessels (**Fig. 20**). On MRI, tumors show variable and inhomogeneous SI on T2-weighted, depending on proportion of fibrous tissue and hemorrhage (T2 hypointense) and myxoid and cystic components (T2 hyperintense). Intralesional and peripheral flow voids are common (**Fig. 21**), reflecting the highly vascular nature.[75–77] The cellular variant of SFT have little fibrous tissue, and is predominantly intermediate to hyperintense signal on T2-weighted, whereas the myxoid variant is extremelyT2 hyperintense Tumors are highly vascular and show marked heterogeneous enhancement after gadolinium administration. A variant of SFT, previously lipomatous hemangiopericytoma, may contain macroscopic fat. Although

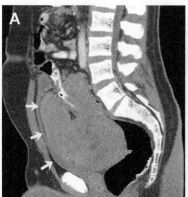
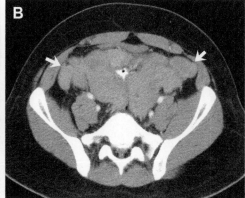

Fig. 19. A 19-year-old man with desmoplastic small round cell tumor. Sagittal and axial contrast-enhanced computed tomography images of the pelvis demonstrate a large soft tissue paravesical mass (*arrows, A*) compressing and displacing bladder anteriorly, encasing the sigmoid colon associated with multiple other peritoneal masses (*arrows, B*) in the lower abdomen.

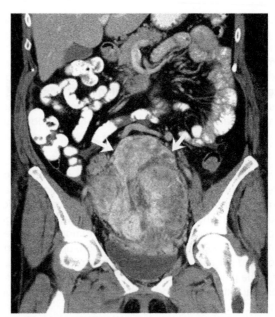

Fig. 20. A 51-year-old woman with solitary fibrous tumor. Coronal reformatted contrast-enhanced computed tomography image of the pelvis demonstrates a large lobulated hypervascular soft tissue mass in the pelvis (*arrows*) with prominent venous collaterals.

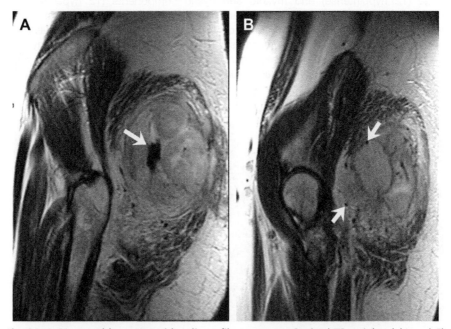

Fig. 21. A 51-year-old woman with solitary fibrous tumor. Sagittal T2-weighted (*A* and *B*) MRIs of the thigh reveal a heterogeneous lobulated high signal intensity mass posterior to the hip joint. There is central T2 hypointense area (*arrow*, A) in the mass correlating with calcification on computed tomography (not shown). There are several linear and serpentine T2 hypointense foci (*arrows*, B) consistent with flow voids.

distinction between benign and malignant SFTs are difficult, large size, heterogeneity, necrosis, bone destruction or organ invasion, and increased uptake on FDG-PET are suspicious for malignancy.[77]

Gastrointestinal Stromal Tumor

GISTs have been added to the classification of the STS for the first time, having previously been classified as tumors of the digestive tract. GIST is most common mesenchymal tumor of the GI tract, with 3000 to 6000 new cases annually in the United States. Pathologically, GIST demonstrates an activating mutation in tyrosine kinase receptors, namely c-kit (CD117) or platelet- derived growth factor receptor-α in 90% of cases.[1] A small subset of indolent gastric GISTs lack these mutations, but demonstrate a loss of function of succinate dehydrogenase, referred to as succinate dehydrogenase-deficient GISTs.[78]

On imaging, GISTs present as large homogeneous or heterogeneous soft tissue masses arising from the bowel wall, with a predominant exophytic or intraluminal component.[79] The stomach is the most common site of origin, followed by the small bowel, esophagus, and rectum. Primary retroperitoneal or mesenteric GISTS are extremely rare. Metastases most frequently involve the liver or peritoneum, although lymph nodal metastases can occur in succinate dehydrogenase-deficient GISTs.[78] GISTs are among the few STS that demonstrate dramatic response to targeted therapy using tyrosine-kinase inhibitors, such as imatinib, which are currently routinely used for neoadjuvant and adjuvant therapy. Response is classically seen as a marked decrease in density with or without size changes.[80] Conversely, resistance is manifested as in increase in density or new and increasing solid components.

UNDIFFERENTIATED/UNCLASSIFIED SARCOMAS

This newly introduced category in the current 2013 WHO classification includes tumors whose tissue of origin cannot be determined by the current techniques and thus cannot be otherwise classified into the existing categories. These tumors currently account for approximately 20% of all sarcomas, and about 25% of these are radiation-associated sarcomas.[1] Undifferentiated/unclassified sarcomas are histologically diverse tumors and may have spindle cell, pleomorphic, round cell, or epithelioid morphology. The largest subtype—undifferentiated pleomorphic sarcoma—are high-grade sarcomas that were previously classified as and better known as malignant fibrous histiocytoma.[26] Unclassified pleomorphic sarcoma typically occur in older patients (50–70 years) presenting as large, painless, well-circumscribed, multinodular, lobulated tumors in the extremities and retroperitoneum. Sometimes, tumors may present with spontaneous hemorrhage or systemic symptoms (giant cell/inflammatory subtypes). On imaging, the findings are varied and nonspecific, depending on the degree of cellularity and the presence of hemorrhage, necrosis, and/or calcification.[2] On MRI, tumors are generally high SI on T2-weighted imaging, heterogeneous on T1-weighted, and demonstrate heterogeneous enhancement (**Figs. 22** and **23**).[81] Calcification/ossification can be seen in 5% to 20% of cases, often in the periphery of the tumor, and is better identified on CT. Osseous involvement, particularly cortical destruction, is seen when abutting the bone.

Intraabdominal/Retroperitoneal Sarcomas

The majority of the intraabdominal sarcomas other than GIST and other rare sarcomas of the abdominal viscera, tend occur in the retroperitoneum. Retroperitoneal sarcomas (RPS) account for 1% to 2% of all solid malignancies and represent 15% of

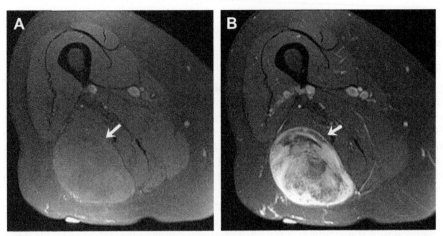

Fig. 22. A 79-year-old woman with unclassified pleomorphic sarcoma, high grade. Axial pre-contrast (*A*) and postcontrast fat-suppressed T1-weighted (*B*) MRIs of the thigh reveal an intramuscular heterogeneous T1 intermediate to high signal intensity mass (*arrows*) with heterogeneous enhancement in the posterior thigh.

all STS.[82] The reported frequencies of RPS in adults varies by studies. Overall, the most frequent RPS histologic types are liposarcomas and leiomyosarcomas. Many of the tumors that were classified previously as malignant fibrous histiocytomas (which was reportedly the third common RPS) are now thought to be dedifferentiated LPS or undifferentiated sarcomas based on immunohistochemistry.[83] Patients with intraabdominal sarcomas present late, because these tumors can grow very large without causing symptoms, and even when symptoms occur, they are frequently nonspecific.

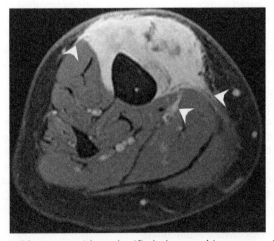

Fig. 23. An 81-year-old woman with unclassified pleomorphic sarcoma. Axial postcontrast fat-suppressed T1-weighted MRI of the leg reveals a heterogeneously enhancing mass in the anterior compartment of the leg, with multiple enhancing taillike extensions (*arrowheads*) along the fascial planes and into the muscle.

Contrast-enhanced CT is the most commonly used modality for identification, localization, and staging of intraabdominal sarcomas, with MRI reserved for specific situations like vascular involvement or neural invasion. Imaging is not reliable to predict the histologic subtypes of most intraabdominal sarcomas, although there are a few exceptions. Bulky exophytic gastric mass without adenopathy should raise the possibility of GIST. The presence of macroscopic fat within the tumor (CT attenuation values of less than −10 Hounsfeld units or high signal on T1-weighted on MRI), suggests the diagnosis of LPS. However, not all LPS demonstrate macroscopic fat on imaging. Dedifferentiated LPS may be composed almost entirely of soft tissue and fluid components, and in those cases, the tumors cannot be reliably differentiated from other types of sarcomas[7] **(Fig. 24)**. Enhancing tumor in the retroperitoneum with nonidentification of the inferior vena cava or tumor within the lumen of the inferior vena cava with luminal expansion is highly suggestive of inferior vena cava LMS[36] (see **Fig. 9**). The presence of multiple peritoneal masses centered in the perivesical region, without distinct site of origin in a young male adult should raise the possibility of desmoplastic small round cell tumor. In a patient presenting with peritoneal sarcomatosis, often seen as of large, spherical, vascular peritoneal implants with minimal ascites, peritoneal spread from GIST, LPS, LMS, sarcomatoid mesothelioma, and desmoplastic small round cell tumor should be suspected.[84]

Imaging has a limited role in predicting the grade of sarcoma and prognosis. In case of LPS, if the tumor is composed of predominantly fat and very little soft tissue, it is likely to be a low-grade tumor, often well-differentiated LPS. However, if the tumor contains predominantly soft tissue/fluid density and with little or no macroscopic fat, it may be a low-, intermediate- or high-grade tumor.[10] Calcification or ossification within an RP LPS has been shown to be a poor prognostic feature.[85] The American Joint Committee on Cancer staging system (7th edition) for STS does not apply to RPS, and currently there is no established staging system for RPS. The main role of

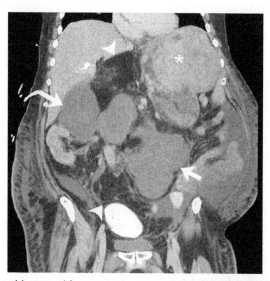

Fig. 24. A 70-year-old man with recurrent retroperitoneal dedifferentiated liposarcoma, 3 years after complete resection. Coronal contrast enhanced computed tomography of the abdomen reveals multifocal intraabdominal masses with areas of soft tissue (*asterisk*), fat (*arrowheads*) and fluid attenuation (*arrow*).

imaging in staging RPS is to determine whether the tumor is localized or if there is evidence of intraabdominal or extraabdominal metastatic disease.

Treatment and imaging follow-up
The definitive treatment for primary intraabdominal sarcomas is surgical resection, with or without preoperative chemotherapy and radiation. In general, up to 75% of RPS resections involve resection of at least 1 contiguous intraabdominal visceral organ (usually kidney, adrenals spleen, or bowel). On imaging, identification of organ involvement and status of the opposite kidney becomes critical. Despite adequate resections, 5- and 10-year survival rates are poor, being 51% and 36%, respectively.[82] This is often owing to local recurrences within the surgical bed, with most occurring within 2 years of primary resection. Detection of local recurrence in LPS is especially difficult because recurrences often mimic normal intraabominal fat on imaging, and recurrent tumors can be heterogeneous with different imaging characteristics than that of the primary tumors[86] (see **Fig. 24**). Regional and distant metastases are also frequent, often involving peritoneal surfaces and liver followed by lungs, soft tissues, and bones. Follow-up imaging is usually performed with CT with the frequency of follow-up often dictated by tumor type, grade, and resection margins. At our institution, imaging is generally performed every 3 to 4 months for 2 years, then every 4 to 6 months for 3 to 5 years, and every 12 months thereafter.

Extremity Soft Tissue Sarcomas

More than 50% of the STS occur in extremities.[87] The most common histologic subtype varies with age[2] (**Table 1**). ESTS usually present as painless, frequently large, palpable soft tissue masses. MRI is the imaging modality of choice of extremity soft tissue tumors and tumorlike masses, owing to its superior tissue contrast and multiplanar capability, without radiation exposure. MRI provides excellent anatomic visualization and characterization of the internal architecture, and accurately defines the extent of tumors and neurovascular involvement. The use of intravenous gadolinium contrast is controversial; at our institution, we routinely perform contrast enhanced MRI. Functional MRI techniques such as diffusion-weighted imaging and dynamic contrast-enhanced MRI are still investigational. Certain MRI features can help in differentiating benign and malignant soft tissue neoplasms and also low-grade and high-grade STS (**Table 2**).

Conventional radiography can be used to detect bone involvement and calcifications; however, it has little role in STS, unlike in bone tumors. Similarly, role of ultrasonography is limited to probable workup of superficial soft tissue masses and guide biopsy. Contrast-enhanced CT is a useful adjunct to MRI, and can aid in the identification of mineralization and osseous involvement, although it is not routinely performed, except in patients with contraindications to MRI and to guide biopsy. PET performed with fluorine18 FDG is used for staging and follow-up of various malignancies, and a number of investigators have studied its use in bone and STS. In a recent metaanalysis, the overall pooled sensitivity and specificity of FDG-PET for detection of all sarcomas were 91% and 85%, respectively, with higher standardized uptake values in sarcomas (range, 0.80–15.43) compared with benign tumors (range, 0.22–1.43).[88]

Treatment and imaging follow-up
The standard of care for ESTS is limb-sparing, function-preserving surgery with negative margins, and often may require complex soft tissue and neurovascular reconstruction.[89] Preoperative tissue diagnosis is the gold standard for diagnosis of STS

Table 1
Clinicopathologic approach to soft tissue sarcomas

Clues to differentiate malignant from benign soft tissue tumors

History of underlying malignancy
Prior therapy including surgery or radiation
Pain - painful mass raises the possibility of inflammatory process
Trauma or anticoagulation - possibility of hematoma or myosistis ossificans
Rate of growth and variations in size (hemangioma, ganglion cyst)
Multiplicity of lesions - possibility of benign processes (lipoma, desmoid, neurofibroma)

Clues to differentiate histologic subtypes of soft tissue sarcomas

Age	0–20 y: Rhabdomyosarcoma
	20–40 y: Alveolar soft part sarcoma, Ewing sarcoma, synovial sarcoma
	40–60 y: Fibrohistiocytic sarcoma, solitary fibrous tumor, MPNST
	>60 y: Liposarcoma, leiomyosarcoma, angiosarcoma, unclassified pleomorphic sarcoma
Location	Skin and superficial dermis: dermatofibrosarcoma protruberans
	Subcutaneous: myxofibrosarcomas and epithelioid sarcomas
	Intermuscular: synovial sarcoma
	Intramuscular: pleomorphic sarcoma, liposarcoma, rhabdomyosarcoma
	Periarticular: synovial sarcoma
	Associated with tendons/aponeuroses: clear cell sarcoma
	Multi-compartmental extension: angiomatous lesions, neurofibromatosis, desmoid fibromatosis, aggressive angiomyxomas
Calcification	Chondroosseous–type tumors (extraskeletal osteosarcoma, ESMC), synovial sarcoma, undifferentiated pleomorphic sarcoma, ossifying fibromyxoid tumors, PEComa
Nodal metastasis	Synovial sarcoma, epithelioid sarcoma, alveolar rhabdomyosarcoma, clear cell sarcoma, extraskeletal Ewing sarcoma, angiosarcoma and alveolar soft part sarcoma

Abbreviations: ESMC, extraskeletal myxoid chondrosarcoma; MPNST, malignant peripheral nerve sheath tumor; PEComa, perivascular epithelioid cell tumor.

(**Box 1**). For preoperative planning in functional limb-sparing resections, it is important to define the extent of tumor (depth and compartment) and relationship of tumor to the adjacent bones and neurovascular bundle. An intracompartmental lesion is one that has not crossed anatomic boundaries such as bone, joint capsule, fascial planes, or tendons. Although MRI is the preferred modality for staging, a recent study of 88 patients with STS has shown that contrast-enhanced CT with CT angiography is comparable with MRI in identifying aggressive lesions and depicting the relationship between tumor and adjacent bones and major vessels.[90] Histologic grade is one of the most important prognostic factors in ESTS outcome, and certain MRI features have been shown to be helpful in differentiating high-grade STS from low-grade tumors (see **Table 2**).[48,91] Although peritumoral T2 hyperintensity is often observed in higher grade sarcomas, it does not imply tumor infiltration in all cases; radiation oncologists often include this region within their planning target volume.[92]

Local recurrence rates after surgery for STS are between 5% and 35% of cases, usually occurring within the first 2 years. Similar to preoperative imaging, MRI is the modality of choice in the postoperative period to distinguish between posttreatment changes and tumor recurrence.[93] In general, recurrences are similar to the primary tumor and often present as T2 hyperintense focal enhancing nodule (**Fig. 25**). Recurrent tumors need to be distinguished from fibrosis, posttreatment inflammatory changes,

Table 2
MRI-based approach to soft tissue sarcomas

Clues to differentiate malignant from benign soft tissue tumors	Lesion size of more than 5 cm Location deep to fascia Irregular margins Heterogeneous signal especially on T1-weighted images Early heterogeneous enhancement with central necrosis
Clues to differentiate high-grade from low-grade sarcomas	Large tumor size Irregular tumor margin Heterogeneous signal intensity on T2-weighted images Peritumoral high signal intensity (peritumoral edema) Peritumoral contrast enhancement Presence of pseudocapsule
Clues to differentiate histologic subtypes of soft tissue sarcomas	
High signal intensity on T1-weighted imaging, which drops in signal on fat suppressed sequences	Adipocytic tumors
Extreme T2 hyperintensity with moderately intense enhancement	Myxoid tumors
Low signal intensity on T2-weighted imaging	Extremely cellular sarcomas, calcification, fibrous tissue (as in low grade fibromyxoid sarcoma) or hemosiderin (pigmented villonodular synovitis)
Flow voids with intense enhancement	Extrapleural solitary fibrous tumor and alveolar soft part sarcoma
T2-hyperintense enhancing curvilinear projection (tail sign)	Myxofibrosarcoma
Bowl of grapes sign Triple sign	Synovial sarcoma

Box 1
Tissue sampling in soft tissue sarcomas

- Gold standard for definitive diagnosis.
- Percutaneous biopsy under image guidance is the preferred method; optimal biopsy site and route depends on the imaging findings.
- Biopsy site should be determined in conjunction with the orthopedic surgeon or surgical oncologist.
- Shortest path between the skin and the lesion should be chosen.
- Target the solid enhancing area, avoiding the cystic, necrotic, or calcified components.
- Avoid a biopsy path that may potentially violate multiple compartments. Biopsy track should be resected during subsequent surgery.
- Limitation of needle biopsies is sampling error; soft tissue sarcomas have a heterogeneous histology.

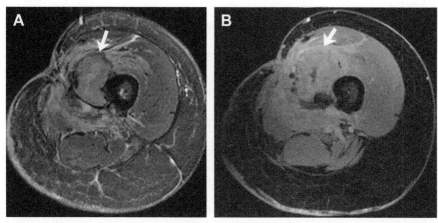

Fig. 25. A 72-year-old woman with recurrent myxofibrosarcoma. Axial short-tau inversion recovery (*A*) and postgadolinium fat-suppressed (*B*) T1-weighted MRIs of the thigh reveal T2 intermediate signal mass in the medial thigh, which enhances after contrast administration (*arrows*). Postoperative changes with edema and non-masslike enhancement in the adjacent muscles are noted medially related to prior resection and radiation.

seroma, and organizing hematoma.[93,94] Metastatic disease is reported in up to 70% of patients with ESTS within the first 2 to 3 years,[95] most commonly to the lungs and bones. Although the first 2 years is the period of highest recurrence risk, follow-up should continue long term because of the persistent risk beyond 5 years. At our institution, imaging of the tumor bed with MRI and distant disease with CT (usually chest CT) is performed every 3 to 4 months for 2 years, then every 4 to 6 months for 3 to 5 years, and yearly thereafter.

Approach to Diagnosis of Soft Tissue Sarcomas: Differentiation of Histologic Types of Soft Tissue Sarcomas

The differentiation between benign and malignant soft tissue tumors as well as differentiating the various histologic subtypes of sarcoma on imaging alone is challenging and requires multidisciplinary approach. In fact, an accurate histologic diagnosis based on imaging alone was reported in only 25% to 30% of cases, although recent numbers may be much higher.[96] However, a combination of patient demographics, pertinent clinical data, location of the mass, multiplicity of lesions, growth pattern, and specific imaging findings may help to narrow down the differential (see **Table 1**). Tissue sampling remains the gold standard for definitive diagnosis and the optimal biopsy site and route depend on the imaging findings and should be determined in conjunction with the surgical or orthopedic oncologists (see **Table 2**).

SUMMARY

STS are heterogeneous malignant tumors with nonspecific imaging features. A combination of clinical, demographic, and imaging characteristics can aid in the diagnosis. Often the imaging findings are indeterminate, and biopsy is performed with the optimal biopsy route discussed with the treating surgeon. Once the diagnosis is made, imaging provides important information regarding the tumor extent, pretreatment planning and surveillance of patients with STS. With advent of advanced imaging and image processing techniques like functional imaging and texture analysis, the role of imaging in the management of STS is anticipated to evolve in the future.

REFERENCES

1. Fletcher CD, Bridge JA, Hogendoorn P, et al. WHO classification of tumours of soft tissue and bone. 4th edition. Geneva (Switzerland): World Health Organization; 2013. p. 305–10.
2. Kransdorf MJ, Murphey MD. Imaging of soft tissue tumors. Philadelphia: Lippincott Williams & Wilkins; 2006.
3. Goldblum JR, Weiss SW, Folpe AL. Enzinger and Weiss's soft tissue tumors. New York: Elsevier Health Sciences; 2013.
4. Jo VY, Fletcher CD. WHO classification of soft tissue tumours: an update based on the 2013 (4th) edition. Pathology 2014;46(2):95–104.
5. Brisson M, Kashima T, Delaney D, et al. MRI characteristics of lipoma and atypical lipomatous tumor/well-differentiated liposarcoma: retrospective comparison with histology and MDM2 gene amplification. Skeletal Radiol 2013;42(5):635–47.
6. Kransdorf MJ, Bancroft LW, Peterson JJ, et al. Imaging of fatty tumors: distinction of lipoma and well-differentiated liposarcoma. Radiology 2002;224(1):99–104.
7. O'Regan KN, Jagannathan J, Krajewski K, et al. Imaging of liposarcoma: classification, patterns of tumor recurrence, and response to treatment. AJR Am J Roentgenol 2011;197(1):W37–43.
8. Bestic JM, Kransdorf MJ, White LM, et al. Sclerosing variant of well-differentiated liposarcoma: relative prevalence and spectrum of CT and MRI features. AJR Am J Roentgenol 2013;201(1):154–61.
9. Murphey MD, Arcara LK, Fanburg-Smith J. From the archives of the AFIP: imaging of musculoskeletal liposarcoma with radiologic-pathologic correlation. Radiographics 2005;25(5):1371–95.
10. Tirumani SH, Wagner AJ, Tirumani H, et al. Is the nonlipomatous component of dedifferentiated liposarcoma always soft tissue on CT? Analysis of CT densities and correlation with rate of growth in 60 patients. Abdom Imaging 2015;40(5):1248–54.
11. Keung EZ, Hornick JL, Bertagnolli MM, et al. Predictors of outcomes in patients with primary retroperitoneal dedifferentiated liposarcoma undergoing surgery. J Am Coll Surg 2014;218(2):206–17.
12. Tirumani SH, Tirumani H, Jagannathan JP, et al. Metastasis in dedifferentiated liposarcoma: predictors and outcome in 148 patients. Eur J Surg Oncol 2015;41(7):899–904.
13. Sung MS, Kang HS, Suh JS, et al. Myxoid liposarcoma: appearance at MR imaging with histologic correlation. Radiographics 2000;20(4):1007–19.
14. Baheti AD, Tirumani SH, Rosenthal MH, et al. Myxoid soft-tissue neoplasms: comprehensive update of the taxonomy and MRI features. AJR Am J Roentgenol 2015;204(2):374–85.
15. Tateishi U, Hasegawa T, Beppu Y, et al. Prognostic significance of MRI findings in patients with myxoid-round cell liposarcoma. AJR Am J Roentgenol 2004;182(3):725–31.
16. Lowenthal D, Zeile M, Niederhagen M, et al. Differentiation of myxoid liposarcoma by magnetic resonance imaging: a histopathologic correlation. Acta Radiol 2014;55(8):952–60.
17. Sheah K, Ouellette HA, Torriani M, et al. Metastatic myxoid liposarcomas: imaging and histopathologic findings. Skeletal Radiol 2008;37(3):251–8.

18. Stevenson JD, Watson JJ, Cool P, et al. Whole-body magnetic resonance imaging in myxoid liposarcoma: a useful adjunct for the detection of extra-pulmonary metastatic disease. Eur J Surg Oncol 2016;42(4):574–80.

19. Seo SW, Kwon JW, Jang SW, et al. Feasibility of whole-body MRI for detecting metastatic myxoid liposarcoma: a case series. Orthopedics 2011;34(11): e748–54.

20. Hoesly PM, Lowe GC, Lohse CM, et al. Prognostic impact of fibrosarcomatous transformation in dermatofibrosarcoma protuberans: a cohort study. J Am Acad Dermatol 2015;72(3):419–25.

21. Bichakjian CK, Olencki T, Alam M, et al. Dermatofibrosarcoma protuberans, version 1.2014. J Natl Compr Canc Netw 2014;12(6):863–8.

22. Riggs K, McGuigan KL, Morrison WB, et al. Role of magnetic resonance imaging in perioperative assessment of dermatofibrosarcoma protuberans. Dermatol Surg 2009;35(12):2036–41.

23. Torreggiani WC, Al-Ismail K, Munk PL, et al. Dermatofibrosarcoma protuberans: MR imaging features. AJR Am J Roentgenol 2002;178(4):989–93.

24. Li X, Zhang W, Xiao L, et al. Computed tomographic and pathological findings of dermatofibrosarcoma protuberans. J Comput Assist Tomogr 2012;36(4):462–8.

25. Zhang L, Liu QY, Cao Y, et al. Dermatofibrosarcoma protuberans: computed tomography and magnetic resonance imaging findings. Medicine (Baltimore) 2015;94(24):e1001.

26. Fletcher CD, Gustafson P, Rydholm A, et al. Clinicopathologic re-evaluation of 100 malignant fibrous histiocytomas: prognostic relevance of subclassification. J Clin Oncol 2001;19(12):3045–50.

27. Sanfilippo R, Miceli R, Grosso F, et al. Myxofibrosarcoma: prognostic factors and survival in a series of patients treated at a single institution. Ann Surg Oncol 2011; 18(3):720–5.

28. Willems SM, Debiec-Rychter M, Szuhai K, et al. Local recurrence of myxofibrosarcoma is associated with increase in tumour grade and cytogenetic aberrations, suggesting a multistep tumour progression model. Mod Pathol 2006;19(3): 407–16.

29. Waters B, Panicek DM, Lefkowitz RA, et al. Low-grade myxofibrosarcoma: CT and MRI patterns in recurrent disease. AJR Am J Roentgenol 2007;188(2):W193–8.

30. Petscavage-Thomas JM, Walker EA, Logie CI, et al. Soft-tissue myxomatous lesions: review of salient imaging features with pathologic comparison. Radiographics 2014;34(4):964–80.

31. Lefkowitz RA, Landa J, Hwang S, et al. Myxofibrosarcoma: prevalence and diagnostic value of the "tail sign" on magnetic resonance imaging. Skeletal Radiol 2013;42(6):809–18.

32. Kaya M, Wada T, Nagoya S, et al. MRI and histological evaluation of the infiltrative growth pattern of myxofibrosarcoma. Skeletal Radiol 2008;37(12):1085–90.

33. Iwata S, Yonemoto T, Araki A, et al. Impact of infiltrative growth on the outcome of patients with undifferentiated pleomorphic sarcoma and myxofibrosarcoma. J Surg Oncol 2014;110(6):707–11.

34. Hartman DS, Hayes WS, Choyke PL, et al. From the archives of the AFIP. Leiomyosarcoma of the retroperitoneum and inferior vena cava: radiologic-pathologic correlation. Radiographics 1992;12(6):1203–20.

35. Cooley CL, Jagannathan JP, Kurra V, et al. Imaging features and metastatic pattern of non-IVC retroperitoneal leiomyosarcomas: are they different from IVC leiomyosarcomas? J Comput Assist Tomogr 2014;38(5):687–92.

36. O'Sullivan PJ, Harris AC, Munk PL. Radiological imaging features of non-uterine leiomyosarcoma. Br J Radiol 2008;81(961):73–81.
37. Gordon RW, Tirumani SH, Kurra V, et al. MRI, MDCT features, and clinical outcome of extremity leiomyosarcomas: experience in 47 patients. Skeletal Radiol 2014;43(5):615–22.
38. Bush CH, Reith JD, Spanier SS. Mineralization in musculoskeletal leiomyosarcoma: radiologic-pathologic correlation. AJR Am J Roentgenol 2003;180(1): 109–13.
39. Saboo SS, Krajewski KM, Zukotynski K, et al. Imaging features of primary and secondary adult rhabdomyosarcoma. AJR Am J Roentgenol 2012;199(6): W694–703.
40. Allen SD, Moskovic EC, Fisher C, et al. Adult rhabdomyosarcoma: cross-sectional imaging findings including histopathologic correlation. AJR Am J Roentgenol 2007;189(2):371–7.
41. Hagiwara A, Inoue Y, Nakayama T, et al. The "botryoid sign": a characteristic feature of rhabdomyosarcomas in the head and neck. Neuroradiology 2001; 43(4):331–5.
42. Freling NJ, Merks JH, Saeed P, et al. Imaging findings in craniofacial childhood rhabdomyosarcoma. Pediatr Radiol 2010;40(11):1723–38 [quiz: 855].
43. Little DJ, Ballo MT, Zagars GK, et al. Adult rhabdomyosarcoma: outcome following multimodality treatment. Cancer 2002;95(2):377–88.
44. Sultan I, Qaddoumi I, Yaser S, et al. Comparing adult and pediatric rhabdomyosarcoma in the surveillance, epidemiology and end results program, 1973 to 2005: an analysis of 2,600 patients. J Clin Oncol 2009;27(20):3391–7.
45. Chikarmane SA, Gombos EC, Jagadeesan J, et al. MRI findings of radiation-associated angiosarcoma of the breast (RAS). J Magn Reson Imaging 2015; 42(3):763–70.
46. Murphey MD, Smith WS, Smith SE, et al. From the archives of the AFIP. Imaging of musculoskeletal neurogenic tumors: radiologic-pathologic correlation. Radiographics 1999;19(5):1253–80.
47. Kamran SC, Howard SA, Shinagare AB, et al. Malignant peripheral nerve sheath tumors: prognostic impact of rhabdomyoblastic differentiation (malignant triton tumors), neurofibromatosis 1 status and location. Eur J Surg Oncol 2013;39(1): 46–52.
48. Zhang Z, Deng L, Ding L, et al. MR imaging differentiation of malignant soft tissue tumors from peripheral schwannomas with large size and heterogeneous signal intensity. Eur J Radiol 2015;84(5):940–6.
49. Wasa J, Nishida Y, Tsukushi S, et al. MRI features in the differentiation of malignant peripheral nerve sheath tumors and neurofibromas. AJR Am J Roentgenol 2010;194(6):1568–74.
50. Bredella MA, Torriani M, Hornicek F, et al. Value of PET in the assessment of patients with neurofibromatosis type 1. AJR Am J Roentgenol 2007;189(4):928–35.
51. Van Herendael BH, Heyman SR, Vanhoenacker FM, et al. The value of magnetic resonance imaging in the differentiation between malignant peripheral nerve-sheath tumors and non-neurogenic malignant soft-tissue tumors. Skeletal Radiol 2006;35(10):745–53.
52. Murphey MD, Gibson MS, Jennings BT, et al. From the archives of the AFIP: imaging of synovial sarcoma with radiologic-pathologic correlation. Radiographics 2006;26(5):1543–65.
53. O'Sullivan PJ, Harris AC, Munk PL. Radiological features of synovial cell sarcoma. Br J Radiol 2008;81(964):346–56.

54. Baheti AD, Tirumani SH, Sewatkar R, et al. Imaging features of primary and metastatic extremity synovial sarcoma: a single institute experience of 78 patients. Br J Radiol 2015;88(1046):20140608.
55. Bixby SD, Hettmer S, Taylor GA, et al. Synovial sarcoma in children: imaging features and common benign mimics. AJR Am J Roentgenol 2010;195(4):1026–32.
56. Stacy GS, Nair L. Magnetic resonance imaging features of extremity sarcomas of uncertain differentiation. Clin Radiol 2007;62(10):950–8.
57. Kransdorf MJ. Malignant soft-tissue tumors in a large referral population: distribution of diagnoses by age, sex, and location. AJR Am J Roentgenol 1995;164(1): 129–34.
58. Suh JS, Cho J, Lee SH, et al. Alveolar soft part sarcoma: MR and angiographic findings. Skeletal Radiol 2000;29(12):680–9.
59. Tian L, Cui CY, Lu SY, et al. Clinical presentation and CT/MRI findings of alveolar soft part sarcoma: a retrospective single-center analysis of 14 cases. Acta Radiol 2016;57(4):475–80.
60. Pang LM, Roebuck DJ, Griffith JF, et al. Alveolar soft-part sarcoma: a rare soft-tissue malignancy with distinctive clinical and radiological features. Pediatr Radiol 2001;31(3):196–9.
61. Viry F, Orbach D, Klijanienko J, et al. Alveolar soft part sarcoma-radiologic patterns in children and adolescents. Pediatr Radiol 2013;43(9):1174–81.
62. McCarville MB, Muzzafar S, Kao SC, et al. Imaging features of alveolar soft-part sarcoma: a report from Children's Oncology Group Study ARST0332. AJR Am J Roentgenol 2014;203(6):1345–52.
63. Sood S, Baheti AD, Shinagare AB, et al. Imaging features of primary and metastatic alveolar soft part sarcoma: single institute experience in 25 patients. Br J Radiol 2014;87(1036):20130719.
64. Wang H, Jacobson A, Harmon DC, et al. Prognostic factors in alveolar soft part sarcoma: a SEER analysis. J Surg Oncol 2016;113(5):581–6.
65. Liu YP, Jin J, Wang WH, et al. A retrospective analysis of lung metastasis in 64 patients with alveolar soft part sarcoma. Clin Transl Oncol 2015;17(10):803–9.
66. Murphey MD, Senchak LT, Mambalam PK, et al. From the radiologic pathology archives: Ewing sarcoma family of tumors: radiologic-pathologic correlation. Radiographics 2013;33(3):803–31.
67. Javery O, Krajewski K, O'Regan K, et al. A to Z of extraskeletal Ewing sarcoma family of tumors in adults: imaging features of primary disease, metastatic patterns, and treatment responses. AJR Am J Roentgenol 2011;197(6):W1015–22.
68. Huh J, Kim KW, Park SJ, et al. Imaging features of primary tumors and metastatic patterns of the extraskeletal Ewing sarcoma family of tumors in adults: a 17-year experience at a single institution. Korean J Radiol 2015;16(4):783–90.
69. Somarouthu BS, Shinagare AB, Rosenthal MH, et al. Multimodality imaging features, metastatic pattern and clinical outcome in adult extraskeletal Ewing sarcoma: experience in 26 patients. Br J Radiol 2014;87(1038):20140123.
70. Mc Auley G, Jagannathan J, O'Regan K, et al. Extraskeletal osteosarcoma: spectrum of imaging findings. AJR Am J Roentgenol 2012;198(1):W31–7.
71. Srinivasan S, Krishnan V, Ali SZ, et al. "Swirl sign" of aggressive angiomyxoma-a lesser known diagnostic sign. Clin Imaging 2014;38(5):751–4.
72. Surabhi VR, Garg N, Frumovitz M, et al. Aggressive angiomyxomas: a comprehensive imaging review with clinical and histopathologic correlation. AJR Am J Roentgenol 2014;202(6):1171–8.
73. Outwater EK, Marchetto BE, Wagner BJ, et al. Aggressive angiomyxoma: findings on CT and MR imaging. AJR Am J Roentgenol 1999;172(2):435–8.

74. Kis B, O'Regan KN, Agoston A, et al. Imaging of desmoplastic small round cell tumour in adults. Br J Radiol 2012;85(1010):187–92.
75. Wignall OJ, Moskovic EC, Thway K, et al. Solitary fibrous tumors of the soft tissues: review of the imaging and clinical features with histopathologic correlation. AJR Am J Roentgenol 2010;195(1):W55–62.
76. Clarencon F, Bonneville F, Rousseau A, et al. Intracranial solitary fibrous tumor: imaging findings. Eur J Radiol 2011;80(2):387–94.
77. Ginat DT, Bokhari A, Bhatt S, et al. Imaging features of solitary fibrous tumors. AJR Am J Roentgenol 2011;196(3):487–95.
78. Tirumani SH, Tirumani H, Jagannathan JP, et al. MDCT features of succinate dehydrogenase (SDH)-deficient gastrointestinal stromal tumours. Br J Radiol 2014; 87(1043):20140476.
79. Tirumani SH, Jagannathan JP, Krajewski KM, et al. Imatinib and beyond in gastrointestinal stromal tumors: a radiologist's perspective. AJR Am J Roentgenol 2013; 201(4):801–10.
80. Tirumani SH, Jagannathan JP, Hornick JL, et al. Resistance to treatment in gastrointestinal stromal tumours: what radiologists should know. Clin Radiol 2013;68(8): e429–37.
81. Tateishi U, Kusumoto M, Hasegawa T, et al. Primary malignant fibrous histiocytoma of the chest wall: CT and MR appearance. J Comput Assist Tomogr 2002; 26(4):558–63.
82. Lewis JJ, Leung D, Woodruff JM, et al. Retroperitoneal soft-tissue sarcoma: analysis of 500 patients treated and followed at a single institution. Ann Surg 1998; 228(3):355–65.
83. Coindre JM, Mariani O, Chibon F, et al. Most malignant fibrous histiocytomas developed in the retroperitoneum are dedifferentiated liposarcomas: a review of 25 cases initially diagnosed as malignant fibrous histiocytoma. Mod Pathol 2003;16(3):256–62.
84. Oei TN, Jagannathan JP, Ramaiya N, et al. Peritoneal sarcomatosis versus peritoneal carcinomatosis: imaging findings at MDCT. AJR Am J Roentgenol 2010; 195(3):W229–35.
85. Tateishi U, Hasegawa T, Beppu Y, et al. Primary dedifferentiated liposarcoma of the retroperitoneum. Prognostic significance of computed tomography and magnetic resonance imaging features. J Comput Assist Tomogr 2003;27(5):799–804.
86. Gupta AK, Cohan RH, Francis IR, et al. CT of recurrent retroperitoneal sarcomas. AJR Am J Roentgenol 2000;174(4):1025–30.
87. Morrison BA. Soft tissue sarcomas of the extremities. Proc (Bayl Univ Med Cent) 2003;16(3):285–90.
88. Bastiaannet E, Groen H, Jager PL, et al. The value of FDG-PET in the detection, grading and response to therapy of soft tissue and bone sarcomas; a systematic review and meta-analysis. Cancer Treat Rev 2004;30(1):83–101.
89. Gronchi A, Lo Vullo S, Colombo C, et al. Extremity soft tissue sarcoma in a series of patients treated at a single institution: local control directly impacts survival. Ann Surg 2010;251(3):506–11.
90. Verga L, Brach Del Prever EM, Linari A, et al. Accuracy and role of contrast-enhanced CT in diagnosis and surgical planning in 88 soft tissue tumours of extremities. Eur Radiol 2015. [Epub ahead of print].
91. White LM, Wunder JS, Bell RS, et al. Histologic assessment of peritumoral edema in soft tissue sarcoma. Int J Radiat Oncol Biol Phys 2005;61(5):1439–45.
92. Bahig H, Roberge D, Bosch W, et al. Agreement among RTOG sarcoma radiation oncologists in contouring suspicious peritumoral edema for preoperative

radiation therapy of soft tissue sarcoma of the extremity. Int J Radiat Oncol Biol Phys 2013;86(2):298–303.

93. James SL, Davies AM. Post-operative imaging of soft tissue sarcomas. Cancer Imaging 2008;8:8–18.

94. Varma DG, Jackson EF, Pollock RE, et al. Soft-tissue sarcoma of the extremities. MR appearance of post-treatment changes and local recurrences. Magn Reson Imaging Clin N Am 1995;3(4):695–712.

95. Pisters PW, Leung DH, Woodruff J, et al. Analysis of prognostic factors in 1,041 patients with localized soft tissue sarcomas of the extremities. J Clin Oncol 1996;14(5):1679–89.

96. Crim JR, Seeger LL, Yao L, et al. Diagnosis of soft-tissue masses with MR imaging: can benign masses be differentiated from malignant ones? Radiology 1992; 185(2):581–6.

Extremity Soft Tissue Sarcoma

Tailoring Resection to Histologic Subtype

Matthew G. Cable, MD, R. Lor Randall, MD*

KEYWORDS

- Sarcoma subtypes • Histologic grade • Resection margin • Representative biopsy
- Extremity sarcoma

KEY POINTS

- The early detection of disease and accurate staging at presentation are the main prognostic factors for overall survival.
- Among malignancies, poorly differentiated sarcoma can appear like poorly differentiated carcinoma and melanoma can mimic many sarcoma types.
- Communication between the pathologist, radiologist, and surgeon can expose nuance between these malignancies and be essential for final diagnosis and staging.
- Many advances have been made in the histologic diagnosis of STS that have, in turn, guided surgical treatment; however, even with the surgical goal of wide resection obtained in most cases, surgeons are still unable to fully cure some patients.

INTRODUCTION

Soft tissue sarcomas (STS) comprise a small group of tumors originating from mesenchymal or connective tissue. Soft tissue tumors as a whole are predominantly benign with a high rate of cure. The few that are malignant sarcomas make up less than 1% of all soft tissue tumors. All STS by definition are malignant, having the capacity to invade adjacent tissues and/or potentially metastasize to distant sites. The annual incidence of STS is estimated to be 5 per 100,000 persons,[1] with the American Cancer Society estimating almost 12,000 new cases in 2015.[2] The National Cancer Database places STS twenty-seventh in overall incidence in the United States, similar to Hodgkin lymphoma and cervical cancer.

STS are found across all demographics with a slight male bias (1:1.2 female/male patients), with incidence increasing after age 55 years and a median overall age of 65 years. This can be deceiving because specific sarcomas can favor younger patients,

The authors have nothing to disclose.
Huntsman Cancer Institute, University of Utah, Salt Lake City, UT, USA
* Corresponding author. Huntsman Cancer Institute, 2000 Circle of Hope, Room 4260, Salt Lake City, UT 84112.
E-mail address: lor.randall@hci.utah.edu

such as Ewing sarcoma and rhabdomyosarcoma existing mostly in the first 2 decades and synovial sarcoma occurring mostly in the third and fourth decades. Although comparatively rare overall, sarcomas still make up 7% of all childhood tumors.[3]

The 5-year survival rate for all STS reported by the Surveillance, Epidemiology, and End Results (SEER) database from 2005 to 2011 is 66%, with an average length of survival after diagnosis of 7 years. The advances in overall survival made with the implementation of chemotherapy and radiation therapy have largely plateaued, and the largest prognostic factors currently are early detection and cancer stage at presentation. Metastasis alone decreases 5-year survival to 16% compared with 84% with localized disease.[4]

Nearly 70% of STS are located in the extremities,[5] and are 4 times more common than sarcomas of the bones and joints.[2] Extremity sarcomas typically carry a better prognosis than tumors located in the retroperitoneum or pelvis.[6] A superficial sarcoma, by definition, is located above the muscle fascia and most of these occur in the extremities.[7] However, only one-third of all extremity STS are superficial.[4]

Typical treatment of extremity STS involves surgical excision with wide margins and adjuvant radiotherapy; that is, limb-sparing multimodal therapy. This generalization overlooks the multitude of factors a surgeon must consider for planning surgical resection margins when dealing with STS. An appreciation of how histology corresponds with tumor biology and surgical anatomic constraints is needed for management of this difficult disease.

HISTOLOGY AS A PROGNOSTIC FACTOR

There is a hierarchy of prognostic factors in STS, with most converging on local recurrence, metastasis, and overall survival. The interplay can get confusing because prognostic factors vary based on endpoint. For example, in extremity STS, the prognostic factors for local recurrence are not necessarily the same as those for metastasis[8]; however local recurrence can itself be a prognostic factor for metastasis.[9]

Histologic grade has an integral role in multiple aspects of STS prognosis, ranging from local recurrence to metastasis and disease specific survival as seen in Kaplan-Meier estimates.[7,10,11] However, the wide-ranging prognostic effect of histologic grade can be underestimated in competing scenarios. This is commonly seen when interpreting the hazard ratio (HR) of histologic grade, such that the HR of one outcome can mask the effect of another. Biau and colleagues[10] elegantly show that high-grade STS has effects on metastasis (HR = 3.47) and local recurrence (HR = 2.16). However the cumulative incidence of local recurrence of STS plateaus over 10 years, with no significant difference between high-grade and low-grade tumors. Death from metastasis precluded local recurrence in patients with high-grade STS but this should not downplay the contribution of high grade on local recurrence. A similar scenario plays out when looking at STS size and local recurrence, with local recurrence of small STS actually overtaking that of larger tumors over time.

Cancer staging partly alleviates this issue by combining several prognostic factors into a single score. Cancer staging has been proven accurate and should be considered in a sarcoma patient workup.[12,13] The staging system developed by the American Joint Committee on Cancer (AJCC) is most widely used. There are 4 prognostic factors that go into determining the sarcoma stage in the AJCC *Cancer Staging Handbook*, 7th edition, including tumor size, nodal involvement, metastasis, and histologic grade (https://cancerstaging.org/). The AJCC stage is prognostic of overall survival in STS (**Fig. 1**).[14]

One notable change between the sixth and seventh editions of the AJCC *Cancer Staging Handbook* was the adoption of the French Federation of Cancer Centres

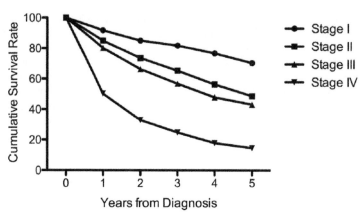

Fig. 1. National Cancer Database (NCDB) figure for survival based on AJCC stage in STS. (*From* Kneisl JS, Coleman MM, Raut CP. Outcomes in the management of adult soft tissue sarcomas. Journal of Surgical Oncology 2014;110:529; with permission.)

Sarcoma Group (FNCLCC) histologic grading system (**Table 1**).[15] A unique aspect of the FNCLCC sarcoma grading system is the large contribution of a tumor differentiation score, which is given to specific STS subtypes. Some STS are given a specific differentiation score (myxoid liposarcoma is always assigned a 2), whereas others are subject to interpretation by the pathologist (angiosarcoma can receive a 1, 2, or 3). Put simply, all malignant sarcomas are not created equal. A well-differentiated

Table 1
French Federation of Cancer Centres Sarcoma Group grading system: definition of parameters

Tumor Differentiation	
Score 1	Sarcomas closely resembling normal adult mesenchymal tissue
Score 2	Sarcomas for which histologic subtyping is certain
Score 3	Undifferentiated and embryonal sarcomas, synovial sarcomas, osteosarcomas, PNET, sarcomas of doubtful type
Mitotic count	
Score 1	0–9 mitoses per 10 high powered fields
Score 2	10–19 mitoses per 10 high powered fields
Score 3	≥20 mitoses per 10 high powered fields
Tumor necrosis	
Score 0	No necrosis
Score 1	<50% tumor necrosis
Score 2	≥50% tumor necrosis
Histologic grade	
Grade 1	Total score 2, 3
Grade 2	Total score 4, 5
Grade 3	Total score 6, 7, 8

From Trojani M, Contesso G, Coindre JM, et al. Soft tissue sarcomas of adults: study of pathologic prognostic variables and definition of histopathological grading system. Int J Cancer 1984;33:37–42; with permission.

leiomyosarcoma with some tumor necrosis and more than 20 mitoses per 10 high-power fields would receive a histologic grade of 2, whereas a synovial sarcoma with no necrosis and no mitotic activity would also receive a histologic grade of 2.

Tumor grading was developed to be applied to STS as a whole but the histologic characteristics of specific sarcoma subtypes often carry different weights. The heterogeneity of STS can range from locally aggressive and nonmetastasizing in desmoid fibromatosis to locally indolent but highly metastatic in alveolar soft parts sarcoma. There are also a few sarcoma subtypes in which grading is not prognostic, such as malignant peripheral nerve sheath tumors.

This being said, more than 75% of all STS are high-grade (excluding benign mesenchymal tumors). This highlights the importance of obtaining an accurate histologic diagnosis in determining tumor grade in extremity STS and tumor grade should never be a substitute for histologic diagnosis.

HISTOLOGIC SUBTYPES WITHIN SOFT TISSUE SARCOMA

The importance of cancer staging cannot be overstated; however, as seen when determining tumor grade, obtaining an accurate tissue diagnosis is paramount. Many different tissue types derive from mesenchymal tissue and there are currently more than 50 histologic subtypes of STS, each with unique prognostic, clinical, and therapeutic features. Because sarcoma management is multimodal, histologic subtype can and should be used to tailor optimum treatment.

Many techniques are used by the musculoskeletal pathologist when determining an STS diagnosis. In addition to traditional staining methods, such as hematoxylin and eosin, the pathologist has an array of diagnostic tools. These include ancillary immunohistochemistry (IHC), flow cytology, and several molecular techniques, such as fluorescence in situ hybridization (FISH) and reverse transcription polymerase chain reaction (RT-PCR) sequencing. There are many characteristic reciprocal chromosomal translocations unique to specific STS that can aid in histologic diagnosis (**Table 2**). If traditional staining methods are not diagnostic, then IHC markers can help to narrow a differential diagnosis within certain tissue types (**Table 3**). Typically a panel of stains is run to help verify tissue of origin. For histology with a broad differential an initial panel of markers might include 2 cytokeratin markers (AE1/AE3 and CAM5.2), 2 melanoma markers (S100 and Sox10), and 2 myogenic markers (SMA and HHF35). A panel of stains for just mesenchymal markers can include vimentin, factor VIII, CD31, CD34, SMA, and desmin. Sarcoma samples can also be dedifferentiated to a point at which they will not stain for characteristic markers. In these situations a multitude of factors, including tumor morphology, location, age, and medical history are taken into account by the orthopedic oncologist and pathologist when determining a histologic diagnosis.

As emphasized when determining tumor grade, 2 STS subtypes may look morphologically similar but have completely different behaviors. Atypical lipoma (atypical lipomatous tumor [ALT]) and well-differentiated liposarcoma are histologically identical lesions that can behave somewhat differently, with the latter having a higher rate of recurrence and risk for dedifferentiation. The difference lies in the location of the lesion that needs to be conveyed to the pathologist because a subcutaneous extremity lesion can be called an atypical lipoma or ALT, whereas well-differentiated liposarcoma is reserved for more deeply seated lesions. The goal for a surgeon is to gain not only a histologic diagnosis but an understanding within that diagnosis of the aggressive (or benign) potential of a particular specimen.

Table 2
Common translocations seen in extremity soft tissue sarcomas

Translocation	Genes Involved	Sarcoma Subtype
t(1;3) (p36.3;q25)	Unknown	Epithelioid hemangioendothelioma
t(1;13) (p36;q14)	PAX7 and FHKR	Alveolar rhabdomyosarcoma
t(1;17) (q32;q21)	Unknown	Bizarre parosteal osteochondromatous proliferation
t(2;13) (q35;q14)	PAX3 and FHKR	Alveolar rhabdomyosarcoma
t(3;12) (q27;q14–15)	HMGA2 and LPP	Lipoma, soft tissue chondroma
t(7;16) (q33;p11)	FUS and CREB3L2	Low-grade fibromyxoid sarcoma
t(9;15) (q22;q11–q21)	TEC/CHN and TCF12	Extraskeletal myxoid chondrosarcoma
t(9;22) (q22–31;q11–q12)	TEC/CHN and EWS	Extraskeletal myxoid chondrosarcoma
t(11;22) (p13;q12)	WT1 and EWS	Desmoplastic small round cell tumor
t(11;22) (q24;q12)	FLI1 and EWS	Ewing sarcoma, PNET
t(12;14) (q14–15;q23–24)	HMGA2/HMGIC and various	Smooth muscle tumors, lipomas
t(12;15) (p13;q25)	ETV6 and NTRK3	Infantile fibrosarcoma
t(12;16) (q13;p11)	CHOP and TLS	Myxoid and round cell liposarcoma
t(12;22) (q13;q12)	ATF1 and EWS	Clear cell sarcoma
t(17;22) (q21–22;q13)	COL1A1 and PDGF beta	Dermatofibrosarcoma protuberans, giant cell fibrosarcoma
t(X;17) (p11.2;q25)	TFE3 and ASPL	Alveolar soft parts sarcoma
t(X;18) (p11.2, q11.2)	SYT and SSX1/SSX2/SSX4	Synovial sarcoma

BIOPSY AND INTERPRETATION

Thankfully, histology gets introduced in a patient's cancer workup relatively early. With few exceptions (ie, lipomas), nearly all extremity soft tissue masses that require surgical excision should and will have biopsies performed before excision. Histology should still factor into the surgeon's plan when obtaining a biopsy because a representative tissue specimen needs to be delivered to the pathologist for a correct diagnosis.

The biopsy tract should be placed so it can be incorporated and excised en bloc with the definitive resection. A longitudinally oriented incision is commonly used and, for extremity lesions, a direct approach with minimal extension into adjacent tissue planes is usually possible for both superficial and deep seated lesions.

Studies have shown core needle biopsies (CNBs) are safe and less invasive than incisional biopsies.[16] However, the accuracy of CNB in comparison with incisional biopsy for obtaining histologic diagnoses specifically in soft tissue musculoskeletal masses remains low (59.5% compared with 77.3%).[17] Extremity STS grade determined by incisional biopsy is also predictive of both metastasis-free survival and disease-free survival, whereas grade determined by CNB is not.[18] The main advantage of incisional biopsy is more tissue available to the pathologist to accommodate a definitive diagnosis and additional cytologic testing, and less chance of obtaining a nonrepresentative sample.

Table 3
Immunohistochemistry markers for soft tissue sarcomas

Cytokeratin	Epithelial marker
CAM5.2 (antibody for CK8 and CK18)	Epithelial marker
AE1/AE3 (pancytokeratin)	Epithelial marker, SS
EMA (epithelial membrane antigen)	Epithelial marker, SS, melanoma
S100	Melanoma and neural crest derivatives
Sox10	Melanoma and neural crest derivatives
HMB45/Melan A	Melanoma, CCS
Desmin	Myogenic tumors (smooth and skeletal muscle)
Muscle specific actin (HHF35)	Myogenic tumors (smooth and skeletal muscle)
SMA	Leiomyosarcoma, myofibroblastic lesions
Myogenin	Immature skeletal muscle (rhabdomyosarcoma), SS
MyoD1	Mature skeletal muscle
H-caldesmon	Smooth muscle tumors
CDK4	Well-differentiated and dedifferentiated liposarcoma
MDM2	Well-differentiated and dedifferentiated liposarcoma
CD31	Vascular
CD34	Vascular, DFSP, SFT, ES, spindle cell tumors, pleomorphic lipoma
ERG	Vascular, highly sensitive, and specific
FLI1	Vascular, EWS
CD20/CD30	lymphoma
CD163/CD68	Histiocytic sarcoma
CD99	EWS, SS, SFT, alveolar rhabdomyosarcoma, mesenchymal chondrosarcoma, lymphoblastic lymphoma
c-kit (CD117)	AML/CML, angiosarcoma, CCS, ES, EWS, melanoma, OGS, rhabdomyosarcoma
MUC4	Low-grade fibromyxoid sarcoma

Abbreviations: AML/CML, acute or chronic myelogenous leukemia; CCS, clear cell sarcoma; DFSP, dermatofibrosarcoma protuberans; ES, epithelioid sarcoma; EWS, Ewing sarcoma; LGFMS, low-grade fibromyxoid sarcoma; OGS, osteosarcoma; SFT, solitary fibrous tumor; SS, synovial sarcoma.

STS can grow to be quite large at presentation, with a median diameter of 5 cm for superficial and 9 cm for deep sarcomas. They are noticed incidentally on imaging or by mass effect because the initial growth for many STS is painless. The tumors tend to push adjacent structures and stay within compartments rather than invade, with the notable exception of myxofibrosarcoma (see later discussion). This means the surgeon can have ample material from which to choose a representative piece.

MRI is the modality of choice for evaluating STS. Tumor margins can be distinguished from surrounding muscle, fat, and potential neurovascular bundles. Although MRI cannot necessarily predict histologic diagnosis or tumor aggressiveness, it does provide indispensable information for biopsy planning. Areas of necrosis, liquefaction, myxoid degeneration, hemorrhage, and fibrosis are typically avoided. Abrupt changes in signal within a mass could indicate dedifferentiation and should be sampled. For many STS the most viable portions are near the periphery of the mass, where adequate nutrients for growth are present. A peripherally obtained biopsy specimen can also evaluate the extent of tumor invasion into adjacent tissues. Sampling only viable tissue can result in a falsely low grade using the FNLCC system (ie, less necrosis) and is acceptable to the alternative of an inadequate biopsy; however, it should be kept in mind the possibility that the tumor will get upgraded on final resection.

Histology interpretation does not necessarily top the list of medical skills for most surgeons, so how should one approach sarcoma histology and apply that information to interpreting a biopsy specimen? Talking directly with a musculoskeletal pathologist is ideal but is not always possible if a specimen is sent to an outside facility. Communication can be reduced to brief emails or telephone conversations, with both parties not necessarily looking at the histology slide at once. Grasping basic trends of sarcoma disease will aid in formulating pertinent questions to ask the surgical pathologist. Surgical pathology reports for different biopsy specimens can often contain the same descriptors, and only by communication can the nuances be teased out (**Table 4**).

Table 4
Clarification topics regarding soft tissue sarcomas biopsy interpretation

Histologic Clarifications	Surgical Clarifications
Dedifferentiated • What degree of dedifferentiation? • Do cells stain for typical IHC markers? • What percentage of the specimen? • Is dedifferentiation common for the presumed diagnosis? • 1 or multiple foci of dedifferentiation?	Anatomic location of resected tissue or biopsy Precise orientation • Cannot be overemphasized • By surgeon to pathologist in operating room • By pathologist to surgeon at handoff • Use of suture tags • 6-color inking • Correlation with imaging
Margins (if present) • Where were margins measured on the specimen? • Are dedifferentiated or aggressive portions close to margins or nutrient vessels? • Thick pseudocapsule or fascia? • Is margin focally or diffusely positive? • Border between normal and abnormal: pushing, cords, or infiltrating single cells • Discrepancy between gross and microscopic assessment?	Relevant structures adjacent to resected tissue • Nerves • Vessels • Fascia • Bone • Joints
Cell morphology • Typical or atypical for presumed diagnosis? • Epithelial or mesenchymal phenotypes (or both)? • Nuclear atypia • Clarify mitotic count if only tumor grade is given • Atypical mitoses present (triple or quadruple asters)?	Tissue appearance before resection or biopsy • Native tumor • Capsule (if present) • Surrounding tissue Prior treatment history • Adjuvant therapy • Trauma or injury • Prior surgery
Necrosis vs apoptosis (if present)	

FROZEN SECTION CONSIDERATIONS

Frozen sections play a unique role in STS, either during the initial biopsy or during definitive resection. Foremost, it requires that a musculoskeletal trained pathologist be available in the surgical or operating room suite. A frozen section should be performed if it will dictate surgical management intraoperatively. An obvious instance is to assess intraoperative margins during definitive resection of an STS, if margins are deemed to be close on gross sectioning. However, frozen sections may also be performed during the initial biopsy with lesions for which imaging is nondiagnostic (**Table 5**). A benign diagnosis can lead to curative marginal excision of the lesion and a malignant diagnosis can result in wound closure with final diagnosis contingent on the permanent sections.

It should be noted that unlike with other cancerous lesions, a questionable soft tissue lesion is more likely to be called malignant on frozen section by the pathologist because this defers to permanent sections and there is minimal risk in a benign lesion being misinterpreted as malignant and being addressed at a later date. The reverse is not true for a malignant sarcoma inappropriately excised with contaminated margins under the supposition of a benign process.[19]

Frozen sections should also be performed to ensure adequacy of tissue given to the pathologist. Heterogeneous sarcomas may require biopsies from multiple locations within the lesion to ensure that the sample is representative. A frozen section containing predominantly scar or reactive tissue, necrosis, or cystic contents may require more tissue for diagnosis by the pathologist. More tissue may also be needed for specific diagnostic techniques, such as flow cytometry or cytogenetics.

Flow cytometry has become essential in the rapid diagnosis of hematological malignancies but has limited use in STS because of the need for single-cell suspensions from the tumor specimen. This being said, flow cytometry is very important in the setting of small round blue cell tumors (Ewing sarcoma, granulocytic or myeloid sarcoma) to rule out leukemia or lymphoma. It is preferred to traditional IHC when monoclonal antibodies will be used or if the sensitivity of a specific antibody is low by IHC (eg, CD45). Flow cytometry is also quantitative, whereas IHC is usually yields a yes or no staining pattern of tissue.

SOFT TISSUE SARCOMAS SUBTYPE GUIDING RESECTION MARGINS

With the diagnosis of STS being made via biopsy, the histology characteristics define the very disease and can guide surgical treatment. Once an accurate histologic diagnosis is made, the decision for surgical resection can be addressed. In certain situations surgery may not be desirable or feasible. The presence of widespread metastasis or poor patient health status may preclude a large resection and warrant palliative tumor debulking. For certain STS seen in the pediatric population, such as

Table 5	
Soft tissue sarcomas that masquerade as well-circumscribed benign processes on imaging	
Sarcoma	**Benign Processes**
Low-grade fibromyxoid sarcoma	Desmoid, cellular myxoma, myxoid neurofibroma
Low-grade myxofibrosarcoma	Intramuscular myxoma, angiomyxoma, benign myxoid processes, nodular fasciitis
Malignant solitary fibrous tumor	Solitary fibrous tumor, nerve sheath tumor, leiomyoma, benign spindle cell tumors
Epithelioid sarcoma	Granuloma anulare, rheumatoid nodule, fibrous histiocytoma, nodular fasciitis
Synovial sarcoma	Vascular malformation, nerve sheath tumor, solitary fibrous tumor
Extraskeletal osteosarcoma	Myositis ossificans, heterotopic ossification, pseudosarcomatous lesions with bone formation

alveolar rhabdomyosarcoma and desmoplastic small round cell tumor, chemotherapy is the mainstay of treatment and surgery can be potentially avoided.

How histology should guide surgical resection is a difficult question because all STS are malignant. The preferred surgical goal for nearly all malignant tumors is a wide resection with adequate margins (excluding well-differentiated liposarcoma). However, once a wide margin is obtained for most extremity STS, histologic grade still independently influences overall survival,[20] in addition to local recurrence and metastasis.[7] If wide resection is desirable for most STS, attention has shifted to how wide a margin is adequate for high-grade STS.

A distinction should be made between a clear margin and a wide margin, with the former definable as no tumor cells seen in contact with the edge of a resected specimen on pathologic testing. Whether a margin is clear or contaminated is plainly visible on histology and is usually a yes or no issue. Margin status has been shown to affect local recurrence.[21,22] However, it is less evident whether margin status alone correlates with overall survival or metastasis.[20,23–26] This is likely because margin status is determined by sampling portions of a tumor resection rather than the entire specimen. A wide margin represents a safety net or confidence interval to accommodate any outlying cells potentially missed on histology. A resected histology specimen can show clear margins but microscopic tumor bed contamination cannot be shown on histology.

The true margin width that maximizes local control is controversial and can vary depending on the aggressiveness of the tumor. What constitutes a wide margin has been debated since the original description of a wide resection by Enneking and colleagues.[27] They described resection of the tumor pseudocapsule with a normal cuff of tissue, and gave no formal measurements. Consensus has varied and tended to decrease over time, as seen with the Scandinavian Sarcoma Group originally considering a wide margin "around 5 cm" but currently "more than 10 mm."[28] Some use 2 cm or equivalent (eg, layer of fascia) as the definition of wide margin but the evidence to support this is spotty at best. Novais and colleagues[20] suggest that only 2 mm is required, showing 47% 5 year overall survival with less than 2 mm margins and 70% with greater than 2 mm margins. No difference was seen in overall survival when distinguishing between 2 mm to 1.9 cm and greater than 2 cm margins. Many studies look at STS as a group and that may mask the more nuanced definition of a wide margin, which depends on STS subtype. King and colleagues[29] showed that in subjects with STS resected with negative margins, 4 of 117 subjects developed local recurrence but 2 of 45 (4.4%) had margins less than 1 mm and 2 of 64 (3.1%) had margins greater than 1 mm. What is more telling is that 3 of the 4 recurrences were either epithelioid sarcoma or myxofibrosarcoma, both very aggressive and infiltrative subtypes of STS.

In many studies it is impossible to determine if tumor aggressiveness or local control is the larger predictor of local recurrence and surgeon dogma often determines the true extent of a wide resection. Surgeon opinion as to what constitutes an optimal resection can vary depending on STS histologic subtype. This variation can be attributed to what a surgeon considers to be a qualitative margin for a given tumor. One method for describing qualitative margins is defined by the International Union Against Cancer, with R0 representing a true negative, R1 a microscopically positive, and R2 a macroscopically incomplete resection. There is, however, no guideline giving a quantitative amount of tissue necessary to obtain each qualitative margin.

A surgical plan for STS should be tailored to the predicted local growth pattern, risk of metastasis, and likely sites of distant spread. STS generally grow along tissue planes rather than traverse them, pushing against adjacent structures but not typically invading. This has large implications when considering surgical margins because certain tumors can spread longitudinally along an entire fascial plane yet remain intra-compartmental, again showing the variability of what can constitute a wide margin.

The margin should be determined based on the type of surrounding tissue, aggressiveness of the tumor, relationships to adjacent neurovascular bundles, and degree of functional impairment. A 1 mm margin (no ink on tumor) is often sufficient for in a low-grade or less aggressive sarcoma with a low potential of microscopic contamination and predictable growth along tissue planes. Conversely, a high-grade sarcoma that aggressively spreads along tissue planes and has a propensity to metastasize might require a wider margin but in reality is often just a few millimeters at its closest point still. Would there be an added benefit of between several millimeters and 1 cm, or would benefit only occur with greater than 2 cm margins? If such a wide margin would prove too morbid, would a margin of several millimeters and adjuvant therapy be preferable to amputation? These are conversations that should be had with every patient but would not be possible without a prior appreciation of the underlying histology for a given STS.

Amputation, compared with limb salvage, is far less common in the current era of sarcoma surgery. Although aggressive histologic subtype certainly plays a role in the decision, the goal in either case is to obtain a clear margin, with amputation being reserved for resections that will result in inadequate margins or a nonfunctional limb.

PLANNED POSITIVE MARGINS

There are some cases in which, according to careful preoperative planning, it is anticipated that a margin may be compromised. These are referred to as planned positive margins, and are very different from unplanned positive margins. Histologically speaking, one would plan for this scenario only if the tumor response could be predicted based on histology. Although histologic necrosis after neoadjuvant therapy can be prognostic in sarcoma of bone, this does not carry over to STS.[30]

Local recurrence is not necessarily guaranteed with residual microscopic disease, as seen in many studies in which the number of contaminated or inadequate margins is often higher than the true number of local recurrences.[20,31] This observation is certainly multifactorial with adjuvant chemotherapy, radiation treatments, and a patient's own inflammatory healing response having large effects on tumor recurrence.

If done appropriately, planned positive margins in conjunction with radiotherapy does not necessarily affect local recurrence.[32,33] It has been shown that marginal resection (R1 resection) after preoperative radiotherapy is equivalent to wide resection in extremity STS.[34] However, a contaminated margin after an unplanned excision carries a worse prognosis, even after wide re-excision, and can be correlated with histologic subtype.[35]

Retaining an incisional biopsy tract can also be interpreted as a planned positive margin. Ideally, a biopsy location is placed as to be incorporated in the eventual surgical incision. This may not always be possible, as often happens in circumstances in which the biopsy is performed by a separate surgeon, or with particularly deep-seated lesions, and may be less critical with needle biopsy tracts as opposed to open biopsy incisions. Leaving a biopsy tract unexcised in a high-grade lesion does not necessarily change the already stringent postoperative surveillance or adjuvant therapy but should still be done with extreme discretion. It has been shown with deep high-grade extremity STS that there is no increase in tumor recurrence or metastasis if a CNB tract is not resected[36]; however, this observation was limited to predominantly pleomorphic undifferentiated sarcomas and liposarcomas.

Table 6
Open phase III trials for soft tissue sarcoma

ClinicalTrials.gov	Title	Location
NCT02451943	A Randomized, Double-Blind, Placebo-Controlled, Phase III Trial Of Doxorubicin plus Olaratumab vs Doxorubicin Plus Placebo in Patients with Advanced or Metastatic Soft Tissue Sarcoma	USA Europe
NCT02449343	A Registered Randomized, Double-Blind, Placebo-Controlled (2:1), Multi-Centered Clinical Trial Of Anlotinib as a Treatment for Soft Tissue Sarcoma (Phase II/III)	China
NCT02379845	Multicenter Randomized, Open-Label Phase Ii/Iii Study, To Compare Efficacy of NBTXR3 Implanted as Intratumor Injection and Activated by Radiotherapy, vs Radiotherapy Alone in Patients With Locally Advanced Soft Tissue Sarcoma (Extremity and Trunk Wall)	Europe Canada
NCT02180867	Pazopanib Neoadjuvant Trial In Non-rhabdomyosarcoma Soft Tissue Sarcomas (PAZNTIS): A Phase II/III Randomized Trial of Preoperative Chemoradiation or Preoperative Radiation Plus or Minus Pazopanib (NSC# 737754)	USA
NCT02120768	Phase III Study of The Role of Barrier Resection in Local Control in Treatment of Extremity Soft Tissue Sarcomas	China
NCT02049905	A Multicenter, Randomized, Open-Label Phase 3 Study to Investigate the Efficacy and Safety of Aldoxorubicin Compared to Investigator's Choice in Subjects with Metastatic, Locally Advanced, or Unresectable Soft Tissue Sarcomas Who Either Relapsed or Were Refractory To Prior Non-adjuvant Chemotherapy	USA Australia Canada Denmark France Hungary Italy Netherlands Poland Russia Spain
NCT01987596	Prospective and Randomized Study of Fixed vs Flexible Prophylactic Administration of Granulocyte Colony-stimulating Factor (G-CSF) in Children With Cancer (Phase III)	USA
NCT01710176	Localized High-Risk Soft Tissue Sarcomas Of The Extremities And Trunk Wall In Adults: An Integrating Approach Comprising Standard Vs Histotype-Tailored Neoadjuvant Chemotherapy (Phase III)	Italy Spain
NCT01692678	Multicenter, Open-label Study of YONDELIS (Trabectedin) in Subjects With Locally Advanced or Metastatic Liposarcoma or Leiomyosarcoma (Phase III)	China
NCT01352117	A Randomized Evaluation Of Antiretroviral Therapy Alone or With Delayed Chemotherapy Vs Antiretroviral Therapy With Immediate Adjunctive Chemotherapy for Treatment Of Limited Stage AIDS-KS in Resource-Limited Settings (REACT-KS) AMC 067 (Phase III)	Brazil Kenya Malawi Peru South Africa Uganda Zimbabwe

(continued on next page)

Table 6 (continued)		
ClinicalTrials.gov	**Title**	**Location**
NCT01223248	A Phase III Randomized Study Comparing Two Dosing Schedules for Hypofractionated Image-Guided Radiation Therapy in Patients With Metastatic Cancer	USA Italy Portugal
NCT00876031	A Randomized Phase-III Trial of the Cooperative Weichteilsarkom Study Group (CWS) for Localized High-Risk Rhabdomyosarcoma and Localized Rhabdomyosarcoma-like Soft Tissue Sarcoma in Children, Adolescents, and Young Adults	Austria Germany Poland Sweden Switzerland
NCT00870701	Randomized Multicentric Phase III Study Comparing Observation vs Post-surgery Radiotherapy After Complete Exeresis With Margins Greater Than or Equal to 1 cm in Soft Tissues Members Sarcoma	France
NCT00334854	Ifosfamide and Doxorubicin, Radiation Therapy, and/or Surgery in Treating Young Patients With Localized Soft Tissue Sarcoma (Phase III)	Austria Belgium Denmark France Ireland Spain Sweden Switzerland UK
NCT00210665	A Multicenter, Open-Label, Single-Arm Study of YONDELIS (trabectedin) for Subjects With Locally Advanced or Metastatic Soft Tissue Sarcoma Who Have Relapsed or Are Refractory To Standard Of Care Treatment (Phase III)	USA Canada Israel

As of May 15, 2015. Excluding retroperitoneal tumors, Ewing, and GIST.

SPECIAL CONSIDERATIONS WITH SPECIFIC SARCOMA SUBTYPES

Clinical studies often group multiple histologic subtypes of extremity STS together due to their extremely low incidence. The number of patients eligible for surgery with curative intent is also diminished by the 14.9% of patients presenting with stage IV disease[37] and by those with unresectable but nonmetastatic disease. The resulting cohort often results in all-inclusive evidence-based recommendations that supersede the nuances of treatment required for individual STS. Entire articles in this series are devoted to certain histologic subtypes (ie, malignant peripheral nerve sheath tumor and liposarcoma) but a few under-recognized extremity STS deserve mentioning here.

Myxofibrosarcoma is notable for invading fascial and anatomic boundaries more often than other histologic subtypes.[1] The pathologic make-up can appear as banal as the day is long, with pleomorphic spindle cells on a myxoid background, yet have a local recurrence rate approaching 60% and metastasis in 15%.[38] IHC may only be positive for vimentin and actin. It is 1 of the few STS in which grade is not predictive of tumor behavior. Myxofibrosarcomas have infiltrative peripheries with long tentacles of cells appreciated on histology that frequently result in positive margins. The appreciable margin is not reliable for surgical resection. Wide margins up to 3 cm or beyond are encouraged, often requiring flaps and vessel reconstruction, and either preceded or followed by (neo) adjuvant radiotherapy.

Several sarcoma subtypes can have myogenic features but this must be interpreted cautiously within this group. In high-grade undifferentiated pleomorphic sarcoma

Table 7
Open randomized phase II trials for soft tissue sarcoma

ClinicalTrials.gov	Title	Location
NCT02367651	A Randomized, Double-Blind, Placebo-Controlled Phase II Study of Pazopanib vs Placebo as Maintenance Therapy for Patients Who Have Not Progressed After First-Line Chemotherapy For Advanced Soft Tissue Sarcoma	N/A
NCT02340884	A Pilot Randomized Controlled Trial of the Promoting Resilience in Stress Management (PRISM) Intervention For Adolescents And Young Adults With Cancer (phase II)	USA
NCT02249949	A Phase II Randomized, Double-Blinded Study of the Peroxisome Proliferator-Activated Receptor Gamma Agonist, Efatutazone vs Placebo in Patients with Previously Treated, Unresectable Myxoid Liposarcoma	N/A
NCT02207309	A Randomized, Double-Blind, Phase II Trial of Pazopanib vs Placebo as Maintenance Therapy in Patients with Retroperitoneal and Visceral High-Risk Soft Tissue Sarcomas Following Prior Neo- and/or Adjuvant Doxorubicin/ Ifosfamide Chemotherapy with Regional Hyperthermia	Germany
NCT02110069	A Randomized Phase 2 Study of Vincristine vs Sirolimus to Treat High Risk Kaposiform Hemangioendothelioma (KHE)	USA
NCT02048371	A Blanket Protocol To Study Oral Regorafenib in Patients with Refractory Liposarcoma, Osteogenic Sarcoma, and Ewing/ Ewing-like Sarcomas (phase II randomized)	USA
NCT01913652	Randomized Phase II Trial of Cabazitaxel or Prolonged Infusional Ifosfamide in Metastatic or Inoperable Locally Advanced Dedifferentiated Liposarcoma	UK
NCT01900743	Activity and Safety of Regorafenib in Patients with Metastatic Soft Tissue Sarcoma Previously Treated with Anthracycline-based Chemotherapy: a Multinational, Randomized, Phase II, Placebo-controlled Trial	Austria France
NCT01861951	A Randomized Phase II Trial Comparing Pazopanib with Doxorubicin as First Line Treatment In Elderly Patients With Metastatic Or Advanced Soft Tissue Sarcoma	Germany Belgium
NCT01593748	A Randomized, Open-label, Phase II, Multicenter Trial of Gemcitabine with Pazopanib or Gemcitabine with Docetaxel in Previously Treated Subjects With Advanced Soft Tissue Sarcoma	USA
NCT01532687	A Randomized, Double-Blind Phase II, Study Of Gemcitabine Alone or in Combination with Pazopanib for Refractory Soft Tissue Sarcoma	Oregon, USA
NCT01391962	A Phase II Trial in Which Patients with Metastatic Alveolar Soft Part Sarcoma are Randomized to Either Sunitinib or Cediranib Monotherapy, with Cross-over at Disease Progression	USA Canada
NCT01337401	A Phase II Trial Of Cediranib In The Treatment Of Patients With Alveolar Soft Part Sarcoma (CASPS)	Australia Spain UK
NCT01303094	Phase II Randomized Trial to Evaluate Two Strategies: Continuing vs Intermittent (Drug-holiday) Trabectedin-regimen in Patients With Advanced Soft Tissue Sarcoma Experiencing Response or Stable Disease After the Sixth Cycle	France

As of June 15, 2015. Excluding retroperitoneal tumors, Ewing, and GIST.

Table 8
Ongoing (but not recruiting) randomized phase II and phase III trials for soft tissue sarcoma

ClinicalTrials.gov	Title	Location
NCT01612481	Phase II Study Evaluating Strategies of Lung Surveillance of Patients Operated of High Grade Soft Tissue Sarcoma: Chest Radiograph vs Chest CT	France
NCT01574716	A Study of the Safety and Efficacy of the Combination of Gemcitabine and Docetaxel in Metastatic Soft Tissue Sarcoma	USA Australia Belgium France Italy Netherlands
NCT01514188	A Multicenter, Randomized, Open-Label Phase 2b Study to Investigate the Preliminary Efficacy and Safety of INNO-206 (Doxorubicin-EMCH) Compared to Doxorubicin in Subjects With Metastatic, Locally Advanced, or Unresectable Soft Tissue Sarcoma	USA Hungary Australia India Romania Russia Ukraine
NCT01440088	A Randomized Phase 3, Multicenter, Open-Label Study Comparing TH-302 in Combination With Doxorubicin vs Doxorubicin Alone in Subjects With Locally Advanced Unresectable or Metastatic Soft Tissue Sarcoma	USA Austria Belgium Canada Denmark France Germany Hungary Israel Italy Poland Russia Spain
NCT01355445	International Randomized Phase II Trial of the Combination of Vincristine and Irinotecan With or Without Temozolomide (VI or VIT) in Children and Adults With Refractory or Relapsed Rhabdomyosarcoma	France
NCT01343277	A Randomized Controlled Study of YONDELIS (Trabectedin) or Dacarbazine for the Treatment of Advanced Liposarcoma or Leiomyosarcoma (Phase III)	USA Australia Brazil New Zealand
NCT01327885	A Randomized, Open-label, Multicenter, Phase 3 Study to Compare the Efficacy and Safety of Eribulin With Dacarbazine in Subjects With Soft Tissue Sarcoma	USA Argentina Australia Austria Belgium Brazil Canada Czech Denmark France Germany Israel Italy Korea Netherlands New Zealand

(continued on next page)

Table 8
(continued)

ClinicalTrials.gov	Title	Location
		Poland
		Romania
		Russia
		Singapore
		Spain
		Thailand
		UK
NCT01303497	Phase II Study, Multicenter, Randomized, Stratified, Evaluating the Efficacy of Weekly Paclitaxel, in Association or Not With Bevacizumab in the Treatment of Metastatic or Locally Advanced Angiosarcomas Not Accessible to Surgery Treatment	France
NCT01288573	A Phase 1/2 Combined Dose Ranging and Randomized, Open-label, Comparative Study of the Efficacy and Safety of Plerixafor in Addition to Standard Regimens for Mobilization of Haematopoietic Stem Cells Into Peripheral Blood, and Subsequent Collection by Apheresis, vs Standard Mobilization Regimens Alone in Pediatric Patients, Aged 1 to <18 Years, With Solid Tumours Eligible for Autologous Transplants	Belgium Czech Denmark France Germany Hungary Israel Italy Netherlands Poland Spain UK
NCT01222715	A Randomized Phase II Trial of Bevacizumab (Avastin) and Temsirolimus (Torisel) in Combination With Intravenous Vinorelbine and Cyclophosphamide in Patients With Recurrent/Refractory Rhabdomyosarcoma	USA Australia Canada New Zealand
NCT01185964	A Phase 1b/2 Randomized Phase 2 Study Evaluating the Efficacy of Doxorubicin With or Without a Human Anti-PDGFRα Monoclonal Antibody (IMC-3G3) in the Treatment of Advanced Soft Tissue Sarcoma	USA
NCT00718484	A Phase II Multicenter, Parallel Group, Randomized Study of Palifosfamide Tris Plus Doxorubicin vs Doxorubicin in Subjects With Unresectable or Metastatic Soft-tissue Sarcoma	USA Italy Romania
NCT00716976	A Randomized Phase III Study of Sodium Thiosulfate for the Prevention of Cisplatin-Induced Ototoxicity in Children	USA Australia Canada
NCT00643565	An Open-label, Multi-center, Randomized Study of the Safety and Effect on Event-free Survival of Bevacizumab in Combination With Standard Chemotherapy in Childhood and Adolescent Patients With Metastatic Rhabdomyosarcoma and Non-rhabdomyosarcoma Soft Tissue Sarcoma (Phase II)	Belgium Brazil Canada Chile Czech France Germany Israel Italy Netherlands Poland Russia Spain UK

(continued on next page)

Table 8 (continued)		
ClinicalTrials.gov	**Title**	**Location**
NCT00484341	NGR016: Randomized Phase II Study Evaluating Two Doses of NGR-hTNF Administered Either as Single Agent or in Combination With Doxorubicin in Patients With Advanced Soft Tissue Sarcoma (STS)	France Italy UK
NCT00354835	Randomized Study of Vincristine, Dactinomycin and Cyclophosphamide (VAC) vs VAC Alternating With Vincristine and Irinotecan (VI) for Patients With Intermediate-Risk Rhabdomyosarcoma (RMS) (Phase III)	USA Australia Canada New Zealand Puerto Rico Switzerland
NCT00346164	Risk-Based Treatment for Non-Rhabdomyosarcoma Soft Tissue Sarcomas (NRSTS) in Patients Under 30 Years of Age (Phase III)	USA Australia Canada New Zealand Puerto Rico
NCT00189137	Phase II Evaluation of Ifosfamide Plus Doxorubicin & Filgrastim vs Gemcitabine Plus Docetaxel & Filgrastim in the Treatment of Localized Poor Prognosis Soft Tissue Sarcoma	USA
NCT00075582	Vincristine, Dactinomycin, and Lower Doses of Cyclophosphamide With or Without Radiation Therapy for Patients With Newly Diagnosed Low-Risk Embryonal/ Botryoid/Spindle Cell Rhabdomyosarcoma (Phase III)	USA Australia Canada New Zealand Puerto Rico Switzerland

As of 6/15/15. Excluding retroperitoneal tumors, Ewing, and GIST.

(UPS), myogenic differentiation does not affect overall survival or disease specific survival.[39] The same is not true of differentiated STS, including leiomyosarcoma and rhabdomyosarcoma, which carry a worse prognosis compared with other STS.[39,40] Retroperitoneal liposarcoma also carries a worse prognosis if myogenic differentiation is present,[41] although this variant rarely occurs in liposarcomas of the extremities.

Certain STS subtypes have a propensity for lymph node metastasis, namely rhabdomyosarcoma, angiosarcoma, clear cell sarcoma, epithelioid sarcoma, and synovial sarcoma. If lymphatic spread is identified quickly without evidence of systemic metastasis, the survival of these patients is similar to patients with localized high-grade sarcomas (>5 cm) of the extremity.[42]

SUMMARY

As previously described, the early detection of disease and accurate staging at presentation are the main prognostic factors for overall survival. This emphasizes the importance of a multidisciplinary team approach in obtaining an accurate and precise histologic diagnosis. Among malignancies, poorly differentiated sarcoma can appear like poorly differentiated carcinoma and melanoma can mimic many sarcoma types. Communication between the pathologist, radiologist, and surgeon can expose nuance between these malignancies and be essential for final diagnosis and staging.

Many advances have been made in the histologic diagnosis of STS that have, in turn, guided surgical treatment. However, even with the surgical goal of wide resection obtained in most cases, surgeons are still unable to fully cure many patients. Clinical trials are now focusing on tailoring adjuvant therapy to histologic subtype, often involving cases with unresectable STS. There are numerous randomized trials currently ongoing and recruiting internationally, reflecting the level of engagement globally at any given time in the current era (**Tables 6–8**).

REFERENCES

1. Gronchi A, Colombo C, Raut CP. Surgical management of localized soft tissue tumors. Cancer 2014;120(17):2638–48.
2. American Cancer Society. American Cancer Society: cancer facts and figures 2015. Atlanta (GA): American Cancer Society; 2015. Available at: http://www.cancer.org/acs/groups/content/@editorial/documents/document/acspc-044552.pdf. Accessed May 18, 2015.
3. Sawamura C, Springfield DS, Marcus KJ, et al. Factors predicting local recurrence, metastasis, and survival in pediatric soft tissue sarcoma in extremities. J Bone Joint Surg Am 2010;468(11):3019–27.
4. Gustafson P. Soft tissue sarcoma. Epidemiology and prognosis in 508 patients. Acta Orthop Scand Suppl 1994;259:1–31.
5. Surveillance, Epidemiology, and End Results (SEER) Program (www.seer.cancer.gov) Research Data (1973-2012). National Cancer Institute, DCCPS, Surveillance Research Program, Surveillance Systems Branch, released April 2015, based on the November 2014 submission.
6. Guadagnolo BA, Zagars GK, Ballo MT, et al. Mortality after cure of soft-tissue sarcoma treated with conservation surgery and radiotherapy. Cancer 2008;113(2):411–8.
7. Lachenmayer A, Yang Q, Eisenberger CF, et al. Superficial soft tissue sarcomas of the extremities and trunk. World J Surg 2009;33(8):1641–9.
8. Pisters PW, Pollock RE. Staging and prognostic factors in soft tissue sarcoma. Semin Radiat Oncol 1999;9(4):307–14.
9. Lewis JJ, Leung D, Casper ES, et al. Multifactorial analysis of long-term follow-up (more than 5 years) of primary extremity sarcoma. Arch Surg 1999;134(2):190–4.
10. Biau DJ, Ferguson PC, Chung P, et al. Local recurrence of localized soft tissue sarcoma: a new look at old predictors. Cancer 2012;118(23):5867–77.
11. Guillou L, Coindre JM, Bonichon F, et al. Comparative study of the National Cancer Institute and French Federation of Cancer Centers Sarcoma Group grading systems in a population of 410 adult patients with soft tissue sarcoma. J Clin Oncol 1997;15(1):350–62.
12. Lahat G, Tuvin D, Wei C, et al. New perspectives for staging and prognosis in soft tissue sarcoma. Ann Surg Oncol 2008;15(10):2739–48.
13. Maki RG, Moraco N, Antonescu CR, et al. Toward better soft tissue sarcoma staging: building on American Joint Committee on Cancer staging systems versions 6 and 7. Ann Surg Oncol 2013;20(11):3377–83.
14. Kneisl JS, Coleman MM, Raut CP. Outcomes in the Management of Adult Soft Tissue Sarcomas. J Surg Oncol 2014;110(5):527–38.
15. Coindre JM. Grading of soft tissue sarcomas: review and update. Arch Pathol Lab Med 2006;130(10):1448–53.
16. Welker JA, Henshaw RM, Jelinek J, et al. The percutaneous needle biopsy is safe and recommended in the diagnosis of musculoskeletal masses. Cancer 2000;89(12):2677–86.

17. Kiatisevi P, Thanakit V, Sukunthanak B, et al. Computed tomography–guided core needle biopsy versus incisional biopsy in diagnosing musculoskeletal lesions. J Orthop Surg 2013;21(2):204–8.
18. Khoja H, Griffin A, Dickson B, et al. Sampling modality influences the predictive value of grading in adult soft tissue extremity sarcomas. Arch Pathol Lab Med 2013;137(12):1774–9.
19. Hollowood K, Fletcher CD. Soft tissue sarcomas that mimic benign lesions. Semin Diagn Pathol 1995;12(1):87–97.
20. Novais EN, Demiralp B, Alderete J, et al. Do surgical margin and local recurrence influence survival in soft tissue sarcomas? Clin Orthop Relat Res 2010;468(11): 3003–11.
21. Sawamura C, Matsumoto S, Shimoji T, et al. What are risk factors for local recurrence of deep high-grade soft-tissue sarcomas? Clin Orthop Relat Res 2012; 470(3):700–5.
22. Stojadinovic A, Leung DH, Hoos A, et al. Analysis of the prognostic significance of microscopic margins in 2,084 localized primary adult soft tissue sarcomas. Ann Surg 2002;235(3):424–34.
23. Trovik CS, Bauer HC. Local recurrence after surgery for soft tissue sarcoma. The Scandinavian Sarcoma Group experience. Acta Orthop Scand Suppl 1999;285: 45–6.
24. Tanabe KK, Pollock RE, Ellis LM, et al. Influence of surgical margins on outcome in patients with preoperatively irradiated extremity soft tissue sarcomas. Cancer 1994;73(6):1652–9.
25. Kolovich GG, Wooldridge AN, Christy JM, et al. A retrospective statistical analysis of high-grade soft tissue sarcomas. Med Oncol 2012 Jun;29(2):1335–44.
26. Potter BK, Hwang PF, Forsberg JA, et al. Impact of margin status and local recurrence on soft-tissue sarcoma outcomes. J Bone Joint Surg Am 2013;95(20):e151.
27. Enneking WF, Spanier SS, Goodman MA. A system for the surgical staging of musculoskeletal sarcoma. 1980. Clin Orthop Relat Res 2003;415:4–18.
28. Trovik CS, Skjeldal S, Bauer H, et al. Reliability of margin assessment after surgery for extremity soft tissue sarcoma: the SSG experience. Sarcoma 2012; 2012:290698.
29. King DM, Hackbarth DA, Kirkpatrick A. Extremity soft tissue sarcoma resections: how wide do you need to be? Clin Orthop Relat Res 2012;470(3):692–9.
30. Menendez LR, Ahlmann ER, Savage K, et al. Tumor necrosis has no prognostic value in neoadjuvant chemotherapy for soft tissue sarcoma. Clin Orthop Relat Res 2007;455:219–24.
31. Turcotte RE, Ferrone M, Isler MH, et al. Outcomes in patients with popliteal sarcomas. Can J Surg 2009;52(1):51–5.
32. Biau DJ, Weiss KR, Bhumbra RS, et al. Monitoring the adequacy of surgical margins after resection of bone and soft-tissue sarcoma. Ann Surg Oncol 2013;20(6): 1858–64.
33. Gerrand CH, Wunder JS, Kandel RA, et al. Classification of positive margins after resection of soft-tissue sarcoma of the limb predicts the risk of local recurrence. J Bone Joint Surg Br 2001;83(8):1149–55.
34. Dagan R, Indelicato DJ, McGee L, et al. The significance of a marginal excision after preoperative radiation therapy for soft tissue sarcoma of the extremity. Cancer 2012;118(12):3199–207.
35. Arai E, Sugiura H, Tsukushi S, et al. Residual tumor after unplanned excision reflects clinical aggressiveness for soft tissue sarcomas. Tumour Biol 2014;35(8): 8043–9.

36. Binitie O, Tejiram S, Conway S, et al. Adult soft tissue sarcoma local recurrence after adjuvant treatment without resection of core needle biopsy tract. Clin Orthop Relat Res 2013;471(3):891–8.

37. Jacobs AJ, Michels R, Stein J, et al. Improvement in overall survival from extremity soft tissue sarcoma over twenty years. Sarcoma 2015;2015:279601.

38. Huang HY, Lal P, Qin J, et al. Low-grade myxofibrosarcoma: a clinicopathologic analysis of 49 cases treated at a single institution with simultaneous assessment of the efficacy of 3-tier and 4-tier grading systems. Hum Pathol 2004;35(5): 612–21.

39. Cipriani NA, Kurzawa P, Ahmad RA, et al. Prognostic value of myogenic differentiation in undifferentiated pleomorphic sarcomas of soft tissue. Hum Pathol 2014; 45(7):1504–8.

40. Stock N, Chateau MC, Collin F, et al. Prognostic value of myogenic differentiation in adult soft tissue sarcomas (STS): a study of 855 cases from the French Sarcoma Group. The Connective Tissue Oncology Society. CTOS 14th Annual Meeting. Available at: http://www.ctos.org/meeting/2008/presentations/thu12_stock.ppt. Accessed August 28, 2015.

41. Gronchi A, Collini P, Miceli R, et al. Myogenic differentiation and histologic grading are major prognostic determinants in retroperitoneal liposarcoma. Am J Surg Pathol 2015;39(3):383–93.

42. Riad S, Griffin AM, Liberman B, et al. Lymph node metastasis in soft tissue sarcoma in an extremity. Clin Orthop Relat Res 2004;426:129–34.

Retroperitoneal Sarcoma
Fact, Opinion, and Controversy

Rebecca A. Gladdy, MD, PhD, FRCSC[a,b,*], Abha Gupta, MD, MSc, FRCPC[c,d],
Charles N. Catton, MD, FRCPC[e,f]

KEYWORDS

- Retroperitoneal sarcoma • Soft tissue sarcoma • Surgery • Local recurrence
- Radiation therapy • Chemotherapy

KEY POINTS

- Retroperitoneal sarcomas (RPS) are rare cancers whose work-up includes detailed radiologic assessment (CT scan of chest/abdomen/pelvis) and expert pathologic review.
- The overall goal of a primary RPS resection is gross resection of tumor with en bloc removal of closely associated/involved viscera and retroperitoneal musculature.
- Neoadjuvant chemotherapy and/or radiation may be key components of the therapeutic armamentarium in patients with RPS especially in chemosensitive subtypes or borderline resectable tumors.
- The predominant pattern of failure in RPS is local recurrence, which occurs in 25% to 50% of patients at 5 years and 35% to 60% at 10 years.
- Long-term surveillance should be in centers of expertise because the decision making for RPS recurrence is complex and warrants multidisciplinary input and access to clinical trials.

FACT

Soft tissue sarcomas (STS) are malignant neoplasms that arise predominately from mesenchymal tissues including fat, muscle, fibrous tissue, and blood vessels.[1] Overall, 15% of STS arise in the retroperitoneum. Retroperitoneal sarcomas (RPS) are rare

Disclosures: The authors have nothing to disclose.
[a] Department of Surgery, Mount Sinai Hospital, University of Toronto, 600 University Avenue, Suite 1225, Toronto, Ontario M5G 1X5, Canada; [b] Department of Surgical Oncology, Princess Margaret Cancer Centre, 610 University Avenue, 3rd Floor, Toronto, Ontario M5G 2M9, Canada; [c] Division of Pediatric Hematology/Oncology, Department of Pediatrics, The Hospital for Sick Children, University of Toronto, Room 9215, Toronto, Ontario M5G 1X8, Canada; [d] Department of Medical Oncology, Princess Margaret Cancer Centre, 610 University Avenue, 5th Floor, Toronto, Ontario M5G 2M9, Canada; [e] Department of Radiation Oncology, University of Toronto, FitzGerald Building, Room 106, 150 College Street, Toronto, Ontario M5S 3E2, Canada; [f] Radiation Medicine Program, Princess Margaret Cancer Centre, 610 University Avenue, 5th Floor, Toronto, Ontario M5G 2M9, Canada
* Corresponding author. Department of Surgery, Mount Sinai Hospital, 600 University Avenue, Suite 1225, Toronto, Ontario M5G 1X5, Canada.
E-mail address: rgladdy@mtsinai.on.ca

tumors with an incidence of 0.5 to 1 cases per 100,000.[2] In general, RPS are sporadic cancers; however, there are several hereditary cancer syndromes associated with STS including Li-Fraumeni and neurofibromatosis type 1. Radiation-associated sarcomas are rare and can arise as a late complication of treatment with a median onset of 10 years.[3,4]

Diagnostic Challenges of Retroperitoneal Sarcomas

One of the challenges in the management of patients with RPS is that most present with advanced disease yet are asymptomatic. It is essential in evaluating an undiagnosed retroperitoneal (RP) mass that other tumors are excluded in particular lymphoma, adenocarcinoma, germ cell tumor, and paraganglioma.[5] After performing a through history and physical examination, obtaining tumor markers (ie, LDH, AFP, βHCG) may aid in making a diagnosis. Although endoscopy is not usually necessary, a percutaneous biopsy may be required for a definitive diagnosis. It is also critical that all patients with RP masses have diagnostic abdominal and pelvic computed tomography (CT) scans performed along with a staging CT chest when malignancy is suspected (**Fig. 1**). MRI is used in cases where CT is contraindicated and/or when it may complement CT, whereas the use of ultrasound alone is discouraged. To date, there is limited utility in use of PET scans in patients with RPS; however, they may be useful in staging other RP tumors, such as lymphoma and adenocarcinoma.

In general, RPS grow by direct local extension into adjacent tissues and structures, often pushing them aside and less commonly invade fascial planes, joints, or bone. They are usually large in size (median size, 20 cm) at presentation.[6] There are more

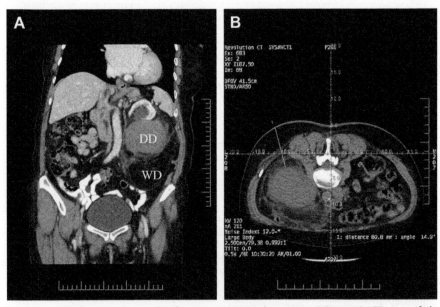

Fig. 1. Establishing the diagnosis of a retroperitoneal sarcoma. Diagnostic CT scan of the abdomen and pelvis demonstrates a retroperitoneal mass with areas suspicious for dedifferentiated (DD) and well-differentiated (WD) liposarcoma (A). A diagnostic biopsy was performed using CT-guidance of the high-grade DD area, which confirmed the diagnosis of liposarcoma (B).

than 80 different histologic subtypes of STS in the retroperitoneum. Liposarcoma (LPS) is the most common (63%), and is further divided into four different subtypes: (1) well-differentiated (WD LPS), (2) dedifferentiated (DD LPS), (3) myxoid round cell (MRC LPS), and (4) pleomorphic. The second most common subtype is leiomyosarcoma (LMS) (19%), which primarily consists of sarcoma of major veins, specifically the inferior vena cava, renal vein, and gonadal vessels. Less frequent RPS subtypes include solitary fibrous tumor (SFT), fibrosarcoma, and malignant peripheral nerve sheath tumor (MPNST). Pathologic diagnoses excluded in this review include benign conditions, such as lipoma, benign peripheral nerve sheath tumors, desmoid, and angiomyolipoma; and visceral sarcomas, such as gastrointestinal stromal tumor, uterine LMS, paratesticular/spermatic cord, or prostatic sarcoma. Histologies including extraosseous Ewing sarcoma, rhabdomyosarcoma, and primitive ectodermal tumors are less common but may be encountered in the retroperitoneum. These generally require special consideration including detailed pathologic assessment and multidisciplinary management strategies.

Some RPS subtypes have diagnostic signatures, however most do not (**Table 1**). For example, malignant fibrous histiocytoma (MFH) is a historical diagnosis and been reclassified as undifferentiated pleomorphic sarcoma.[7] Undifferentiated pleomorphic sarcoma has emerged as a less common subtype in the retroperitoneum because most high-grade poorly differentiated sarcomas are diagnosed as DD LPS based on positive MDM2 immunohistochemistry confirmed by fluorescent in situ hybridization. Expert pathologic review is essential in managing patients with sarcoma, which includes an extensive immunohistochemical panel plus access to standardized molecular diagnostic tests when applicable. Whether this assessment is done preoperatively with a percutaneous biopsy as a standard of care is still debated; however, this approach is endorsed in most but not all sarcoma expert centers (discussed in the opinion section). The use of intraoperative biopsy for an RP mass that is incidentally discovered or not fully worked up preoperatively is discouraged because this is often nondiagnostic and may involve disruption of tumor planes.[5]

The current staging for STS from the American Joint Committee on Cancer 7th edition incorporates histologic grade and TNM status.[8] The most significant change to the 7th edition is the downstaging of nodal disease from stage IV to stage III, although lymph node involvement is uncommon in STS (5%–15%).[9] TNM staging has limited

Table 1
Common soft tissue sarcoma subtypes in the retroperitoneum with diagnostic markers

Histology	Frequency (%)	Immunohistochemistry	Molecular
Liposarcoma	63	MDM2, CDK4, p16	MDM2 amplification
Leiomyosarcoma	19	Smooth muscle actin, desmin, H-caldesmin	Not applicable
Solitary fibrous tumour	6	CD34, CD99, BCL2, STAT6	NAB2-STAT6 fusion product
Malignant peripheral nerve sheath tumour	3	S100, SOX10, CD56, CD57, PGP9.5	Not applicable
Undifferentiated pleomorphic sarcoma	2	Not applicable	Not applicable
Other	7	Diagnosis-dependent	Diagnosis-dependent

Data from Gronchi A, Strauss DC, Miceli R, et al. Variability in patterns of recurrence after resection of primary retroperitoneal sarcoma (RPS): a report on 1007 patients from the Multi-institutional Collaborative RPS Working Group. Ann Surg 2016;263(5):1002–9.

use in patients with RPS because almost all RPS are greater than 5 cm in size and by definition are deep.[6] An alternate means of prognosticating survival in resected RPS was derived by analyzing population-based data, which defined grade, invasion of adjacent structures, and histologic subtype as better predictors of outcome than American Joint Committee on Cancer staging, yet this has not been widely adapted.[10] It is, however, universally accepted that grade is the most important prognostic factor in STS. The most widely used grading system is from the French three-tiered system, which is based on assigning a score for tumor differentiation (1–3), mitotic activity (1–3), and necrosis (0–2).[11] Alternatively, sarcoma-specific nomograms have been developed and validated to predict postoperative survival[12,13] and subtype-specific survival.[14]

Management of Primary Retroperitoneal Sarcomas

The cornerstone of treatment in primary RPS is surgical resection. Although the use of neoadjuvant chemotherapy and radiation therapy (RT) is not universally agreed on because of lack of level one evidence (discussed in the controversies section), neoadjuvant therapies may be key components of the therapeutic armamentarium especially in chemosensitive subtypes or borderline resectable tumors (**Fig. 2**). Thus, it has been advocated that patients with RPS be managed and treatment decisions rendered at expert sarcoma centers where the multidisciplinary team consists of dedicated sarcoma pathologists, diagnostic radiology, surgical oncology, medical oncology, and radiation oncology (discussed in the opinion section). Furthermore, the extensive surgical procedures performed in patients with RPS require advanced supportive care by anesthesia, intensive care, and/or interventional radiology.

The overall goal of a primary RPS resection is gross resection of tumor with en bloc removal of closely associated/involved viscera and RP musculature. Resection should also include complete removal of all ipsilateral RP fat in patients with LPS. The role of more extended RP resection has been advocated by several centers but remains controversial (discussed in the section on extended RPS resections). The anatomic constraints of the retroperitoneum render margin-negative excisions more technically challenging than for STS at other sites.[15] Overall, grossly incomplete resection is discouraged, because it may not be beneficial. Preoperative planning may also include a differential renal scan to anticipate renal dysfunction postoperatively if a nephrectomy is likely. Additionally, assessment and optimization of the patient's nutritional and performance status before surgery is important to mitigate perioperative complications because the large size of RPS can impair adequate nutritional intake and/or is associated with deconditioning.

The best chance of a curative outcome is at the primary resection; thus detailed surgical planning and expertise is required to perform multivisceral resections with reconstruction while minimizing microscopically positive margins.[15] Viscera commonly resected in RPS include colon, kidney, pancreas, spleen, diaphragm, small bowel, duodenum, liver, bladder, with resection of psoas, iliacus musculature, and/or abdominal wall.[6] Select cases require resection and reconstruction of major vascular structures (interior vena cava, aorta, and/or iliac vessels) and less commonly include vertebral or pelvic bony resection. Another complex surgical issue is extension of the RPS into other anatomic compartments, such as crossing the inguinal ligament into the scrotum or adductor compartment of the thigh or posterior extension out of the sciatic notch. These technically challenging cases therefore may require involvement of multidisciplinary surgical teams including uro-oncology, orthopedic oncology, vascular surgery, and/or plastic surgery. Generally accepted criteria for RPS unresectability

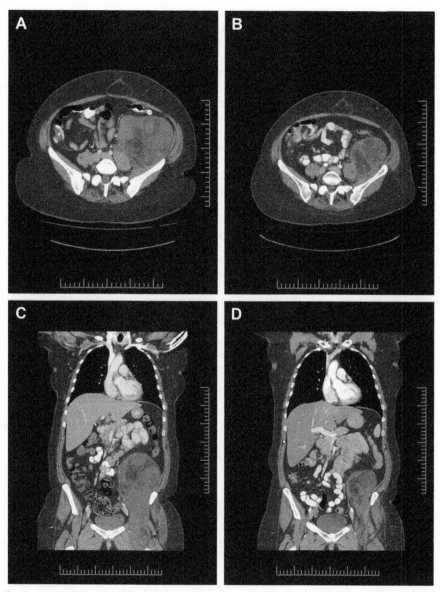

Fig. 2. Response to neoadjuvant chemotherapy and radiation in RPS. Diagnostic CT scan of an RPS extending into the adductor canal (*A, C*). A diagnosis of myxoid-round cell liposarcoma (FUS-CHOP gene fusion positive) was established with a preoperative biopsy. Cytoreduction was achieved with the administration of five cycles of doxorubicin and ifosfamide followed by 25 fractions of radiation therapy as observed on the preoperative CT scan (*B, D*). Surgical resection of the RPS with complete psoas and iliacus resection and transection of the femoral nerve was performed with preservation of the sigmoid colon, ureter, and iliac vessels.

include diffuse metastases, peritoneal implants, or extensive/circumferential involvement of the superior mesenteric artery (SMA) or superior mesenteric vein (SMV).

Given the large size of most RPS (>20 cm), the ability to achieve and accurately pathologically assess microscopically clear (R0) margins is limited.[16] Although R0 resections have been reported to be associated with decreased abdominal recurrence and improved overall survival (OS) by multivariate analysis in a series by Bonvalot and colleagues,[17] this has not been replicated in other series.[18,19] Thus, most RPS centers of excellence report gross margin clearance (R0 and R1) compared with grossly incomplete resections (R2) (**Table 2**).[20]

With the complexity of surgery undertaken in patients with RPS, the morbidity and mortality associated with these procedures with and without neoadjuvant therapies is increasingly recognized as an important index of quality of care. Although 30-day mortality in patients with RPS from single institutional series (1.4%–3.0%)[21,22] or combined multicenter experience (1.9%)[6] is consistent with outcomes in other major oncologic abdominal procedures, major perioperative morbidity is common. Specifically, the 30-day morbidity in 1007 primary RPS from the Multi-institutional Collaborative RPS Working Group, which combined the experience of eight international sarcoma centers,[6] reported grade 3 events in 12.7% of patients, whereas grade 4 events occurred in 5.2% of patients as defined by Common Terminology Criteria for

Table 2
Recurrence rates in retroperitoneal sarcoma series

Author, Year	Number Resected	Margin (%) R0/R1 vs R2	Median Follow-up (mo)	Local Recurrence (%)	Distant Recurrence (%)	Notes
Gronchi et al,[6] 2016	1007	95	58	5-y 26 10-y 35	5-y 21 10-y 22	8 expert centers
Tan et al,[4] 2016	632	90	90	5-y 39	5-y 24	Single expert center
Gronchi et al,[25] 2015	377	96	44	5-y 24	5-y 22	2 expert centers
Smith et al,[21] 2015	362	96	26	3-y LRFS 98 WD LPS 57 DD LPS 80 LMS	5-y DRFS 46 100 WD LPS 86 DD LPS 65 LMS	Single expert center
Toulemonde et al,[29] 2014	511	76	78	5-y LRFS 46	—	12 French sarcoma centers
Keung et al,[36] 2014	119	80	74	5-y LRFS 15	5-y DRFS 33	Single expert center DD LPS only
Bonvalot et al,[22] 2010	249	93	37	5-y 22	5-y 24	2 expert centers
Gronchi et al,[52] 2009	193	89	58	5-y LR Recent cohort 28 Early cohort 48	5-y DR Recent cohort 22 Early cohort 13	Single expert center
Lewis et al,[19] 1998	231	80	28	5-y LRFS 59	5-y DRFS 79	Single expert center

Abbreviations: DR, distant recurrence; DRFS, distant recurrence-free survival; LR, local recurrence; LRFS, local recurrence-free survival.

Adverse Events.[23] Part of the controversy in performing extended resections is that these procedures are associated with increased morbidity including high reoperative rates (12%), which are usually performed for anastomotic leakage or postoperative bleeding.[22] With extended resection, factors associated with increased morbidity include three or more organs resected, major vascular resection, gastrectomy, and/or duodenectomy.[22] Finally, there are limited data to address the concern that preoperative RT is associated with increased perioperative morbidity. Thus, the morbidity and toxicity data being compiled in the ongoing phase III multicenter STRASS (Study of Preoperative Radiotherapy Plus Surgery Versus Surgery Alone for Patients with RPS) sponsored by the European Organization for Research and Treatment of Cancer (NCT01344018) should be informative.[24]

Outcomes and Recurrence in Retroperitoneal Sarcomas

OS rates for primary RPS treated with curative intent range from 39% to 70% at 5 years and 20% to 64% at 10 years from series with long-term follow-up (**Table 3**).[5,6,10,25–27] Predictive factors associated with survival include age, tumor size, completeness of resection, grade, and multifocality.[6]

The predominant pattern of failure in RPS is local recurrence (LR), which occurs in 25% to 50% of patients at 5 years and 35% to 60% at 10 years (see **Table 2**).[4,17,19,25] The median time to LR ranges from 24 to 41 months.[25,28] Factors associated with LR include age, size, completeness of resection, grade, tumor rupture, multifocality, administration of RT, and histologic subtype.[6,29] With long-term follow-up from prospective databases at single institutions and a recently established RPS consortium (Trans-Atlantic RPS Working Group), there is a better appreciation that histologic subtype directs patterns of failure. Specifically, in a study of 675 patients with primary RPS, DD LPS had a high LR rate of 58% at 5 years and 62% at 15 years compared

Table 3
Survival rates in retroperitoneal sarcoma series

Author, Year	Number Resected	Primary RPS (%)	Median Follow-up (mo)	Survival (%)	(Neo) Adjuvant Therapy (%)	
					Chemotherapy	Radiation
Gronchi et al,[6] 2016	1007	100	58	OS 5-y 67 10-y 46	18.2	32
Tan et al,[4] 2016	632	100	90	DSD 5-y 31	18	8
Gronchi et al,[25] 2015	377	100	44	OS 5-y 64	32	31
Smith et al,[21] 2015	362	100	26	DSS 3-y 81	3	8
Smith et al,[26] 2014	40	73	73	OS 5-y 70 10-y 64	—	100
Toulemonde et al,[29] 2014	511	100	78	OS 5-y 66	17	29
Keung et al,[36] 2014	119	100	74	OS 5-y 42	12.6	28
Bonvalot et al,[22] 2010	249	100	37	OS 5-y 64	37	36
Gronchi et al,[52] 2009	288	67	58	OS 10-y 36	32	31
Bonvalot et al,[17] 2009	374	100	52	OS 5-y 57	34	32
van Dalen et al,[27] 2007	115	100	122	OS 5-y 39	18	16
Lewis et al,[19] 1998	231	100	28	OS 5-y 54	—	—

Abbreviations: DSD, disease-specific death; DSS, disease-specific survival.

with WD LPS and MRC LPS, which had 39% and 60% incidence of LR at 5 and 15 years, respectively.[4] Furthermore, LR was uncommon in patients with SFT (8%) and, interestingly, all LR in MPNST patients occurred within 3 years.

The development of distant recurrence (DR) occurs in 21% to 24% patients at 5 years and 22% patients at 10 years (see **Table 2**). The median OS post-DR is 20 months.[25,30] Predictive factors associated with DR include size, grade, multifocality, and subtype. Metastasis most commonly occurs in the lung (30%) and liver (5%–10%); other sites of RPS DR include bone, RP fat, mediastinum, and soft tissue.[31] Although LR rates are low in LMS (10%–20% at 5 years), DR occurs in 58% of high-grade LMS at 10 years and is the main cause of sarcoma-specific death.[4,25,31] Other STS associated with high DR rates at 10 years are SFT (41%) and DD LPS (28%), whereas MPNST and WD LPS have limited DR rates of 15% and 8%, respectively.

Patients with RPS should be surveyed for their lifetime because late recurrence (>20 years) occurs.[32] Because the risk of recurrence is most highly associated with tumor grade, guidelines for RPS surveillance are stratified as follows: low-grade, CT chest/abdomen/pelvis every 6 months for first 2 to 3 years then yearly thereafter; and high-grade, CT chest/abdomen/pelvis every 4 months for first 2 to 3 years, then every 6 months for next 2 years and then annually.[33] Ideally, long-term surveillance should be in centers of expertise because the decision making to manage recurrence is complex and ongoing clinical trials should be available. Furthermore, to better understand RPS outcomes, ongoing clinical assessment and data collection are critical in determining which interventions are beneficial to patients long-term.

OPINION
Are Diagnostic Biopsies Standard of Care in Patients with Retroperitoneal Sarcomas?

Whether a diagnostic biopsy should be performed on all patients with RPS is still debated. Advocates cite that initiation of neoadjuvant therapies and surgical planning is optimally executed once the sarcoma subtype has been established and the diagnosis of either a benign RP tumor or carcinoma has been excluded.[33] When performing a diagnostic biopsy, detailed imaging should be obtained before tumor manipulation. Biopsies should be performed using CT or ultrasound image-guidance to target tissue most concerning for high-grade features while avoiding necrotic areas using a large-bore needle (16 or 18 gauge) with a covering sheath (see **Fig. 1**). Multiple cores (at least four) should be obtained to limit sampling error and provide adequate tissue for detailed histologic and molecular diagnosis. Fine-needle aspiration is not typically advised. Laparoscopic or open biopsies are only indicated if repeated percutaneous biopsies are not diagnostic. The main concern about preoperative biopsy is that there is a theoretic risk of tumor rupture; however, there is no evidence to support this notion.[34] Although imaging may be adequate to infer a diagnosis of high-grade LPS, biopsy can also play a role in determining the extent of or need for resection of low-grade LPS versus other benign conditions including lipoma and myelolipoma. Thus, as data emerge that outcome is related to RPS histologic subtype,[4,25] the ability for sarcoma surgeons to plan more limited resections based on favorable biology (SFT) and/or implement neoadjuvant therapy for chemosensitive subtypes (LMS, MRC LPS) reinforces the consideration for preoperative biopsy.

Retroperitoneal Sarcomas Should Be Managed at Expert High-Volume Multidisciplinary Centers

Outside of specialized centers, there remains limited experience with RPS. As with other complex abdominal procedures (ie, pancreatoduodenectomy),[35] there is emerging evidence that a wide range of outcomes including OS are improved in patients with sarcoma who are treated with specialist care compared with those that are not. Evidence to support care in high-volume centers is two-fold. First, in a recent RPS study, tumor integrity (either ruptured or transected) was an important predictor of progression-free survival and OS in the management of patients with primary DD LPS.[36] Tumor compromise was likely a surrogate of surgical expertise because this retrospective study included procedures performed by nonsarcoma surgeons. Second, the National Institute for Health and Care Excellence in the United Kingdom published guidelines were generated using expert literature review, which reinforced the benefits derived from expert care.[37] Another evidence-based systemic review of the literature was performed by Cancer Care Ontario and also concluded that outcomes in patients with sarcoma were improved in a high-volume center with multidisciplinary management.[38] Finally, analysis of survival and functional outcomes in high- versus low-volume centers in the Florida Cancer Data System demonstrated an OS survival benefit in patients with RPS treated at a high-volume center.[39]

Adjuvant Radiotherapy Should Be Given Preoperatively if at All

Because the main clinical challenge in RPS is LR, determining whether adjuvant RT is beneficial in patients with RPS has been an area of ongoing investigation. In contrast to extremity STS, where the role of adjuvant RT has been established in clinical trials,[40–42] evidence to support its routine use in patients with RPS is limited (discussed in section on controversies–role of RT). Although prospective clinical trials have reported that preoperative external beam RT is well tolerated by most patients,[43] it is still unclear if RT improves OS and/or LRFS. The addition of perioperative brachytherapy in RPS, however, is associated with increased toxicity and no survival benefit with long-term follow-up.[26] Thus, current consensus guidelines support the delivery of external beam RT preoperatively in patients with RPS because this is associated with less toxicity as the in situ tumor frequently displaces sensitive small bowel, the target volume definition is much more accurate, the risk of intraoperative tumor seeding is theoretically reduced, and a preoperative dose of 50 Gy is well tolerated compared with 60 to 66 Gy in the postoperative setting.[44]

Management of Recurrent Disease

After RPS recurs, the lifetime chance of cure is considered limited.[25,45] Approximately 9% to 27% of recurrences present with synchronous LR and DR, which is associated with poor (median, 12 months) survival.[6,17,25] If patients recur with local disease only and resection is technically feasible without excessive morbidity, this should only be considered when there has been a long disease-free interval. These factors are present, however, in a minority of recurrences. In a study by Gronchi and colleagues[25] only 21 patients (27%) of first recurrences underwent surgery, which was completely resected in 18 patients.[25] Factors predictive of survival for patients undergoing resection of a first recurrence include grade, multifocality, and tumor growth rate.[28,46,47] Management of recurrences may also include a period of observation to determine tumor biology, especially in asymptomatic patients. The use of RT and/or chemotherapy should also be considered preoperatively in borderline resectable or chemosensitive subtypes. Further recurrences become more challenging to completely resect, and with each recurrence survival diminishes while morbidity increases.[19] Although debulking surgery is not generally recommended, surgical palliation may provide some symptom relief in select patients.[48]

The management of metastatic RPS is complex and multidisciplinary input is critical to establish goals of care of curative-intent resection or palliation. The literature on resection of metastatic disease is confounded by patient selection and therefore treatment decisions should be considered on case-by-case basis. Five-year OS up to 40% has been reported after pulmonary metastasectomy[49]; however, there are limited data regarding hepatic metastasectomy.[50,51] Although palliative chemotherapy is not associated with improved survival but may reduce tumor size to relieve symptoms, its role in patients with asymptomatic metastasis is unclear. Finally, palliative RT is effective management for painful metastasis.

CONTROVERSY
Role of Extended Resection for Retroperitoneal Sarcomas

The rationale for extended RPS resections is to achieve wider margins by performing a compartmental resection similar to what is performed for extremity STS. In two independent studies published in 2009, this aggressive surgical approach, which included resection of uninvolved structures, was reported to be associated with improved local control.[17,52] However, this potential advance in RPS management was tempered by concerns that included limited patient follow-up, which would impact cumulative LR incidence; retrospective data collection; selective organ resection; increased perioperative morbidity; and high rates of reoperation without improvement in OS.[53] Although follow-up studies provided morbidity data[22] and improved local control rates, which is most evident in patients with low-grade tumors,[54] the routine use of extended compartmental resection has not translated into RPS surgical practice.[16,55] What has emerged from this active debate is a collaborative effort in improving the quality of surgery and care in patients with RPS as demonstrated by consensus guidelines in RPS management from the Trans-Atlantic RPS Working Group[5] with publication of combined primary RPS outcomes,[6] a technical consideration position paper in RPS surgery from E-Surge,[15] and the ongoing multicenter accrual of patients in the STRASS trial, which should be completed in 2016.

Role of Radiotherapy

Generally, it is agreed that any RT used should be administered neoadjuvantly in patients with RPS that are be considered for curative intent surgery because it is well tolerated and has limited toxicity (discussed in the opinion section on adjuvant RT). Several retrospective studies have suggested that (neo) adjuvant RT reduces the risk of LR in RPS.[17,52,56–58] In a recent subgroup analysis of 1007 RPS, a durable high local control rate was observed in a single center that had administered higher rates of RT (70%); however, this was also associated with an increased rate of organ resection. The limitation in translating the use of RT in patients with RPS is that there are no high level evidence data that demonstrate the use of RT improves survival. In the phase III randomized STRASS trial,[24] the primary study outcome is to determine if there is a difference in abdominal recurrence-free survival between patients with RPS undergoing curative surgery alone and those undergoing preoperative RT followed by curative-intent surgery. Secondary end points include determining if there is a difference in metastasis-free survival, abdominal LR-free interval, OS, assessment of tumor response to RT, and assessment of the toxicity profile of preoperative RT. To date 192 of the planned 256 patients have been accrued across 11 European countries and three North American sites with completion of the second interim safety analysis, which did not identify any safety or compliance concerns. In the absence of level one evidence, preoperative RT remains an important consideration in patients with RPS because local control continues to be a challenge and it is generally well tolerated.

Role of Chemotherapy

Adjuvant chemotherapy is not routinely recommended in high-grade STS because of lack of sufficient evidence that it improves OS.[59] However, neoadjuvant chemotherapy may be beneficial for chemosensitive histologies (LMS and MRC LPS) or borderline resectable tumors where cytoreduction may enhance the ability to achieve a gross resection and potentially limit the need to resect critical structures (see **Fig. 2**).[60] With a goal of maximal cytoreduction preoperatively, combination therapy with doxorubicin plus ifosfamide may be considered over single-agent doxorubicin because of relative higher response rates in the former (26% vs 14%; $P<.0006$).[61] Although distant failures are less common in RPS than extremity STS, systemic therapy may still be considered in those where resection of LR is not feasible or deemed not beneficial.[30] In addition to doxorubicin-based therapy, trabectedin[62] or gemcitabine (alone or in combination with docetaxel)[63] may be reasonable alternatives worth considering. Otherwise options are limited and inclusion in clinical trials should be considered.

Quality of Life and Survivorship

Although cancer-specific outcomes for RPS have been steadily emerging from experienced centers, there has been a paucity of information on patient-reported and functional outcomes in comparison with other STS sites, such as extremity.[64] Most recently, the Milan group reported long-term outcomes in RPS, which focused on chronic pain, hernia formation, renal impairment, and sexual function.[65] Unfortunately, one of the limitations of the study was that only data from long-term survivors could be obtained. As with other complex pelvic/abdominal surgical procedures,[66,67] functional outcomes are important metrics of care in patients with RPS in the short and intermediate term. For the first time, health-related quality of life studies using general cancer quality of life assessment tools (European Organization for Research and Treatment of Cancer QLQ-30) with gastric (STO22) and colorectal cancer (CR29) modules are part of prospective data collection in the STRASS trial and are being assessed at baseline, 1 year, and 5 years after randomization. However, specific tools that address RPS-specific concerns do not exist and thus studies with qualitative interviews to define patient experience may aid in defining and developing an RPS-focused health-related quality of life questionnaire.

SUMMARY

Once the diagnosis of RPS is established, detailed imaging and multidisciplinary discussion should guide treatment including surgical resection and in select cases, neoadjuvant therapy. LR is common in RPS and is associated with grade, histologic subtype, completeness of resection, and size. Although the role of preoperative RT is not yet defined, an ongoing international phase III trial should yield data on RPS-specific outcomes including recurrence-free survival, toxicity, and quality of life. As guidelines to standardize RPS patient management emerge, expert pathologic assessment and management in centers of excellence are benchmarks of quality of care. The efficacy of current chemotherapy is limited and thus there is a critical need to understand the molecular basis of sarcoma so that new drug therapies are developed. Finally, multicenter clinical trials are needed to limit opinion and controversy in this complex and challenging disease.

REFERENCES

1. Goldblum J, Weiss R, Sharon W, et al. Folpe Enzinger and Weiss' soft tissue tumors. 6th edition. Philadelphia: Saunders/Elsevier; 2014.

2. Cormier JN, Gronchi A, Pollock RE. Soft tissue sarcomas. In: Brunicardi FC, editor. Schwartz's principles of surgery. New York: McGraw-Hill; 2015. p. 1465–94.

3. Gladdy RA, Qin LX, Moraco N, et al. Do radiation-associated soft tissue sarcomas have the same prognosis as sporadic soft tissue sarcomas? J Clin Oncol 2010; 28:2064–9.

4. Tan MC, Brennan MF, Kuk D, et al. Histology-based classification predicts pattern of recurrence and improves risk stratification in primary retroperitoneal sarcoma. Ann Surg 2016;263(3):593–600.

5. Trans-Atlantic RPS Working Group. Management of primary retroperitoneal sarcoma (RPS) in the adult: a consensus approach from the Trans-Atlantic RPS Working Group. Ann Surg Oncol 2015;22:256–63.

6. Gronchi A, Strauss DC, Miceli R, et al. Variability in patterns of recurrence after resection of primary retroperitoneal sarcoma (RPS): a report on 1007 patients from the Multi-institutional Collaborative RPS Working Group. Ann Surg 2016; 263(5):1002–9.

7. Fletcher CD, Bridge JA, Hogendoorn P, et al. WHO classification of tumours of soft tissue and bone. 4th edition. Lyon (France): International Agency for Research on Cancer; 2014.

8. Edge SBBD, Compton CC, Fritz AG, et al. AJCC (American Joint Committee on Cancer). Cancer staging manual. 7th edition. New York: Springer; 2010.

9. Fong Y, Coit DG, Woodruff JM, et al. Lymph node metastasis from soft tissue sarcoma in adults. Analysis of data from a prospective database of 1772 sarcoma patients. Ann Surg 1993;217:72–7.

10. Nathan H, Raut CP, Thornton K, et al. Predictors of survival after resection of retroperitoneal sarcoma: a population-based analysis and critical appraisal of the AJCC staging system. Ann Surg 2009;250:970–6.

11. Coindre JM. Pathology and grading of soft tissue sarcomas. Cancer Treat Res 1993;67:1–22.

12. Kattan MW, Leung DH, Brennan MF. Postoperative nomogram for 12-year sarcoma-specific death. J Clin Oncol 2002;20:791–6.

13. Gronchi A, Miceli R, Shurell E, et al. Outcome prediction in primary resected retroperitoneal soft tissue sarcoma: histology-specific overall survival and disease-free survival nomograms built on major sarcoma center data sets. J Clin Oncol 2013;31:1649–55.

14. Dalal KM, Kattan MW, Antonescu CR, et al. Subtype specific prognostic nomogram for patients with primary liposarcoma of the retroperitoneum, extremity, or trunk. Ann Surg 2006;244:381–91.

15. Bonvalot S, Raut CP, Pollock RE, et al. Technical considerations in surgery for retroperitoneal sarcomas: position paper from E-Surge, a master class in sarcoma surgery, and EORTC-STBSG. Ann Surg Oncol 2012;19:2981–91.

16. Raut CP, Swallow CJ. Are radical compartmental resections for retroperitoneal sarcomas justified? Ann Surg Oncol 2010;17:1481–4.

17. Bonvalot S, Rivoire M, Castaing M, et al. Primary retroperitoneal sarcomas: a multivariate analysis of surgical factors associated with local control. J Clin Oncol 2009;27:31–7.

18. Singer S, Antonescu CR, Riedel E, et al. Histologic subtype and margin of resection predict pattern of recurrence and survival for retroperitoneal liposarcoma. Ann Surg 2003;238:358–70 [discussion: 70–1].

19. Lewis JJ, Leung D, Woodruff JM, et al. Retroperitoneal soft-tissue sarcoma: analysis of 500 patients treated and followed at a single institution. Ann Surg 1998; 228:355–65.

20. Kirane A, Crago AM. The importance of surgical margins in retroperitoneal sarcoma. J Surg Oncol 2016;113(3):270–6.

21. Smith HG, Panchalingam D, Hannay JA, et al. Outcome following resection of retroperitoneal sarcoma. Br J Surg 2015;102:1698–709.

22. Bonvalot S, Miceli R, Berselli M, et al. Aggressive surgery in retroperitoneal soft tissue sarcoma carried out at high-volume centers is safe and is associated with improved local control. Ann Surg Oncol 2010;17:1507–14.

23. Common Terminology Criteria for Adverse Events (CTCAE) v3.0. Available at: http://ctep.cancer.gov/protocolDevelopment/electronic_applications/docs/ctcaev3.pdf. Accessed May 30, 2016.

24. Available at: https://clinicaltrials.gov/ct2/show/NCT01344018. Accessed May 30, 2016.

25. Gronchi A, Miceli R, Allard MA, et al. Personalizing the approach to retroperitoneal soft tissue sarcoma: histology-specific patterns of failure and postrelapse outcome after primary extended resection. Ann Surg Oncol 2015;22:1447–54.

26. Smith MJ, Ridgway PF, Catton CN, et al. Combined management of retroperitoneal sarcoma with dose intensification radiotherapy and resection: long-term results of a prospective trial. Radiother Oncol 2014;110:165–71.

27. van Dalen T, Plooij JM, van Coevorden F, et al. Long-term prognosis of primary retroperitoneal soft tissue sarcoma. Eur J Surg Oncol 2007;33:234–8.

28. Grobmyer SR, Wilson JP, Apel B, et al. Recurrent retroperitoneal sarcoma: impact of biology and therapy on outcomes. J Am Coll Surg 2010;210:602–8, 8–10.

29. Toulmonde M, Bonvalot S, Meeus P, et al. Retroperitoneal sarcomas: patterns of care at diagnosis, prognostic factors and focus on main histological subtypes: a multicenter analysis of the French Sarcoma Group. Ann Oncol 2014;25:735–42.

30. Toulmonde M, Bonvalot S, Ray-Coquard I, et al. Retroperitoneal sarcomas: patterns of care in advanced stages, prognostic factors and focus on main histological subtypes: a multicenter analysis of the French Sarcoma Group. Ann Oncol 2014;25:730–4.

31. Gladdy RA, Qin LX, Moraco N, et al. Predictors of survival and recurrence in primary leiomyosarcoma. Ann Surg Oncol 2013;20:1851–7.

32. Brennan MF, Antonescu CR, Moraco N, et al. Lessons learned from the study of 10,000 patients with soft tissue sarcoma. Ann Surg 2014;260:416–21 [discussion: 21–2].

33. ESMO/European Sarcoma Network Working Group. Soft tissue and visceral sarcomas: ESMO Clinical Practice Guidelines for diagnosis, treatment and follow-up. Ann Oncol 2014;25(Suppl 3):iii102–12.

34. Wilkinson MJ, Martin JL, Khan AA, et al. Percutaneous core needle biopsy in retroperitoneal sarcomas does not influence local recurrence or overall survival. Ann Surg Oncol 2015;22:853–8.

35. Birkmeyer JD, Finlayson SR, Tosteson AN, et al. Effect of hospital volume on in-hospital mortality with pancreaticoduodenectomy. Surgery 1999;125:250–6.

36. Keung EZ, Hornick JL, Bertagnolli MM, et al. Predictors of outcomes in patients with primary retroperitoneal dedifferentiated liposarcoma undergoing surgery. J Am Coll Surg 2014;218:206–17.

37. Improving outcomes for people with sarcoma. 2014. Available at: http://www.nice.org.uk/guidance/csg9. Accessed May 30, 2016.

38. EVIDENCE-BASED SERIES #11–9: Multidisciplinary Specialist Care for Sarcoma. 2010. Available at: https://www.cancercare.on.ca/common/pages/UserFile.aspx?fileId=83391. Accessed May 30, 2016.

39. Gutierrez JC, Perez EA, Moffat FL, et al. Should soft tissue sarcomas be treated at high-volume centers? An analysis of 4205 patients. Ann Surg 2007;245:952–8.

40. Rosenberg SA, Tepper J, Glatstein E, et al. The treatment of soft-tissue sarcomas of the extremities: prospective randomized evaluations of (1) limb-sparing surgery plus radiation therapy compared with amputation and (2) the role of adjuvant chemotherapy. Ann Surg 1982;196:305–15.

41. Yang JC, Chang AE, Baker AR, et al. Randomized prospective study of the benefit of adjuvant radiation therapy in the treatment of soft tissue sarcomas of the extremity. J Clin Oncol 1998;16:197–203.

42. Pisters PW, Harrison LB, Leung DH, et al. Long-term results of a prospective randomized trial of adjuvant brachytherapy in soft tissue sarcoma. J Clin Oncol 1996;14:859–68.

43. Pawlik TM, Pisters PW, Mikula L, et al. Long-term results of two prospective trials of preoperative external beam radiotherapy for localized intermediate- or high-grade retroperitoneal soft tissue sarcoma. Ann Surg Oncol 2006;13:508–17.

44. Baldini EH, Wang D, Haas RL, et al. Treatment guidelines for preoperative radiation therapy for retroperitoneal sarcoma: preliminary consensus of an international expert panel. Int J Radiat Oncol Biol Phys 2015;92:602–12.

45. Gyorki DE, Brennan MF. Management of recurrent retroperitoneal sarcoma. J Surg Oncol 2014;109:53–9.

46. Tseng WW, Madewell JE, Wei W, et al. Locoregional disease patterns in well-differentiated and dedifferentiated retroperitoneal liposarcoma: implications for the extent of resection? Ann Surg Oncol 2014;21:2136–43.

47. Park JO, Qin LX, Prete FP, et al. Predicting outcome by growth rate of locally recurrent retroperitoneal liposarcoma: the one centimeter per month rule. Ann Surg 2009;250:977–82.

48. Yeh JJ, Singer S, Brennan MF, et al. Effectiveness of palliative procedures for intra-abdominal sarcomas. Ann Surg Oncol 2005;12:1084–9.

49. Billingsley KG, Burt ME, Jara E, et al. Pulmonary metastases from soft tissue sarcoma: analysis of patterns of diseases and postmetastasis survival. Ann Surg 1999;229:602–10 [discussion: 10–2].

50. Pawlik TM, Vauthey JN, Abdalla EK, et al. Results of a single-center experience with resection and ablation for sarcoma metastatic to the liver. Arch Surg 2006; 141:537–43 [discussion: 43–4].

51. DeMatteo RP, Shah A, Fong Y, et al. Results of hepatic resection for sarcoma metastatic to liver. Ann Surg 2001;234:540–7 [discussion: 7–8].

52. Gronchi A, Lo Vullo S, Fiore M, et al. Aggressive surgical policies in a retrospectively reviewed single-institution case series of retroperitoneal soft tissue sarcoma patients. J Clin Oncol 2009;27:24–30.

53. Pisters PW. Resection of some – but not all – clinically uninvolved adjacent viscera as part of surgery for retroperitoneal soft tissue sarcomas. J Clin Oncol 2009;27:6–8.

54. Gronchi A, Miceli R, Colombo C, et al. Frontline extended surgery is associated with improved survival in retroperitoneal low- to intermediate-grade soft tissue sarcomas. Ann Oncol 2012;23:1067–73.

55. Crago AM. Extended surgical resection and histology in retroperitoneal sarcoma. Ann Surg Oncol 2015;22:1401–3.

56. Stoeckle E, Coindre JM, Bonvalot S, et al. Prognostic factors in retroperitoneal sarcoma: a multivariate analysis of a series of 165 patients of the French Cancer Center Federation Sarcoma Group. Cancer 2001;92:359–68.

57. Catton CN, O'Sullivan B, Kotwall C, et al. Outcome and prognosis in retroperitoneal soft tissue sarcoma. Int J Radiat Oncol Biol Phys 1994;29:1005–10.
58. Kelly KJ, Yoon SS, Kuk D, et al. Comparison of perioperative radiation therapy and surgery versus surgery alone in 204 patients with primary retroperitoneal sarcoma: a retrospective 2-institution study. Ann Surg 2015;262:156–62.
59. Pervaiz N, Colterjohn N, Farrokhyar F, et al. A systematic meta-analysis of randomized controlled trials of adjuvant chemotherapy for localized resectable soft-tissue sarcoma. Cancer 2008;113:573–81.
60. Patrikidou A, Domont J, Cioffi A, et al. Treating soft tissue sarcomas with adjuvant chemotherapy. Curr Treat Options Oncol 2011;12:21–31.
61. Judson I, Verweij J, Gelderblom H, et al. Doxorubicin alone versus intensified doxorubicin plus ifosfamide for first-line treatment of advanced or metastatic soft-tissue sarcoma: a randomised controlled phase 3 trial. Lancet Oncol 2014; 15:415–23.
62. Demetri GD, von Mehren M, Jones RL, et al. Efficacy and safety of trabectedin or dacarbazine for metastatic liposarcoma or leiomyosarcoma after failure of conventional chemotherapy: results of a phase III randomized multicenter clinical trial. J Clin Oncol 2016;34(8):786–93.
63. Ducoulombier A, Cousin S, Kotecki N, et al. Gemcitabine-based chemotherapy in sarcomas: a systematic review of published trials. Crit Rev Oncol Hematol 2016; 98:73–80.
64. Davis AM, O'Sullivan B, Bell RS, et al. Function and health status outcomes in a randomized trial comparing preoperative and postoperative radiotherapy in extremity soft tissue sarcoma. J Clin Oncol 2002;20:4472–7.
65. Callegaro D, Miceli R, Brunelli C, et al. Long-term morbidity after multivisceral resection for retroperitoneal sarcoma. Br J Surg 2015;102:1079–87.
66. Phukan R, Herzog T, Boland PJ, et al. How Does the level of sacral resection for primary malignant bone tumors affect physical and mental health, pain, mobility, incontinence, and sexual function? Clin Orthop Relat Res 2016;474(3):687–96.
67. Davidge KM, Eskicioglu C, Lipa J, et al. Qualitative assessment of patient experiences following sacrectomy. J Surg Oncol 2010;101:447–50.

Sarcomas of the Breast with a Spotlight on Angiosarcoma and Cystosarcoma Phyllodes

Katherine Thornton, MD

KEYWORDS

• Sarcoma • Breast • Angiosarcoma • Cystosarcoma • Phyllodes

KEY POINTS

• Breast sarcomas are a distinct tumor group and should be treated differently than breast carcinomas.

• Angiosarcomas as a subgroup are aggressive neoplasms and one of the more common subgroups identified in breast sarcomas.

• Cystosarcoma phyllodes, often not included in sarcoma reviews, are a unique tumor group and should be approached in a similar fashion to breast sarcomas.

INTRODUCTION

Breast sarcomas are a diverse group of neoplasms arising from the nonepithelial components of the breast. Because of the heterogeneity of the histologic subtypes, it is always difficult to lump them into one overarching consensus review. They comprise less than 1% of breast cancer and less than 5% of all sarcomas.[1,2] Annual incidence has been estimated at approximately 45 new cases per 10 million women.[3] There is mounting concern that this will increase over time given the common use of adjuvant radiation for breast carcinoma. Despite the diversity of subtypes, it is important to separate breast sarcomas out as a unique tumor group in an effort to highlight the divergent clinical course from breast carcinoma and encourage the importance of referring patients to a multidisciplinary sarcoma team when logistically feasible.

SUBTYPES AND RISK FACTORS

By and large, all histologic subtypes of sarcoma have the possibility of arising in the breast. Some of the more common subtypes include undifferentiated pleomorphic

Disclosures: Novartis Speaker's Bureau, and Advisory role to Jannsen Pharmaceuticals.
Center for Sarcoma and Bone Oncology, Dana-Farber Cancer Institute, 450 Brookline Avenue, D2105, Boston, MA 02115, USA
E-mail address: katherinea_thornton@dfci.harvard.edu

high-grade sarcoma, myxofibrosarcoma, angiosarcoma, and spindle cell sarcoma. Other subtypes (leiomyosarcoma, Ewing, rhabdomyosarcoma, synovial sarcoma, chondrosarcoma, and extraosseous osteosarcoma) have also been reported in smaller case series or case reports; however, these are exceedingly rare.[4,5] In general, with the exception of cystosarcoma phyllodes and primary or secondary breast angiosarcoma, when encountering a soft tissue sarcoma in the breast, the first course of action should be to exclude the possibility of another primary source that has metastasized to the breast.[6]

The two most commonly described risk factors for breast sarcoma include radiation, typically as a treatment for a previous malignancy (ie, mantle radiation for Hodgkin disease or breast carcinoma) and lymphedema (Steward-Treves syndrome).[7] Cahan and colleagues[8] in 1948 defined the criteria for postradiation sarcoma. The requirements are (1) evidence of an initial distinct malignant tumor different from the subsequent sarcoma, (2) development of the second malignant tumor in an irradiated field, (3) long interval between irradiation and development of sarcoma, and (4) histological confirmation of sarcoma. Occupational exposure to vinyl chlorides has been linked to hepatic angiosarcoma,[9] and artificial breast implants have been implicated but are controversial.[10,11] TP53 mutation can predispose to sarcomas in general, with some occurring in the breast.[12] Despite the possible causes, most breast sarcomas present without any obvious predisposing factor.

Radiation-associated sarcomas of the breast can develop after a wide range of time intervals, with a cumulative incidence of 0.3% at 15 years after radiation treatment reported in a case series of patients diagnosed between 1973 and 1997.[13] Whether this will decrease over time with improvement in radiation techniques and with dose reductions, or conversely, increase, as radiation is used more frequently and operations become more conservative, remains to be seen. Various subtypes have been reported in postradiation breast sarcomas, but angiosarcoma seems to be one of the most common. The median time to occurrence after radiation ranges from 5 to 8 years with a wide range of 1 to 16 years reported.[13–15] The risk increases with higher dose of radiation, exposure during childhood, concurrent dose of chemotherapy, and preexisting genetic conditions, such as BRCA-1 mutation.[16–18]

DIAGNOSIS AND STAGING

Diagnosis of breast sarcomas is made histologically by a percutaneous biopsy. Core biopsy is generally preferred to fine-needle aspiration, which will typically yield insufficient material.[19] Punch biopsies may be sufficient for radiation-associated angiosarcoma, which is typically a cutaneous sarcoma. For local staging, breast mammography, ultrasound, and breast MRI are most commonly used. In mammography, microcalcifications are not seen as frequently as in breast carcinomas; therefore, MRI may be a better modality.[20]

The 10-year overall survival of breast sarcomas was 62% in one series[21]; the 5- and 10-year relapse-free survival was 47% and 42% in another series whereby patients did not have distant metastases at presentation.[22] It is difficult to lump such a heterogeneous tumor group together and derive any meaningful data with regard to overall survival. But in various retrospective case series and reports, characteristics like histology, margin status, size, depth of tumor, and grade seem to be the overall driving prognostic factors.[5,21,23,24]

TREATMENT

The treatment paradigm for breast sarcoma has mirrored that of its soft tissue counterparts with the main objective being surgical resection with wide margins. This treatment may require a mastectomy depending on the size and infiltration of the tumor; extent of surgery is histology dependent. Unlike breast carcinomas, lymph node metastasis is not common, with few notable exceptions, including epithelioid sarcomas and angiosarcomas. In a retrospective case series including 34 lymph node dissections for breast sarcomas, none were positive.[25] Conversely, in a series of 28 patients with breast angiosarcoma who underwent axillary lymph node dissection as part of their primary surgery, 2 (7%) had positive lymph nodes.[26,27]

Chemotherapy for breast sarcomas, similar to their extremity and retroperitoneal counterparts, has remained controversial. In locally advanced cases, neoadjuvant chemotherapy and/or radiation may be warranted to decrease tumor size and subsequently allow for a margin negative resection.[28] Caution should be advised, however, when using chemotherapy to try to reduce size to perform lumpectomy versus mastectomy. As responses to chemotherapy are highly variable, the risk of rendering a resectable patient unresectable is not negligible.[28] This risk is particularly troublesome given the close proximity to the chest wall. Invasion into the underlying muscle and bone may necessitate a more morbid surgery.[29]

The data supporting or refuting adjuvant chemotherapy in breast sarcoma are exceedingly controversial. Advocates supporting the use for adjuvant chemotherapy in soft tissue sarcoma (STS) have often turned towards the sarcoma meta-analyses, which compared adjuvant chemotherapy versus observation in resected localized STS. The more recent meta-analysis reviewing 18 phase III trials was an update on an earlier meta-analysis analyzing 14 trials. At the time of the initial publication, there did not seem to be an overall survival advantage. However, there was a significant improvement in time to local and distant recurrence and overall recurrence-free survival, with a trend toward improved overall survival.[30] Critics of the article centered on the lack of adequate dosing and the utilization of single-agent doxorubicin. The updated article incorporated 4 more eligible studies using ifosfamide, and the results this time suggested a statistically significant survival advantage. Whether this was due to a larger sample size, narrowing the confidence intervals, or dose intensification with use of multiagent regimens is unknown. The evidence was most significant in extremity sarcomas. However, caution is always advised when interpreting subgroup analyses in a meta-analysis.[31] A more recent, retrospective, single-institution study evaluating adjuvant chemotherapy over a 10-year period also found a benefit to adjuvant chemotherapy with a median disease-free survival of 29.6 months compared with 7.8 months and a median overall survival of 67.0 months versus 33.7 months in treated versus untreated patients.[32] Interpreting these data is always troublesome given the retrospective pooled data and the heterogeneity of tumor types involved. Retrospective data, heterogeneity of histologic sub-types, coupled with the dosing regimens used, makes relying on these data as support to use chemotherapy challenging.

More recently, Le Cesne and colleagues[33] published a pooled analysis of 2 STBSG (Soft Tissue and Bone Sarcoma Group)-European Organization for Research and Treatment of Cancer (EORTC) phase III clinical trials specifically evaluating the use of adjuvant chemotherapy in soft tissue sarcoma. The data were pooled with the intent of prospectively identifying whether there were any small patient subgroups deriving benefit from adjuvant chemotherapy, given the disparities in previous findings.[34,35] The investigators concluded that chemotherapy was not associated with a better overall survival in younger patients or in any histologic subgroup. The 2 consecutive EORTC studies are the largest adjuvant studies published to date. Both studies failed to demonstrate any advantage of adjuvant chemotherapy on overall survival. However, as has been the case with other adjuvant studies, there does seem to be an advantage to recurrence free survival (RFS).

The take-home message, once again, is that there seems to be no reliable take-home message. The EORTC data suggest, given no overall survival advantage, adjuvant chemotherapy should not be considered as standard of care. Counseling patients at high risk for recurrence regarding the variation of opinions and using adjuvant chemotherapy in the context of a clinical trial is advised.

TALE OF 2 BREAST SARCOMAS
Cystosarcoma Phyllodes

Phyllodes tumor is a rare neoplasm that accounts for 1% of all breast cancer in women.[36] Phyllodes tumors are often excluded from discussion of other breast sarcomas given the epithelial component that is present. However, given the similar clinical course and survival characteristics between the two entities, cystosarcoma phyllodes are included in this discussion.

The median age at presentation is typically the mid-40s.[36–38] The tumors are often large and can occasionally reach sizes of up to 40 cm in diameter. Rates of recurrence vary significantly depending on the series, with distant metastases occurring in a minority of patients, and generally occurring in those with borderline or malignant grading. Metastases to the lymph nodes in one institutional case series were observed in fewer than 5% of patients.[39] Johannes Müller initially described phyllodes tumors as cystosarcoma phyllodes in 1838.[40] The current World Health Organization (WHO) classification was established in 2003.[41] They are composed of biphasic stromal and glandular elements. The WHO classification distinguishes 3 histologic subtypes of phyllodes tumors: benign, borderline, and malignant, which account for 58.4% to 74.6%, 15.0% to 16.1%, and 9.3% to 31.0% of all phyllodes tumors, respectively.[39] The grading system is based on degree of stromal hypercellularity, mitoses, cytologic atypia, and degree of stromal overgrowth.[42]

The behavior of most benign phyllodes tumors is fairly indolent. Local recurrences can occur in approximately 10% to 17% of patients,[43] with metastases exceedingly rare. However, the more borderline and malignant variants carry a significant chance of metastases. Surgical resection remains the most important treatment, with tumor histology dictating whether excision, wide local excision, or mastectomy is favored.[43,44] All patients should be followed prospectively following primary treatment. Although benign phyllodes tumors have low metastasis potential, it is still possible; therefore, patients should be followed for local recurrence as well as distant surveillance. Malignant phyllodes should be followed similar to a high-grade sarcoma with chest imaging every 3 to 4 months for 2 years, every 6 months out to 5 years, and annually thereafter. Bone scan should be considered as case reports of bone-only metastases exist.[45]

In one large case series out of China, the researchers found that younger patients were more likely to develop local recurrence, with a median age of 33 years. Whether this was biology or extent of surgery was not commented on.[39] Despite the difference in local recurrence, there was not an age-related difference in distant metastasis and overall survival. Their findings suggest that in younger patients, discussions about wider local excisions or mastectomy should be performed. In other larger series, this correlation did not hold true.[46] Similar to other extended case series that found local recurrence rates ranging from 12.2% to 32.0%, 10% of patients developed distant metastases. However, of those that developed distant metastases, approximately 25% were classified as having malignant phyllodes at diagnosis.[39]

The most frequent site of metastases is soft tissue, followed by lungs, thoracic cavity, bones, and pleura. The thoracic cavity and soft tissue lesions likely arose from local recurrences into adjacent tissues. Margin status cannot be overemphasized. The National Comprehensive Cancer Network's "Breast Cancer" version 1.2016 (http://www.nccn.org) delineates a surgical margin of 1 cm as adequate.

As is the case with many other soft tissue sarcomas, there are varying opinions on whether adjuvant chemotherapy adds any benefit to breast sarcomas and in general is not recommended outside of a clinical trial.[44,46]

Unfortunately, large randomized prospective studies of radiation therapy in phyllodes tumors are lacking; therefore, there are no definitive guidelines. In general, in cases whereby adequate margins are difficult to obtain, and local recurrence would result in significant morbidity, radiation may be considered following the same guidelines applied to soft tissue sarcoma.[47,48]

Angiosarcoma

Angiosarcomas affecting the breast are typically divided into 2 broad categories: primary (arising de novo in the breast) and secondary (typically the after effect of prior breast irradiation). The so-called Stewart-Treves syndrome or angiosarcoma arising from prior lymphedema would occur usually in the upper arm as a result of lymph node dissections that were performed during radical mastectomies. With more conservative management of breast carcinoma, including breast conservation surgery and smaller radiation fields, one does not encounter Stewart-Treves syndrome as often.[15,49]

Angiosarcoma arising in the setting of prior radiation therapy mainly involves the skin, with or without local invasion of subjacent breast tissue.[50] As more patients undergo breast-conserving surgeries with the addition of adjuvant radiation, the incidence may be increasing. The prognosis of secondary breast angiosarcoma is dismal and seems to be independent of tumor grade.[7,51]

In a single-institution retrospective case series published by the Mayo clinic, the investigators found that, although secondary angiosarcoma and primary angiosarcoma occur in 2 distinct patient populations, their outcomes are similar. Most series report an overall survival of approximately 18 to 36 months. However, the Mayo patients had an overall median survival of 3 years. Although secondary angiosarcoma was more likely to be high grade in their review, the median tumor size and median survival were similar.[51]

In several case series of breast angiosarcomas, histologic grade seemed to play an important role. However, Nascimento and colleagues[49] noted that the tumors in their retrospective case series were evenly distributed among the 3 different histologic grades. Most were treated by mastectomy with only a minority of the patients receiving any form of adjuvant treatment. Although the rate of local recurrence was moderate, the rate of distant metastases was quite high, with approximately 60% of the patients developing metastatic disease. In contrast to older studies, there was no histologic grade correlation with patient outcomes.

D'Angelo and colleagues,[7] in a retrospective series evaluating clinical characteristics, prognostic factors, and treatment outcomes with surgery and chemotherapy in patients with radiation-associated angiosarcoma of the breast, found a median disease-specific survival (DSS) of 2.97 years. Their 1-, 2-, and 5-year DSS was 84%, 66%, and 47%, respectively, which was worse than other previously reported series. Not surprisingly, their study suggested age and depth were independent predictors of DSS, with tumors that invade the underlying muscularis layers behaving more aggressively. However, somewhat surprisingly, and contrary to an earlier retrospective case series by the MD Anderson group, they did not identify margin status as a predictor of local recurrence; instead only depth was associated. Regardless of the type of resection, the local recurrence rates tend to be high in all the series. The 1-year local RFS was 55% in the D'Angelo study. However, in a smaller study reported by Monroe and colleagues,[52] the 1-year local recurrence rate was 84%, though most of those patients did not undergo mastectomy.

In conclusion, the behavior of breast sarcomas can be as divergent as that of the more benign phyllodes tumors on one end of the spectrum and the more aggressive angiosarcoma on the other. Given the heterogeneity and rarity of the tumors, patients should be referred to centers with sarcoma multidisciplinary teams. Along with the clinical expertise found at such centers, it also allows for more standardization of data and the possibility of patients to be enrolled in clinical trials.

REFERENCES

1. Holm M, Aggerholm-Pedersen N, Mele M, et al. Primary breast sarcoma: a retrospective study over 35 years from a single institution. Acta Oncol 2016;55(5): 584–90.
2. Voutsadakis IA, Zaman K, Leyvraz S. Breast sarcomas: current and future perspectives. Breast 2011;20(3):199–204.
3. Sheth GR, Cranmer LD, Smith BD, et al. Radiation-induced sarcoma of the breast: a systematic review. Oncologist 2012;17(3):405–18.
4. Ogundiran TO, Ademola SA, Oluwatosin OM, et al. Primary osteogenic sarcoma of the breast. World J Surg Oncol 2006;4:90.
5. Adem C, Reynolds C, Ingle JN, et al. Primary breast sarcoma: clinicopathologic series from the Mayo Clinic and review of the literature. Br J Cancer 2004;91(2): 237–41.
6. Lim SZ, Ong KW, Tan BK, et al. Sarcoma of the breast: an update on a rare entity. J Clin Pathol 2016;69(5):373–81.
7. D'Angelo SP, Antonescu CR, Kuk D, et al. High-risk features in radiation-associated breast angiosarcomas. Br J Cancer 2013;109(9):2340–6.
8. Cahan WG, Woodard HQ, Higinbotham NL, et al. Sarcoma arising in irradiated bone; report of 11 cases. Cancer 1948;1(1):3–29.
9. McLaughlin JK, Lipworth L. A critical review of the epidemiologic literature on health effects of occupational exposure to vinyl chloride. J Epidemiol Biostat 1999;4(4):253–75.
10. Balzer BL, Weiss SW. Do biomaterials cause implant-associated mesenchymal tumors of the breast? Analysis of 8 new cases and review of the literature. Hum Pathol 2009;40(11):1564–70.
11. Brinton LA. The relationship of silicone breast implants and cancer at other sites. Plast Reconstr Surg 2007;120(7 Suppl 1):94S–102S.
12. Birch JM, Alston RD, McNally RJ, et al. Relative frequency and morphology of cancers in carriers of germline TP53 mutations. Oncogene 2001;20(34):4621–8.
13. Yap J, Chuba PJ, Thomas R, et al. Sarcoma as a second malignancy after treatment for breast cancer. Int J Radiat Oncol Biol Phys 2002;52(5):1231–7.
14. Kirova YM, Feuilhade F, Calitchi E, et al. Radiation-induced sarcoma after breast cancer. Apropos of 8 cases and review of the literature. Cancer Radiother 1998; 2(4):381–6 [in French].
15. Cozen W, Bernstein L, Wang F, et al. The risk of angiosarcoma following primary breast cancer. Br J Cancer 1999;81(3):532–6.
16. Karlsson P, Holmberg E, Samuelsson A, et al. Soft tissue sarcoma after treatment for breast cancer–a Swedish population-based study. Eur J Cancer 1998;34(13): 2068–75.

17. Rubino C, Shamsaldin A, Lê MG, et al. Radiation dose and risk of soft tissue and bone sarcoma after breast cancer treatment. Breast Cancer Res Treat 2005; 89(3):277–88.
18. Guibout C, Adjadj E, Rubino C, et al. Malignant breast tumors after radiotherapy for a first cancer during childhood. J Clin Oncol 2005;23(1):197–204.
19. Lum YW, Jacobs L. Primary breast sarcoma. Surg Clin North Am 2008;88(3): 559–70.
20. Yang WT, Hennessy BT, Dryden MJ, et al. Mammary angiosarcomas: imaging findings in 24 patients. Radiology 2007;242(3):725–34.
21. Zelek L, Llombart-Cussac A, Terrier P, et al. Prognostic factors in primary breast sarcomas: a series of patients with long-term follow-up. J Clin Oncol 2003;21(13): 2583–8.
22. McGowan TS, Cummings BJ, O'Sullivan B, et al. An analysis of 78 breast sarcoma patients without distant metastases at presentation. Int J Radiat Oncol Biol Phys 2000;46(2):383–90.
23. Fields RC, Aft RL, Gillanders WE, et al. Treatment and outcomes of patients with primary breast sarcoma. Am J Surg 2008;196(4):559–61.
24. Bousquet G, Confavreux C, Magné N, et al. Outcome and prognostic factors in breast sarcoma: a multicenter study from the rare cancer network. Radiother Oncol 2007;85(3):355–61.
25. Barrow BJ, Janjan NA, Gutman H, et al. Role of radiotherapy in sarcoma of the breast–a retrospective review of the M.D. Anderson experience. Radiother Oncol 1999;52(2):173–8.
26. Vorburger SA, Xing Y, Hunt KK, et al. Angiosarcoma of the breast. Cancer 2005; 104(12):2682–8.
27. Sher T, Hennessy BT, Valero V, et al. Primary angiosarcomas of the breast. Cancer 2007;110(1):173–8.
28. Reynoso D, Subbiah V, Trent JC, et al. Neoadjuvant treatment of soft-tissue sarcoma: a multimodality approach. J Surg Oncol 2010;101(4):327–33.
29. Quadros CA, Vasconcelos A, Andrade R, et al. Good outcome after neoadjuvant chemotherapy and extended surgical resection for a large radiation-induced high-grade breast sarcoma. Int Semin Surg Oncol 2006;3:18.
30. Tierney JF, Stewart LA, Parmar MKB. Adjuvant chemotherapy for localised resectable soft-tissue sarcoma of adults: meta-analysis of individual data. Sarcoma meta-analysis collaboration. Lancet 1997;350(9092):1647–54.
31. Pervaiz N, Colterjohn N, Farrokhyar F, et al. A systematic meta-analysis of randomized controlled trials of adjuvant chemotherapy for localized resectable soft-tissue sarcoma. Cancer 2008;113(3):573–81.
32. Brunello A, Rizzato MD, Rastrelli M, et al. Adjuvant chemotherapy for soft tissue sarcomas: a 10-year mono-institutional experience. J Cancer Res Clin Oncol 2016;142(3):679–85.
33. Le Cesne A, Ouali M, Leahy MG, et al. Doxorubicin-based adjuvant chemotherapy in soft tissue sarcoma: pooled analysis of two STBSG-EORTC phase III clinical trials. Ann Oncol 2014;25(12):2425–32.
34. Woll PJ, Reichardt P, Le Cesne A, et al. Adjuvant chemotherapy with doxorubicin, ifosfamide, and lenograstim for resected soft-tissue sarcoma (EORTC 62931): a multicentre randomised controlled trial. Lancet Oncol 2012;13(10):1045–54.
35. Bramwell V, Rouesse J, Steward W, et al. Adjuvant CYVADIC chemotherapy for adult soft tissue sarcoma–reduced local recurrence but no improvement in survival: a study of the European Organization for Research and Treatment of Cancer Soft Tissue and Bone Sarcoma Group. J Clin Oncol 1994;12(6):1137–49.

36. Guillot E, Couturaud B, Reyal F, et al. Management of phyllodes breast tumors. Breast J 2011;17(2):129–37.
37. Ben Hassouna J, Damak T, Gamoudi A, et al. Phyllodes tumors of the breast: a case series of 106 patients. Am J Surg 2006;192(2):141–7.
38. Kraemer B, Hoffmann J, Roehm C, et al. Cystosarcoma phyllodes of the breast: a rare diagnosis: case studies and review of literature. Arch Gynecol Obstet 2007; 276(6):649–53.
39. Wei J, Tan YT, Cai YC, et al. Predictive factors for the local recurrence and distant metastasis of phyllodes tumors of the breast: a retrospective analysis of 192 cases at a single center. Chin J Cancer 2014;33(10):492–500.
40. Lee BJ, Pack GT. Giant Intracanalicular myxoma of the breast: The so-called cystosarcoma phyllodes mammae of Johannes Muller. Annals of Surgery 1931;93(1): 250–68.
41. Reinfuss M, Mituś J, Smolak K, et al. Malignant phyllodes tumours of the breast. A clinical and pathological analysis of 55 cases. Eur J Cancer 1993;29A(9):1252–6.
42. Mishra SP, Tiwary SK, Mishra M, et al. Phyllodes tumor of breast: a review article. ISRN Surg 2013;2013:361469.
43. Tan BY, Acs G, Apple SK, et al. Phyllodes tumours of the breast: a consensus review. Histopathology 2016;68(1):5–21.
44. Chaney AW, Pollack A, McNeese MD, et al. Primary treatment of cystosarcoma phyllodes of the breast. Cancer 2000;89(7):1502–11.
45. El Ochi MR, Toreis M, Benchekroun M, et al. Bone metastasis from malignant phyllodes breast tumor: report of two cases. BMC Clin Pathol 2016;16:4.
46. Macdonald OK, Lee CM, Tward JD, et al. Malignant phyllodes tumor of the female breast: association of primary therapy with cause-specific survival from the Surveillance, Epidemiology, and End Results (SEER) program. Cancer 2006; 107(9):2127–33.
47. Khosravi-Shahi P. Management of non metastatic phyllodes tumors of the breast: review of the literature. Surg Oncol 2011;20(4):e143–8.
48. August DA, Kearney T. Cystosarcoma phyllodes: mastectomy, lumpectomy, or lumpectomy plus irradiation. Surg Oncol 2000;9(2):49–52.
49. Nascimento AF, Raut CP, Fletcher CD. Primary angiosarcoma of the breast: clinicopathologic analysis of 49 cases, suggesting that grade is not prognostic. Am J Surg Pathol 2008;32(12):1896–904.
50. Morgan EA, Kozono DE, Wang Q, et al. Cutaneous radiation-associated angiosarcoma of the breast: poor prognosis in a rare secondary malignancy. Ann Surg Oncol 2012;19(12):3801–8.
51. Scow JS, Reynolds CA, Degnim AC, et al. Primary and secondary angiosarcoma of the breast: the Mayo Clinic experience. J Surg Oncol 2010;101(5):401–7.
52. Monroe AT, Feigenberg SJ, Mendenhall NP. Angiosarcoma after breast-conserving therapy. Cancer 2003;97(8):1832–40.

Management of Sarcoma Metastases to the Lung

Christopher S. Digesu, MD[a], Ory Wiesel, MD[a],
Ara A. Vaporciyan, MD[b], Yolonda L. Colson, MD, PhD[a],*

KEYWORDS

- Sarcoma • Pulmonary metastasectomy • Thoracic surgery • Prognostic factors
- VATS • SBRT

KEY POINTS

- Sarcoma is a rare, heterogeneous disease with a common propensity to metastasize to the lungs.
- With careful patient selection, pulmonary metastasectomy improves survival when compared with historical controls.
- Many favorable prognostic factors have been identified, including long disease-free interval and complete (R0) resection.
- Video-assisted thoracoscopic surgery is increasingly used in highly select patients with favorable prognostic characteristics.
- Extensive resection for large or recurrent metastatic sarcomas can be safely performed in some patients.

INTRODUCTION

Sarcoma comprises a heterogeneous group of histologic subtypes with a propensity to metastasize to the lungs. Isolated pulmonary metastases occur in as many as 20% of patients diagnosed with soft tissue sarcoma and as many as 40% in those with a primary bone sarcoma.[1,2] Although historically pulmonary metastasis represented advanced disease and the need for palliation, surgical resection for control of disease burden has become a mainstay of therapy and a potentially curative option for those with resectable pulmonary metastasis. The role for surgery continues to evolve with the introduction of adjunctive therapies, including radiofrequency ablation; advanced

This work was supported with funding from the National Institutes of Health (R01EB017722-01A1, T32 CA009535).
[a] Division of Thoracic Surgery, Department of Surgery, Brigham and Women's Hospital, Harvard Medical School, 15 Francis Street, Boston, MA 02155, USA; [b] Division of Surgery, Department of Thoracic and Cardiovascular Surgery, The University of Texas MD Anderson Cancer Center, 1515 Holcombe Boulevard, Box 1489, Houston, TX 77030, USA
* Corresponding author.
E-mail address: ycolson@partners.org

radiation therapy, such as stereotactic body radiation therapy (SBRT); and complex salvage operations. These advances have driven the need for complex multidisciplinary care, particularly with the inclusion of a thoracic surgeon.[3] Resection of metastatic pulmonary sarcoma has been reported since the late 1800s; however, the first isolated resection of metastatic foci occurred in 1926 by Divis.[4] Despite this, there have been no published randomized controlled trials comparing surgery with systemic therapy or radiation for metastatic sarcoma, though significant research, particularly with the formation of the International Registry of Lung Metastases (IRLM), indicates that pulmonary metastasectomy (PM), when it can be performed, is associated with improved outcomes.[4,5]

Many of the original reports of PM for sarcoma were small case series pointing toward improved overall survival with resection in eligible patients when compared with historical controls. For example, one center noted a high incidence of patients with osteosarcoma developing lung metastases follow extremity amputation. A system for iterative complete surgical resection of pulmonary metastases in these patients was developed, with some patients requiring up to 9 thoracotomies. Five-year survival in this center's cohort significantly increased from 0% to 32%.[4,6]

The IRLM was formed in the 1990s as a consortium of high-volume centers performing PM for a variety of malignancies, including sarcoma. In a long-term follow-up study from the IRLM, 5206 patients underwent metastasectomy with 42% having sarcoma as the primary tumor. Most patients underwent open thoracotomy or sternotomy and had an overall survival of 31% at 5 years and 26% at 10 years. Patients with sarcoma, however, were more likely to recur (64%) as opposed to those with epithelial (46%) or germ cell (26%) metastases. Favorable outcomes were reported in those with a longer disease-free interval (DFI), small number of nodules, and complete resection.[5]

Guidelines for physicians and surgeons in the treatment of metastatic pulmonary sarcoma have been proposed dating back to Ehrenhaft and colleagues[7] in 1958; however, the lack of randomized controlled trials has limited their overall utility. Rusch and colleagues[8] concluded that patients should meet the following criteria: control of the primary tumor; ability to resect metastatic disease completely; ability of patients to tolerate pulmonary resection; absence of extrathoracic metastases; and absence of better alternative systemic therapies. The indications for resection of metastatic sarcoma to the lung continue to evolve as more studies examine the use of minimally invasive surgery, the utility of aggressive resections, and alternate therapies, such as SBRT.

In this article, the authors review the prognostic factors associated with improved survival following pulmonary metastasectomy for sarcoma, preoperative evaluation, surgical techniques and management, long-term follow-up, and the complex management of large tumors and recurrent disease.

PROGNOSTIC FACTORS

Although the primary source of sarcoma may be highly variable and includes both indolent and aggressive subtypes, several characteristics have been identified to inform patients' prognosis and treatment plan. It is again important to note that these characteristics have largely been identified based on single-center, retrospective reviews that, although generally consistent, may be subject to bias from the pathologic heterogeneity of sarcomas, multiple adjuvant therapies involved, and careful case selection by surgeons.[9] In addition, although the characteristics may be useful in guiding the surgeon as well as the rest of the multidisciplinary team, they do not preclude patients from undergoing PM, especially in those with limited disease. With this in mind, many of the prognostic factors characterized include the histology of the primary sarcoma, DFI, number of lesions in the lung, a surgeon's ability to obtain a complete resection, the responsiveness to chemotherapy, and lymph node status. A summary of recent articles examining some of these factors can be found in **Table 1**.

Histology

Nearly 100 different histologic subtypes of sarcoma with varying grades of differentiation have been identified.[10] Sarcoma is generally divided into the broad categories of soft tissue and primary bone with undifferentiated pleomorphic sarcoma and primary bone being the most likely to metastasize to the lung.[2,11] Among soft tissue sarcomas, undifferentiated pleomorphic sarcoma (formerly malignant fibrous histiocytoma) is the most common histology (25%), followed by leiomyosarcoma (18%), synovial sarcoma (10%), and liposarcoma (10%).[12] Similar to osteosarcoma, soft tissue sarcomas arising on the extremities are more likely to metastasize to the lung than those arising from the viscera.[13] There is also an increase in frequency of metastasis associated with increasing histologic grade.[14] Survival varies widely in accordance with the many different histologic subtypes. Blackmon and colleagues[15] demonstrated a median survival following resection for osteosarcoma, malignant fibrous histiocytoma, synovial sarcoma, and leiomyosarcoma as 28.9, 16.7, 30.2, and 41.8 months, respectively.

Disease-Free Interval

DFI is defined as the time from the treatment of the primary lesion to the development of pulmonary metastases. DFI has been a clear prognostic indicator for many years and in nearly all studies. The IRLM showed that patients (including all primary sources of tumor) with a DFI of 0 to 11 months had a median survival of 29 months as opposed to patients with a DFI greater than 36 months when the median survival is 49 months.[5] In a recent retrospective review of 120 patients with pulmonary metastases specifically from sarcoma, Dosset and colleagues[12] confirmed the results of the IRLM (**Fig. 1**).

Number of Metastatic Foci

Patients are at risk for developing multiple pulmonary lesions in the setting of metastatic sarcoma. Although several early studies demonstrated the number of metastatic lesions was inversely correlated with survival outcomes, larger studies, including a single-center study by Billingsley, did not show a significant difference in survival between patients with less than 4 lesions and those with greater than 4 lesions.[1,12,16] There is no universal consensus on what represents the maximum number of lesions, and likely the decision to proceed with surgery should be considered within the context of patients clinical status and whether a complete resection is possible.

Completeness of Resection

Complete (R0) resection of metastatic foci is associated with improved outcomes in most studies and is widely considered a requirement before proceeding with PM.[1,4,16,17] Early reports suggested a true R0 resection may only be obtainable in as many as 30% of patients with soft tissue sarcoma metastases; however, more advanced imaging and improved surveillance have likely resulted in resection of smaller lesions with fewer intraoperative surprises.[1] Although complete resection is the ultimate goal, treatment strategies are emerging that focus on complete control of disease. For instance, in a patient with multiple lesions some may be controlled with chemotherapy (no growth detected on serial imaging), whereas others may

page 724 Digesu et al

Table 1
Pulmonary metastasectomy for sarcoma: a select review of recent series dedicated to pulmonary metastasectomy for sarcoma from 2009 to 2015

Study	Sample Size	Histologic Subset[a]	OS	DFI	Completeness of Resection[b]	Preoperative chemotherapy	VATS (%)
Dossett et al,[12] 2015	120	• Undifferentiated pleomorphic (25%) • Osteosarcoma (18%) • Leiomyosarcoma (18%)	5-y survival: 44%	MOS <12 mo: 43 mo MOS >12 mo: 93 mo (P = .004)	R0 MOS: 29.6 mo R1/2 MOS: 6.3 mo (P = .002)	22%	63
Blackmon et al,[15] 2009	234	• Osteosarcoma (19.5%) • Leiomyosarcoma (17.5%) • MFH (14.1%)	5-y survival: 26%	N/A	N/A	100%	1.7
Smith et al,[17] 2009	94	• Leiomyosarcoma (22%) • Synovial sarcoma (18%) • MFH (16%)	5-y survival: 15%	MOS <25 mo: 13.5 mo MOS >25 mo: 32 mo (P = .001)	R0 MOS: 22 mo R1 MOS: 11.5 mo (P<.0001)	MOS yes: 12 mo MOS no: 16 mo (P = .2)	N/A
Gossot et al,[33] 2009	113	• Synovial sarcoma (21.7%) • MFH (20%) • Osteosarcoma (15%)	5-y survival: 52.5%	N/A	N/A	N/A	27.4
Reza et al,[60] 2014	145	• Leiomyosarcoma (24%) • Osteosarcoma (16%) • Synovial sarcoma (16%)	5-y survival: 42%	Mean DFI 30.4 ± 39.4 mo	5-y OS R0: 42%	77.1%	25.5
Kim et al,[61] 2011	97	• Osteosarcoma (17.5%) • MFH (15.4%) • Leiomyosarcoma (13.4%)	5-y survival: 50.1%	5-y OS <12 mo: 21% 5-y OS >12 mo: 65% (P<.0001)	5-y OS R0: 54% (P = .004)	N/A	18.6
Mizuno et al,[62] 2013	52	• Osteosarcoma (42%) • MFH (14%) • Liposarcoma (12%)	5-y survival: 50.9%	5-y OS <12 mo: 17.2% 5-y OS >12 mo: 38.3% (P = .003)	5-y OS R0: 54.2% (P<.001)	N/A	59
Garcia Franco et al,[2] 2010	52	• Osteosarcoma (59.6%) • Ewing sarcoma (23.1%) • Chondrosarcoma (3.8%)	5-y survival: 31%	5-y OS <20 mo: ~20% 5-y OS >20 mo: ~42% (P = .03)	N/A	N/A	19
Raciborska et al,[63] 2015	38	Ewing sarcoma (100%)	3-y survival: 60.7%	N/A	N/A	100%	0

Abbreviations: MFH, malignant fibrous histiocytoma; MOS, median overall survival; N/A, not available; OS, overall survival; VATS, video-assisted thoracoscopic surgery.
[a] Three most common histologic subtypes.
[b] R0 is equivalent to complete resection or negative margins.

Overall Survival at 12 Months DFI After Initial Resection

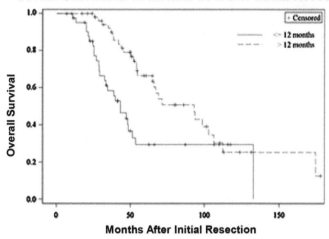

Fig. 1. Kaplan-Meier curve showing overall survival of patients PM from sarcoma stratified by DFI greater than 12 months or 12 months or less. (*From* Dossett LA, Toloza EM, Fontaine J, et al. Outcomes and clinical predictors of improved survival in a patient undergoing pulmonary metastasectomy for sarcoma. J Surg Oncol 2015;112(1):105; with permission.)

enlarge over time. In this case, the surgeon, in conjunction with a multidisciplinary team, may decide only to resect uncontrolled lesions, thus, saving healthy lung parenchyma. Similarly, strategies combining surgery and SBRT are being used, highlighting the importance of individualizing care to achieve control of disease.[18]

Response to Chemotherapy

Although the need for neoadjuvant chemotherapy is controversial, response to chemotherapy is generally a positive prognostic factor when considering PM, whereas progression on chemotherapy is associated with worse outcomes. Stephens and colleagues[19] examined patients who were started on chemotherapy after presentation with a synchronous metastasis, multiple pulmonary metastases, or short DFI. Patients with progression followed by PM (defined as an increase in size or number of nodules while on chemotherapy) had a 4-fold increased risk of death, and none were alive at 5 years.

PREOPERATIVE EVALUATION
Preoperative Imaging

Most patients with metastatic sarcoma initially present with an extrapulmonary primary tumor. Nearly a third of patients are discovered to have a synchronous pulmonary lesion at the time of presentation, and the rest are found to have pulmonary metastasis at a later date. Thus, surveillance chest imaging is routine for patients with sarcoma.[1] Computed tomography (CT) is the standard of care for staging of disease (for intermediate- or high-grade tumors) and for preoperative planning for metastatic sarcoma. High contrast between air in the lungs and soft tissue structures allows for detection of small pulmonary nodules. Metastatic foci typically appear as discrete soft tissue densities with smooth borders as opposed to the classic spiculated appearance of primary non–small cell lung cancer.[20] Osteosarcoma metastases may appear as benign calcified pulmonary nodules, though as many as 40% of osteosarcoma lesions are not calcified.[21] CT is more sensitive than F18-fluorodeoxyglucose PET (FDG-PET) imaging for sarcomas with only 44% of metastatic sarcoma demonstrating FDG avidity.[22] There is some evidence, however, that FDG-PET may be useful in detecting recurrence.[23]

Preoperative Pulmonary Testing

Many patients with metastatic sarcoma will develop recurrent disease; therefore, careful consideration of patients' preoperative pulmonary functional status must be undertaken. Among those enrolled in the IRLM, 20% of the 5206 patients underwent repeat resection and 5% underwent 3 or more procedures.[5] Assessment of the percent-predicted forced expiratory volume in the first second of expiration and diffusing capacity of the lungs for carbon monoxide (DLCO) in patients undergoing repeat resections for pulmonary metastases demonstrated a 10.8% and 9.7% loss, respectively, 3 months following surgery. The need for postresection chemotherapy or bilateral procedures was a predictor for worse lung function following metastasectomy.[24]

Timing of Surgery

The timing of surgery has been debatable as some surgeons take an aggressive approach with resection soon after identification of pulmonary metastases and others allow for a diagnostic interval between identification and resection. Allowing an interval between detection and PM may provide the surgeon with clues to the tumor doubling time as well as to whether patients will respond or progress while on chemotherapy.[19] For patients with few pulmonary lesions and a long DFI, the decision to proceed directly with PM is more clearly indicated, whereas patients with multiple new or rapidly growing metastases are less likely to gain benefit particularly if chemotherapy is not effective in preventing new lesions from appearing.[25]

SURGICAL TECHNIQUE AND MANAGEMENT
Open Technique

Early on, surgical therapy for sarcoma metastases was based on gaining adequate access and visualization in order to perform a complete resection, including removal of any occult or residual disease. Standard posterolateral thoracotomy provided excellent visualization and allowed the surgeon to examine the entire pleural surface.[26] Bilateral lesions, however, are not uncommon, with some surgeons performing either 2-staged thoracotomies or median sternotomy for access to the bilateral chest cavities, although sternotomy can be particularly difficult for access to the lower lobes or posterior hilum. Some surgeons may also perform a clamshell incision or bilateral anterior thoracotomy. In children, bilateral anterior thoracotomies provided adequate access to the lower lobes with similar perioperative outcomes to standard posterolateral thoracotomy.[27–29] Newer trends include limited skin incisions, particularly with video-assisted thoracoscopic surgery (VATS), and muscle-sparing approaches when open thoracotomy is performed.[26]

Video-Assisted Thoracoscopic Surgery

VATS was introduced in the early 1990s as a minimally invasive alternative to open thoracotomy. VATS has become an increasingly popular method for pulmonary resection given many studies indicating shorter hospital stays and decreased postoperative lengths of stay while reducing perioperative morbidity and mortality.[30,31] Given that the IRLM study reported a 16% increase in the number of metastatic nodules found at the time of resection, there was a significant concern that even more occult metastases would be missed in the absence of bimanual palpation.[5] Ellis and colleagues[32] demonstrated that when thoracotomy was performed, significantly more nodules were palpated and resected than were identified on preoperative CT (3.24 vs 2.12, P = .001). Furthermore, significantly more of these nodules were confirmed as malignant on final pathologic analysis (2.40 vs 1.60, P = .01). Some argue that missing these additional small nodules identified only by direct bimanual lung palpation may not be clinically relevant and may not have a significant impact on overall survival and recurrence-free survival. Gossot and colleagues[33] questioned the need for traditional open thoracotomy and aggressive initial resection, as many patients will relapse requiring reoperation and a repeat thoracotomy is often technically more difficult. On retrospective analysis of patients eligible for wedge resection with less than 2 small lesions (<30 mm), no significant difference was shown among patients undergoing VATS versus open thoracotomy in either 5-year overall survival (52.5% vs 34.0%, P = .2) or 3-year disease-free survival (26.4% vs 24.8%, P = .74). It is important to note that most of the 113 patients who received a thoracotomy were more likely to have larger lesions. This finding represents selection bias and highlights the careful selection of patients for thoracoscopy. With this in mind, several new studies (albeit with mixed tumor histologies) do support the increasing the use of VATS in select patients for pulmonary metastasectomy.[34–36] The controversy of open versus VATS resection for PM for sarcoma highlights the importance of careful patient selection and understanding disease behavior. The surgeon must balance the minimization of perioperative morbidity through the use of VATS with the risk of potentially inadequate access to often multiple and possibly deep nodules and, thus, failing to obtain a true R0 resection.

Extent of Resection

Although many studies have indicated better outcomes with complete resection and negative margins, there is little evidence that performing an anatomic resection (ie, segmentectomy or lobectomy) provides additional benefit as long as an R0 resection is achieved.[37] This circumstance is in contrast to primary lung cancer whereby a larger anatomic resection results in improved staging and a lower risk of recurrence.[38] Given the tendency of metastatic sarcoma to recur and, thus, the need for additional pulmonary resections, parenchyma-sparing approaches to preserve pulmonary reserve are critically important. For lesions that are technically challenging to remove via wedge resection because of lesion location, segmentectomy may offer an advantage for achieving an R0 resection while sparing lung parenchyma and maintaining adequate lung function.[37–39]

Lymph Node Sampling

Lymphadenectomy is not the standard of care of patients with pulmonary metastases as the significance of nodal involvement is unclear, and lymph node involvement is rare in sarcoma.[17,40] Lo Faso and colleagues[34] found nodal involvement in only 20% of patients, and involvement was not significantly associated with an overall difference in survival. In the only study in which a systematic mediastinal and hilar lymph node dissection was performed, Pfannschmidt and colleagues[41] found thoracic lymph node involvement in 20.3% of patients with sarcoma and an improved median survival for N0 patients (47.0 months for N0 and 18.3 months for N1, P = .036). Lymphadenectomy has not been studied in a prospective randomized study, and the additional dissection needed may increase the difficulty of subsequent resection.

ADJUNCTIVE THERAPIES
Whole Lung Irradiation

Whole-lung irradiation (WLI) is generally not performed in metastatic sarcoma with the exception of Ewing sarcoma, which is uniquely radiosensitive. WLI for Ewing sarcoma demonstrates improved survival and little short- and long-term toxicity.[42,43]

Radiofrequency Ablation

In one retrospective study, 29 patients with metastatic sarcoma to the lung underwent CT-guided radiofrequency ablation for treatment of a total of 47 pulmonary lesions. The 3-year survival rate was 65.2% (95% confidence interval 0.42–0.81) with a median disease-free survival of 7 months. Although no major complications were reported, 68.7% of patients did develop a pneumothorax from the procedure, with half requiring intervention.[44]

Stereotactic Body Radiation Therapy

SBRT is a short period of external high-dose, focused radiation therapy and is associated with minimal side effects.[45] Many sarcoma subtypes have traditionally been considered radioresistant; however, the emergence of SBRT is changing this paradigm with some evidence pointing toward a different radiobiology associated with the high-dose, hypofractionated SBRT.[46] In one center, SBRT was administered for the treatment of sarcoma metastases to the lung in cases of indolent or progressive disease, bilateral disease, multiple synchronous lesions, or in patients with contraindications to surgery. A significant response was recorded in 96% of patients, and no severe toxicity events were recorded.[47] Long-term results using SBRT for sarcoma metastases are lacking; however, several studies have shown a 5-year overall survival ranging from 50.0% to 60.5%.[47,48]

LONG-TERM FOLLOW-UP

Long-term survival for patients with soft tissue sarcoma following PM has been reported as low as 14%, though newer studies indicate that the 5-year overall survival for such patients is closer to 30% to 50%.[2,14,49,50] Although survival rates are improving with new therapeutic modalities, recurrence remains as high 83%.[12] Thus, long-term and likely lifelong follow-up and surveillance is a necessity, despite controversy as to the optimal follow-up interval and imaging modality for surveillance.[51] If recurrence is discovered, patients with recurrent pulmonary metastases have undergone repeat resection with favorable outcomes.[52] With the potential for long-term survival, the cost-effectiveness of pulmonary metastasectomy is substantial particularly when compared with chemotherapy alone ($14,357 per life-year gained for PM vs $104,210 for chemotherapy alone).[53]

COMPLEX MANAGEMENT

With only small case series reported, the decision to perform an extended or large resection for pulmonary metastases is challenging. The IRLM reported a 3% pneumonectomy rate, with these patients having the highest perioperative mortality rate.[5] Casiraghi and colleagues[54] studied the role of extended pulmonary metastasectomy in 29 patients (20.7% had metastatic sarcoma) in whom chest wall, diaphragm, extensive vascular resection and reconstruction, sleeve pulmonary resection, or pneumonectomy were performed. Extended resections were found to have acceptable 30-day morbidity and mortality (38% vs 0%, respectively). Mody and

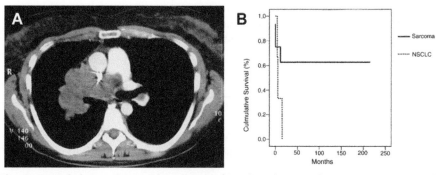

Fig. 2. Extended resections with support of cardiopulmonary bypass in patients with sarcoma. (*A*) Contrast chest CT of patient with leiomyosarcoma invading pulmonary arteries. (*B*) Survival following extensive resection of sarcoma versus non–small cell lung cancer (NSCLC) on cardiopulmonary bypass. (*From* Wiebe K, Baraki H, Macchiarini P, et al. Extended pulmonary resection of advanced thoracic malignancies with support of cardiopulmonary bypass. Eur J Cardiothorac Surg 2006;29(4):572–5; with permission.)

colleagues[55] reported on a large case series of extended resection for tumor invading the thoracic spine and requiring vertebrectomy. Sarcoma was present in 9 of the 32 cases with 82% achieving an R0 resection.

In a systemic review, Migliore and colleagues[56] summarized the current studies done for extended resection of pulmonary metastasis, specifically pneumonectomy or completion pneumonectomy, confirming it is feasible and justified in select cases (large tumor yet amenable to complete resection, long DFI, and so forth). Furthermore, using an aggressive approach to resect all metastases present (irrespective of the number of metastases and including repeat resections for all recurrences) resulted in a 5-year survival ranging from 19% to 52%. Advanced tumors with invasion into the mediastinum affecting the heart and greater vessels have also been resected; despite requiring cardiopulmonary bypass, favorable outcomes have been reported, which are surprisingly superior to those obtained with extended resections for non–small cell lung cancer (**Fig. 2**).[57]

NOVEL THERAPY-ISOLATED LUNG PERFUSION

Den Hengst and colleagues[58] recently reported the results of a phase II clinical trial of pulmonary metastasectomy with isolated lung perfusion (ILuP) using melphalan, an alkylating chemotherapeutic agent. The investigators studied 20 patients with sarcoma metastasis and showed an improved local pulmonary control without mortality and with comparable morbidity with historical PM. Follow-up from the initial phase I study using melphalan ILuP demonstrated an overall survival of 54.8% with no long-term pulmonary toxicity.[59]

SUMMARY

Although sarcoma is a relatively rare disease, pulmonary metastases are a common occurrence among those with sarcoma. Treatment requires a multidisciplinary approach that typically involves the medical oncologist and thoracic surgeon. Despite an absence of randomized data, evidence exists in support of the surgical resection of metastatic sarcoma to the lung parenchyma, specifically in patients with favorable prognostic factors. Long-term results have demonstrated improved survival when compared with historical controls, though recurrence is common and lifelong surveillance is required. With evolving indications for surgery and new adjunctive therapies, the overall treatment of pulmonary metastases from sarcoma continues to improve.

REFERENCES

1. Billingsley KG, Burt ME, Jara E, et al. Pulmonary metastases from soft tissue sarcoma analysis of patterns of disease and postmetastasis survival. Ann Surg 1999;229(5):602–12.
2. Garcia Franco CE, Torre W, Tamura A, et al. Long-term results after resection for bone sarcoma pulmonary metastases. Eur J Cardiothorac Surg 2010;37(5): 1205–8.
3. National Institute for Health and Care Excellence (NICE). Guidance on cancer services. Improving outcomes for people with sarcoma. The manual. The National Institute for Health and Care Excellence (NICE); 2006. Available at: https://www. nice.org.uk/guidance/csg9.
4. Pastorino U. History of the surgical management of pulmonary metastases and development of the international registry. Semin Thorac Cardiovasc Surg 2002; 14(1):18–28.
5. Pastorino U, Buyse M, Friedel G, et al. Long-term results of lung metastasectomy: prognostic analyses based on 5206 cases. J Thorac Cardiovasc Surg 1997; 113(1):37–9.
6. Beattie EJ, Harvey JC, Marcove, et al. Results of multiple pulmonary resections for metastatic osteogneic sarcoma after two decades. J Surg Oncol 1991; 46(3):154–5.
7. Ehrenhaft JL, Lawrence MS, Sensenig DM. Pulmonary resection for metastatic lesions. AMA Arch Surg 1958;77(4):606–12.
8. Rusch VW. Pulmonary metastasectomy current indications. Chest 1995;107(6 Suppl):322S–31S.
9. Treasure T, Macbeth F. Doubt about effectiveness of lung metastasectomy for sarcoma. J Thorac Cardiovasc Surg 2015;149(1):93–4.
10. Fletcher CM, Bridge JA, Mertens F. World Health Organization classification of tumours of soft tissue and bone. 4th edition. Lyon (France): IARC Press; 2013.
11. Kager L, Zoubek A, Potschger U, et al. Primary metastatic osteosarcoma: presentation and outcome of patients treated on neoadjuvant Cooperative Osteosarcoma Study Group protocols. J Clin Oncol 2003;21:2011–8.
12. Dossett LA, Toloza EM, Fontaine J, et al. Outcomes and clinical predictors of improved survival in a patient undergoing pulmonary metastasectomy for sarcoma. J Surg Oncol 2015;112(1):103–6.
13. Gadd MA, Casper ES, Woodruff JM, et al. Development and treatment of pulmonary metastases in adult patients with extremity soft tissue sarcoma. Ann Surg 1993;218:705–12.
14. Temple LK, Brennan MF. The role of pulmonary metastasectomy in soft tissue sarcoma. Semin Thorac Cardiovasc Surg 2002;14(1):35–44.
15. Blackmon SH, Shah N, Roth JA, et al. Resection of pulmonary and extrapulmonary sarcomatous metastases is associated with long-term survival. Ann Thorac Surg 2009;88(3):877–84.
16. Casiraghi M, De Pas T, Maisonneuve P, et al. A 10-year single-center experience on 708 lung metastasectomies: the evidence of the "International Registry of Lung Metastases". J Thorac Oncol 2011;6(8):1373–8.

17. Smith R, Pak Y, Kraybill W, et al. Factors associated with actual long-term survival following soft tissue sarcoma pulmonary metastasectomy. Eur J Surg Oncol 2009; 35(4):356–61.

18. Frakulli R, Salvi F, Balestrini D, et al. Stereotactic radiotherapy in the treatment of lung metastases from bone and soft-tissue sarcoma. Anticancer Res 2015; 35(10):5581–6.

19. Stephens EH, Blackmon SH, Correa AM, et al. Progression after chemotherapy is a novel predictor of poor outcomes after pulmonary metastasectomy in sarcoma patients. J Am Coll Surg 2011;212(5):821–6.

20. Klippenstein DL, Lamonica DM. Preoperative imaging for metastasectomy. Surg Oncol Clin N Am 2007;16(3):471–92.

21. Ciccarese F, Bazzocchi A, Ciminari R, et al. The many faces of pulmonary metastases of osteosarcoma: retrospective study of 283 lesions submitted to surgery. Eur J Radiol 2015;84(12):2679–85.

22. Johnson GR, Zhuang H, Khan J, et al. Roles of positron emission tomography with fluorine-18-deoxyglucose in the detection of local recurrent and distant metastatic sarcoma. Clin Nucl Med 2003;28(10):815–20.

23. Fortes DL, Allen MS, Lowe VJ, et al. The sensitivity of 18F-fluorodeoxyglucose positron emission tomography in the evaluation of metastatic pulmonary nodules. Eur J Cardiothorac Surg 2008;34(6):1223–7.

24. Welter S, Cheufou D, Ketscher C, et al. Risk factors for impaired lung function after pulmonary metastasectomy: a prospective observational study of 117 cases. Eur J Cardiothorac Surg 2012;42:e22–7.

25. Kruger M, Schmitto JD, Wiegmann B, et al. Optimal timing of pulmonary metastasectomy – Is a delayed operation beneficial or counterproductive? Eur J Surg Oncol 2014;40(9):1049–55.

26. Pastorino U, Valente M, Muscolino G, et al. Muscle-sparing antero-lateral thoracotomy for pulmonary or mediastinal resection. In: Motta G, editor. Lung Cancer. Frontiers in science and treatment. Genova (Italy): Grafica LP; 1994. p. 337–41.

27. Abbo O, Guatta R, Pinnagoda K, et al. Bilateral anterior sternothoracotomy (clemshell incision): a suitable alternative for bilateral lung sarcoma metastasis in children. World J Surg Oncol 2014;12:233.

28. Zarroug AE, Hamner CE, Pham TH, et al. Bilateral staged versus bilateral simultaneous thoracotomy in the pediatric population. J Pediatr Surg 2006;41:647–51.

29. Kaifi JT, Gusani NJ, Deshaies I, et al. Indications and approach to surgical resection of lung metastases. J Surg Oncol 2010;102(2):187–95.

30. Kirby TJ, Mack MJ, Landreneau RJ, et al. Lobectomy-video assisted thoracic surgery versus muscle-sparing thoracotomy. A randomized trial. J Thorac Cardiovasc Surg 1995;109(5):997–1001.

31. Falcoz PE, Puyraveau M, Thomas PA, et al. Video-assisted thoracoscopy surgery versus open lobectomy for primary non-small-cell lung cancer: a propensity-matched analysis of outcome from the European Society of Thoracic Surgeon database. Eur J Cardiothorac Surg 2016;49(2):602–9.

32. Ellis MC, Hessman CJ, Weerasinghe R, et al. Comparison of pulmonary nodule detection rates between preoperative CT imaging and intraoperative lung palpation. Am J Surg 2011;201(5):619–22.

33. Gossot D, Radu C, Girard P, et al. Resection of pulmonary metastases from sarcoma: can some patients benefit from a less invasive approach? Ann Thorac Surg 2009;87(1):238–43.

34. Lo Faso F, Solaini L, Rosalba L, et al. Thoracoscopic lung metastasectomies: a 10-year, single-center experience. Surg Endosc 2013;27:1938–44.

35. Carballo M, Maish MS, Jaroszewski DE, et al. Video-assisted thoracic surgery (VATS) as a safe alternative for the resection of pulmonary metastases: a retrospective cohort study. J Cardiothorac Surg 2009;4:13.

36. Cheang MY, Herle P, Pradhan N, et al. Video-assisted thoracoscopic surgery versus open thoracotomy for pulmonary metastasectomy: a systematic review. ANZ J Surg 2015;85(6):408–13.

37. Berry MF. Role of segmentectomy for pulmonary metastases. Ann Cardiothorac Surg 2014;3(2):176–82.

38. Keenan RJ, Landreneau RJ, Maley RH Jr, et al. Segmental resection spares pulmonary function in patients with stage I lung cancer. Ann Thorac Surg 2004; 78:228–33.

39. Leshnower BG, Miller DL, Fernandez FG, et al. Video-assisted thoracoscopic surgery segmentectomy: a safe and effective procedure. Ann Thorac Surg 2010;89:1571–6.

40. Fong Y, Coit DG, Woodruff JM, et al. Lymph node metastasis from soft tissue sarcoma in adults. Analysis of data from a prospective database of 1772 sarcoma patients. Ann Surg 1993;217(1):72–7.

41. Pfannschmidt J, Klode J, Muley T, et al. Nodal involvement at the time of pulmonary metastasectomy: experiences in 245 patients. Ann Thorac Surg 2006;81(2): 448–54.

42. Paulussen M, Ahrens S, Burdach S, et al. Primary metastatic (stage IV) Ewing tumor: survival analysis of 171 patients from the EICESS studies. European Intergroup Cooperative Ewing Sarcoma Studies. Ann Oncol 1998;9:275–81.

43. Casey DL, Alektiar KM, Gerber NK, et al. Whole lung irradiation for adults with pulmonary metastases from Ewing sarcoma. Int J Radiat Oncol Biol Phys 2014; 89(5):1069–75.

44. Palussiere J, Italiano A, Descat E, et al. Sarcoma lung metastases treated with percutaneous radiofrequency ablation: results from 29 patients. Ann Surg Oncol 2011;18:3771–7.

45. Rusthoven KE, Kavanagh BD, Burri SH, et al. Multi-institutional phase I/II trial of stereotactic body radiation therapy for lung metastases. J Clin Oncol 2009; 27(10):1579–84.

46. Brown JM, Carlson DJ, Brenner DJ. The tumor radiobiology of SRS and SBRT: are more than the 5 Rs involved? Int J Radiat Oncol Biol Phys 2014;88:254–62.

47. Navarria P, Ascolese AM, Cozzi L. Stereotactic body radiation therapy for lung metastases from soft tissue sarcoma. Eur J Cancer 2015;51(5):668–74.

48. Soyfer V, Corn BW, Shtraus N, et al. Single-institution experience of SBRT for lung metastases in sarcoma patients. Am J Clin Oncol 2014. [Epub ahead of print].

49. Predina JD, Puc MM, Bergey MR, et al. Improved survival after pulmonary metastasectomy for soft tissue sarcoma. J Thorac Oncol 2011;6(5):913–9.

50. van Geel AN, Pastorino U, Jauch KW, et al. Surgical treatment of lung metastases: the European Organization for Research and Treatment of Cancer-Soft Tissue and Bone Sarcoma Group study of 255 patients. Cancer 1996;77(4): 675–82.

51. Lord HK, Salter DM, MacDougall RH, et al. Is routine chest radiography a useful test in the follow up of all adult patients with soft tissue sarcoma? Br J Radiol 2006;79(946):799–800.

52. Toussi MS, Bagheri R, Dayani M, et al. Pulmonary metastasectomy and repeat metastesectomy for soft-tissue sarcoma. Asian Cardiovasc Thorac Ann 2013; 21(4):437–42.
53. Porter GA, Cantor SB, Walsh GL, et al. Cost-effectiveness of pulmonary resection and systemic chemotherapy in the management of metastic soft tissue sarcoma: a combined analysis from the University of Texas M.D. Anderson and Memorial Sloan-Kettering Cancer Centers. J Thorac Cardiovasc Surg 2004;127(5): 1366–72.
54. Casiraghi M, Maisonneuve P, Brambilla D, et al. The role of extended pulmonary metastasectomy. J Thorac Oncol 2015;10(6):924–9.
55. Mody GN, Bravo Iniguez C, Armstrong K, et al. Early surgical outcomes of en bloc resection requiring vertebrectomy for malignancy invading the thoracic spine. Ann Thorac Surg 2016;101(1):231–7.
56. Migliore M, Jakovic R, Hensens A, et al. Extending surgery for pulmonary metastasectomy: what are the limits? J Thorac Oncol 2010;5(6 Suppl 2):S155–60.
57. Wiebe K, Baraki H, Macchiarini P, et al. Extended pulmonary resection of advanced thoracic malignancies with support of cardiopulmonary bypass. Eur J Cardiothorac Surg 2006;29(4):571–7.
58. den Hengst WA, Hendriks JM, Balduyck B, et al. Phase II multicenter clinical trial of pulmonary metastasectomy and isolated lung perfusion with melphalan in patients with resectable lung metastases. J Thorac Oncol 2014;9(10):1547–53.
59. den Hengst WA, Van Putte BP, Hendriks JM, et al. Long-term survival of a phase I clinical trial of isolated lung perfusion with melphalan for resectable lung metastases. Eur J Cardiothorac Surg 2010;38(5):621–7.
60. Reza J, Sammann A, Jin C, et al. Aggressive and minimally invasive surgery for pulmonary metastasis of sarcoma. J Thorac Cardiovasc Surg 2014;147(4): 1193–200.
61. Kim S, Ott HC, Wright CD, et al. Pulmonary resection of metastatic sarcoma: prognostic factors associated with improved outcomes. Ann Thorac Surg 2011; 92(5):1780–6.
62. Mizuno T, Taniguchi T, Ishikawa Y, et al. Pulmonary metastasectomy for osteogenic and soft tissue sarcoma: who really benefits from surgical treatment? Eur J Cardiothorac Surg 2013;43(4):795–9.
63. Raciborska A, Bilska K, Rychlowska-Pruszynska M, et al. Management and follow-up of Ewing sarcoma patients with isolated lung metastases. J Pediatr Surg 2015. [Epub ahead of print].

Combined Therapy of Gastrointestinal Stromal Tumors

Piotr Rutkowski, MD, PhD[a],*, Daphne Hompes, MD, PhD[b]

KEYWORDS

- Gastrointestinal stromal tumor • Neoadjuvant therapy • Adjuvant therapy • Imatinib
- Surgery

KEY POINTS

- Preoperative (neoadjuvant) therapy in locally advanced GIST may facilitate resection with microscopically clear margins, decrease the risk of perioperative tumor spill, and decrease extent and morbidity of the surgical procedure.
- Existing evidence-based clinical practice guidelines suggest adjuvant imatinib for at least 36 months for patients with high-risk GIST (tumor >5 cm in size with high mitotic rate [>5 mitoses/50 high-power fields] or tumor rupture or a risk of recurrence that is >50%).
- Surgical removal of residual disease during imatinib treatment may allow for complete remission (in approximately 20%) in selected patients with GIST after response to therapy, probably prolonging durable remission.
- The time of the implementation of surgical treatment warrants further studies; mutilating surgery in metastatic GIST should be avoided, as systemic therapy is the mainstay of treatment in this setting and surgery is only adjunctive to tyrosine kinase inhibitors therapy.

INTRODUCTION: GASTROINTESTINAL STROMAL TUMORS GENERAL OVERVIEW

Gastrointestinal stromal tumors (GIST) are the most common mesenchymal neoplasms of the gastrointestinal tract. Morphologically and clinically they are a heterogeneous group of tumors, with a biological behavior that is difficult to predict, ranging from clinically benign to malignant. Radical surgery is the treatment of choice in primary resectable GIST. Nevertheless, approximately 40% to 50% of patients will develop recurrent or metastatic disease after curative resection.[1–4] Understanding

Disclosure: P. Rutkowski has received honoraria from Novartis and Pfizer, and served as a member of Advisory Board for Novartis and Bayer. D. Hompes has nothing to disclose.
[a] Department of Soft Tissue, Bone Sarcoma and Melanoma, Maria Sklodowska-Curie Memorial Cancer Center, Institute of Oncology, Roentgena 5, Warsaw 02-781, Poland; [b] Department of Surgical Oncology, University Hospitals Gasthuisberg Leuven, Herestraat 49, Leuven 3000, Belgium
* Corresponding author.
E-mail address: piotr.rutkowski@coi.pl

the molecular mechanisms of their pathogenesis demonstrated that most GISTs are associated with activating, constitutive, mutually exclusive mutations of 2 genes: *KIT* and *PDGFRA* (platelet-derived growth factor receptor-α). These are the early oncogenic events during GIST development and result in overexpression and activation of oncoproteins KIT and PDGFR.[2,5–8] A significant subset of GIST is still diagnosed at a locally advanced, unresectable and/or disseminated stage of disease. Metastases preferably occur in the peritoneal cavity and/or the liver.[3,5] Conventional cytotoxic chemotherapy treatment is ineffective in advanced cases of GIST. Radiotherapy is also of limited value in the management of GIST, mainly because these tumors are often located in close proximity with dose-limiting vital organs.[3,5] However, advances in the understanding of molecular mechanisms of GIST pathogenesis have recently resulted in the development of a treatment modality that has become a model of targeted therapy in oncology. Imatinib mesylate is a tyrosine kinase inhibitor of KIT, BRC/ABL fusion protein, FMS (receptor for colony stimulating factor 1), Abl-related gene, and PDGFR-alpha and PDGFR-beta. It has revolutionized the treatment of advanced GIST and was the first effective nonsurgical treatment in inoperable and/or metastatic cases.[1,2,5–8] Current survival in advanced GIST is strikingly superior to historical clinical data, with a reported median overall survival (OS) of 5 to 6 years[4,9] and median progression-free survival (PFS) ranging from 2 to 3 years.[10–13] In case of progression during imatinib treatment (which is mainly related to occurrence of new secondary *KIT/PDGFRA* mutations) there are currently several therapeutic strategies, such as escalation of the dose of imatinib to 800 mg daily, surgical removal of focally progressive lesions, and therapy with registered second-line drug sunitinib malate and third-line drug regorafenib (both are multitargeted tyrosine kinase inhibitors with anti-angiogenic properties).[14–18] Recently, imatinib has been registered for adjuvant therapy in patients after resection of primary GIST with high risk of recurrence based on the results of 2 randomized trials (ACOSOG Z9001 and Scandinavian Sarcoma Group XVIII = SSGXVIII/AIO).[19,20] Currently in selected cases of locally advanced GISTs, a strategy of neoadjuvant imatinib therapy has become a common approach.

In this review article we have focused on the evolving role of combined therapy with surgery and tyrosine kinase inhibitors in GIST management.

RISK ASSESSMENT OF PRIMARY GASTROINTESTINAL STROMAL TUMORS

The treatment of choice in primary, resectable, localized GISTs is radical surgery with negative margins, but virtually all GISTs are associated with a risk of recurrence, and approximately 40% of patients with potentially curative resections will ultimately develop recurrent or metastatic disease.[2–4] The identification of the risk factors for recurrence after primary surgery is crucial for reliable prognosis, follow-up schedule, and the selection of patients who may potentially benefit from the adjuvant therapy, aiming for a decrease in disease recurrences. The main criteria of aggressive behavior of GISTs are based on the presence of invasion of adjacent structures and/or the presence of metastases (overtly malignant cases), as well as on primary tumor site, size, and mitotic index.[21] Several risk-stratification systems have been proposed in the recent years. In 2001, a Consensus Conference held at the National Institutes of Health (NIH) provided the first evidence-based definition and a practical scheme for the risk assessment in the clinical course of this disease. The risk categorization was based on evaluation of the tumor size and mitotic rate (evaluated per 50 high-powered fields [HPF] or mm^2) as the most reliable prognostic factors.[22–24] Additional analysis in patients with primary tumor after complete macroscopic resection confirmed the significance of tumor anatomic location as the independent prognostic factor. Miettinen and Lasota created the classification for risk assessment in gastric, duodenal, intestinal, and rectal GISTs (National Comprehensive Cancer Network-American Forces Institute of Pathology [NCCN-AFPI]),[2,21,25–28] which constituted the basis for new staging system of American Joint Committee on Cancer (**Table 1**).[29,30] It combines 3 crucial features (ie, size, site of origin, and mitotic index) and it reflects the fact that gastric GISTs show a much lower rate of aggressive behavior than jejunal and ileal GISTs of comparable size and/or mitotic rate.[21,27,28] Recently it was established that tumor rupture (spontaneous or iatrogenic) is an additional important risk factor strongly associated with the increased recurrence rates.[4,31] Therefore, in 2008 Joensuu and colleagues[32–34] proposed another simplified classification system based on 4 prognostic factors (tumor size, site, mitotic count, and the presence of tumor rupture). Furthermore, completeness of resection is an independent prognostic risk factor; rather obviously patients with resectable primary GIST who undergo R0 resection have a significantly longer survival than patients undergoing incomplete resection.[4,35,36]

Taking into account that some of prognostic features (such as mitotic index and tumor size) are continuous (not categorical) variables, prognostic nomograms for prediction of tumor were developed.[37–39] Joensuu and colleagues'[32] prognostic contour maps resulting from nonlinear modeling may be appropriate for estimation of individualized outcomes. The comparison of different classification systems shows that patients with intermediate risk have a clinical course more similar to the low-risk group, which implies that only the high-risk patients would likely benefit from adjuvant therapy after primary tumor resection.[32]

In addition to the clinicopathological factors mentioned previously, *KIT* and *PDGFRA* mutational status may also have a prognostic significance in primary GIST. However, currently available data are insufficient to incorporate the kinase mutation status into the risk stratification of primary tumors. Several studies have indicated a more favorable prognosis for patients carrying exon 11 point mutations or insertions, as well as *PDGFRA* exon 18 mutations, whereas tumors harboring *KIT* exon 9 duplications as well as *KIT* exon 11 deletions (especially involving codons 557 and/or 558 or in homozygous state) were associated with more aggressive behavior.[40–47] Recent analysis of clinicopathologic and molecular data from 1056 patients with localized GIST who underwent surgery with curative intention (R0/R1) and were registered in the European Contica GIST database confirmed the independent prognostic significance of the *KIT* deletions involving codons 557 and/or 558, especially in GIST of gastric origin.[24] Population-based series of patients with primary

Table 1
Relevant risk parameters for primary gastrointestinal stromal tumor including molecular data

Parameters	Lower Risk	Higher Risk
Surgery	R0	R1, tumor rupture
Localization	Stomach	Small or large intestine
Size (cm)	≤5	>5
Mitotic index	≤5/50 HPF	>5/50 HPF
Gene mutation	PDGFRA	KIT, wild-type (nn-PDGFRA, non-KIT)
Type of *KIT* mutation	Duplications/insertions in exon 11	Exon 11 deletions (especially involving codons 557–558), exon 9

Abbreviations: HPF, high-power field; PDGFRA, platelet-derived growth factor receptor-α.

resectable GIST confirmed more favorable outcomes of PDGFRA mutations and KIT exon 11 duplication mutations or deletions of 1 codon.[48] Further developments in molecular analysis (such as inclusion genomic index) may further optimize the individual risk assessment and inclusion criteria for adjuvant therapy after primary tumor resection.[49]

PRIMARY LOCALIZED GASTROINTESTINAL STROMAL TUMORS
Neoadjuvant Strategy

Locally advanced GISTs are defined as those tumors that can potentially benefit from neoadjuvant treatment with imatinib through a decrease in size and vulnerability. If the tumor is localized at a critical anatomic site, such as the gastroesophageal junction, juxtapancreatic duodenum, or lower rectum, the surgical procedure can be downsized from an extensive multiorgan or full-organ resection to a more limited surgical procedure, without compromising local radicality. Very large tumors also can be potential candidates for preoperative therapy, because they tend to be extremely fragile and hypervascular, with a substantial risk of intraoperative rupture and/or bleeding.

Thus, based on the spectacular activity of imatinib on metastatic GIST, neoadjuvant therapy seems an attractive treatment strategy in locally advanced and/or marginally resectable GIST. Although current European (European Society of Medical Oncology [ESMO]) and US (NCCN) guidelines recommend this neoadjuvant strategy in selected cases,[50,51] it seems that is not yet fully implemented in routine practice. This neoadjuvant cytoreductive and tumor cell inactivating treatment in localized GIST aims to facilitate resection with microscopically clear margins, to decrease the extent and morbidity of the surgical procedure, and to minimize tumor micrometastases, thus increasing the patient's chance for cure.[52,53] Neoadjuvant therapy can reduce the need for extensive, multiorgan resections and diminish the intraoperative risk of rupture of devitalized tumor and spillage of active tumor cells into the peritoneal cavity (which is closely related to the risk of disease dissemination). Furthermore, it decreases the necessity of blood transfusions as a consequence of intraoperative tumor bleeding.[54,55] **Fig. 1** illustrates a locally advanced gastric GIST, detected due to gastrointestinal bleeding, which responded to imatinib 400 mg daily, resulting in a significant shrinkage of tumor. This enabled a complete tumor removal via wedge resection.

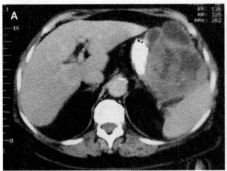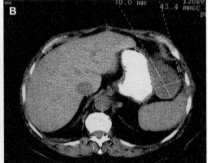

Fig. 1. CT images demonstrating response of locally advanced gastric GIST detected due to gastrointestinal bleeding with significant shrinkage of tumor allowing for complete tumor removal via wedge resection. (*A*) Before and (*B*) after treatment with imatinib (400 mg daily).

When used as a neoadjuvant treatment, imatinib is administered until maximal response is achieved. The duration of treatment can vary between 6 and 12 months. Usually, after 6 to 9 months, when 2 consecutive images (mostly computed tomography [CT]) show no further tumor regression, this is considered the point of maximal response. At that moment, a plateau in tumor shrinkage is reached, whereas the risk of developing secondary resistance to imatinib therapy is still very low.[56–58] A study by Tirumani and colleagues[59] confirmed that the best response to neoadjuvant imatinib is reached after approximately 28 weeks of treatment, with a plateau response at 34 weeks. Therefore, continuation of imatinib beyond this time span is probably not beneficial.

To avoid missing the optimal timing for surgery, careful response assessment should be undertaken. In selected cases, especially if mutational status was not determined in advance, this assessment should include imaging with PET/CT, as this modality may more adequately predict short-term treatment responses. Moreover, there is clear evidence that treatment with imatinib should always be followed by surgical resection. In the BFR-14 trial, Blesius and colleagues[60] demonstrated that patients with potentially resectable GIST who are treated with imatinib alone (ie, without resection) have a similar disease-free survival (DFS) and OS to that of patients with metastatic GIST. Thus, imatinib cannot replace surgery.

Imatinib can generally be stopped safely the day before surgery and restarted (when indicated) as soon as postoperative oral food intake is restored.[55,61,62] However, some centers prefer to stop the drug 1 week before surgery and do not restart it until 1 week after surgery.

Although preoperative therapy has become a common approach in individualized GIST cases, formal evidence from clinical trials regarding the outcome of neoadjuvant treatment with imatinib is limited.[53,63] Several articles report on small series of patients treated with imatinib before tumor resection, but they often have a mixed population of patients with primary, nonmetastatic GIST, as well as patients with metastatic GIST operated for residual disease.[57,61,64–77] The largest cohort of patients with GIST treated with neoadjuvant imatinib followed by resection was a series of 161 patients from 10 sarcoma centers of the European Organisation for Research and Treatment of Cancer (EORTC) Soft Tissue and Bone Sarcoma Group (STBSG). This study reported excellent safety data and long-term results, with a 5-year DFS (calculated from date of resection) and OS (calculated from start of preoperative imatinib) of 65% and 87%, respectively.[53] Only 1% of patients progressed during preoperative therapy. Microscopically radical resection (R0) was obtained in 83.2% of cases. Postoperative complications were recorded in 15% of cases, but only 3% required surgical intervention. One patient died postoperatively after total gastrectomy. Tielen and colleagues[78] analyzed a series of 57 patients with locally advanced GIST treated with neoadjuvant imatinib, with a median treatment duration of 8 months. Microscopically radical resection (R0) was possible in 84% of patients. Five-year DFS and OS of 77% and 88% were reported, respectively. Median tumor size of 12.2 cm before treatment was reduced to 6.2 cm after imatinib treatment. No tumor rupture was recorded.[78] Goh and colleagues[69] analyzed 37 patients preoperatively treated with imatinib, and concluded that radical resection was possible in 33 (89%) cases. Postoperative complications were recorded in only 4 (11%) of cases. A Dutch study presented data of 57 patients with locally advanced GIST who underwent surgery after a median time of 8 months of treatment with imatinib.[78] Tumor perforation did not occur in any of the patients and R0 resection was achieved in 84% of cases. Forty-four patients did not develop recurrence during follow-up. Recent reports indicate the possibility of successful laparoscopic resection of locally advanced gastric or esophageal GIST treated with neoadjuvant imatinib.[79,80]

Only 3 small, nonrandomized phase II trials are available evaluating neoadjuvant therapy with imatinib in locally advanced GIST (**Table 2**).[81–85] In the Radiation Therapy Oncology Group (RTOG), the National Cancer Institute, and the American College of Radiology Imaging Network (ACRIN)–RTOGS-0132/ACRIN 6665 phase II trial, 31 patients with primary, localized GIST received imatinib at the dosage of 600 mg daily preoperatively for 8 to 12 weeks and in case of objective response or stable disease they underwent elective surgery, followed by 2 years of adjuvant imatinib.[81] Results of this trial confirmed the safety of this approach and a high percentage of relapse-free survival was observed after surgery.[82] Two-year DFS and OS rates were 83% and 93%, respectively,[81] but discontinuation of adjuvant imatinib decreased the outcome to 5-year DFS and OS rates of 57% and 77%, respectively.[82] This study may have also identified gene expression signatures that are predictive for response to imatinib.[86] The German phase II CST1571-BDE43 study is the largest trial on neoadjuvant treatment with imatinib. After 6 months of imatinib, only 1 patient was inoperable at planned surgery and 26 (64%) of 41 patients had less extensive surgery than initially planned before administration of imatinib.[83]

These results imply that neoadjuvant therapy with imatinib increases the possibility of complete tumor resection and decreases the need for extensive and/or multivisceral resections. The median time of preoperative imatinib in the EORTC STBSG data was 10 months.[53] With longer neoadjuvant therapy, approximately 80% of cases demonstrate objective response to imatinib therapy. This is higher than the response rates reported in the phase II RTOG 0132 trial,[81] in which a maximum of 12 weeks of preoperative imatinib only was used. Goh and colleagues[69] as well as Doyon and colleagues[87] reported similar data. Furthermore, neoadjuvant imatinib seems to be a safe treatment strategy. In the EORTC STBSG series only 3% of patients were reported to require surgical reintervention due to postoperative complications.[53]

The proper candidates for preoperative imatinib are those patients who may benefit from tumor downstaging before operation; that is, patients in whom preoperative therapy with imatinib enables an organ-sparing resection with negative margins, avoiding mutilating surgery, intraoperative tumor rupture, and/or extensive blood loss (**Box 1**). Obviously, this neoadjuvant strategy is especially attractive in surgically demanding tumor sites, such as distal rectum, gastroesophageal junction, duodenum or esophagus, where preservation of vital functions is pivotal.[53,55,88] Resection of advanced primary tumors at these sites may be related to significant morbidity and functional defects. In some selected cases, downstaging of the primary tumor may sometimes even allow laparoscopic surgery instead of open surgery through an extensive midline laparotomy. Of course, these patients must be selected carefully by multidisciplinary assessment to optimize clinical outcomes. Before starting neoadjuvant therapy, a biopsy is obligatory (preferentially core-needle biopsy) and ideally the selection process should also be based on tumor genotyping results. The assessment of molecular status before neoadjuvant therapy is obligatory according to current ESMO guidelines,[50] but this may sometimes be difficult on a small biopsy sample. Nevertheless, it is clear now that the presence of primary gain-of-function mutations in *KIT* or *PDGFRA* genes strongly correlates with outcome of imatinib therapy in advanced GIST. The mutational status of the primary tumor is related to PFS and it predicts the probability of response to imatinib. Tumors harboring exon 11 *KIT* mutations demonstrate the best response to imatinib (70%–85% objective response rate) and these patients have the longest overall and PFS.[89–92] On the other hand, several clinical and laboratory studies confirmed that tumors with exon 18 *PDGFRA* D842V mutations are insensitive to imatinib, whereas other *PDGFRA*-mutant GIST show variable response.[89,93] In GIST harboring exon 18 *PDGFRA* D842V mutations (which are relatively frequent in the

Table 2
Summary of trials and major series with neoadjuvant imatinib therapy in GIST

| | Eligibility Criteria | Trial Design | Patient Numbers, n | Endpoints and Results | | | | |
				DFS/RFS	OS	ORR	PFS	Toxicity/SAE
Phase II RTOG-S0132/ACRIN 6665[82]	Cohort A: Locally advanced GIST ≥5 cm Cohort B: potentially resectable metastatic/recurrent GIST KIT-positive	Nonrandomized Neo-adj. imatinib 600 mg/d. for 8–12 wk and adj. imatinib for 2 y [R0 resection: 67%]	Total: n = 52 Cohort A: n = 30 Cohort B: n = 22	5-y. RFS: 57%	2-y. OS: 92% 5-y. OS: 77%	—	2-y. PFS: 80.5%	Grade 3: 29% Grade 4: 16% Grade 5: 4%
Phase II MD Anderson Cancer Center[85]	GIST at size ≥1 cm KIT-positive	Nonrandomized Neo-adj. imatinib 600 mg/d. for 3, 5 or 7 d and adj. imatinib for 2 y	n = 19	1-y. DFS: 94% 2-y. DFS: 87%	—	—	—	—
Phase II APOLLON CST1571-BDE43[83]	Locally advanced GIST KIT-positive	Nonrandomized Neo-adj. imatinib 400 mg/d. for 6 mo [R0 resection: 87%]	n = 41	3-y. RFS: 85%	Mean OS: 74.9 mo Mean OS: 83%	—	Mean PFS: 67% Mean TTP: 64 mo	—
EORTC STBSG collaborative series[53]	Locally advanced, nonmetastatic GISTs KIT-positive	Retrospective study Neo-adj. imatinib 400 mg/d. for median time of 40 wk [range: 6–190 wk] [R0 resection: 83%]	n = 161	5-y. DFS: 65%	5-y. OS: 87% 5-y. DSS: 95% Median OS: 104 mo	80%	—	—

Abbreviations: adj, adjuvant; DFS, disease-free survival; DSS, disease-specific survival; GIST, gastrointestinal stromal tumor; neo-adj, neoadjuvant; OS, overall survival; RFS, recurrence-free survival; TTP, time to progression.

Box 1
Current recommendations for preoperative imatinib therapy

- Locally advanced tumor, not a priori amenable for surgery without mutilating/multivisceral operation (eg, abdominal-perineal resection, pelvic evisceration, Whipple procedure, esophagogastric resection)

- When a negative resection margin of the organ of origin is difficult to obtain, a high risk of tumor rupture can be expected or complication due to the extensive surgery can be foreseen

- When function-sparing resection, minimizing the extent of surgery and reducing postoperative morbidity and mortality can be expected after tumor shrinkage (wedge resection instead of total gastrectomy with splenectomy, local excision instead of Whipple procedure, one cavity approach instead of abdominal-thoracic resection).

---

stomach) neoadjuvant treatment with imatinib is futile, as these tumors are not sensitive to this drug. Furthermore, it has been demonstrated that patients with advanced and metastatic GIST harboring *KIT* exon 9 mutations may benefit from an increased imatinib dose (escalated to 800 mg daily).[91,92] This indicates that patients with this mutation may be undertreated, when applying standard 400-mg daily dosage, but so far no clinical trial explored the outcome of an increased imatinib dose in this subset of patients in a neoadjuvant setting.

Based on assessment of size, location, and mitotic index, most primary GISTs treated with preoperative imatinib are considered high-risk or intermediate-risk tumors. This makes them candidates for adjuvant treatment with imatinib. According to current guidelines, imatinib should be administered postoperatively for 36 months (see also the next section). The EORTC STBSG series demonstrated the significant difference in DFS in favor of patients receiving imatinib, especially in patients with small-bowel GIST, who have an intrinsically higher risk of developing recurrence.[32]

Adjuvant Strategy

Postoperative recurrence of moderate and high-risk GIST is frequently observed. This led to the idea of using imatinib as an adjuvant treatment after primary surgery to prevent or delay recurrence and thus prolong survival. In 2008, imatinib was registered for use in adjuvant therapy after resection of primary GIST at significant risk of relapse. This was based on the results of clinical trials demonstrating a significant reduction in the risk of recurrence.[19] However, the data did not provide a clear guidance as to optimal duration of treatment.

The role of imatinib in the adjuvant treatment setting has been evaluated in several phase II and III clinical trials: ACOSOG Z9000 and Z9001 (conducted by the American College of Surgeons Oncology Group), SSGXVIII/AIO (conducted by the Scandinavian Sarcoma Group and the Sarcoma Group of the Arbeitsgemeinschaft Internistische Onkologie XVIII), RTOG S0132 (conducted by the Radiation Therapy Oncology Group), and EORTC 62024 (conducted by the European Organization for Research and Treatment of Cancer) (**Table 3**).[82,94–99] Data from the ACOSOG Z9001 phase III study, comparing 1 year of adjuvant therapy with imatinib 400 mg daily to placebo in patients after R0 resection of GIST of at least 3 cm in diameter, have shown a significant reduction in the risk of recurrence from 17% to 2% at 1 year (20 months of follow-up; $P = .0001$, hazard ratio = 0.35).[94] The treatment was well tolerated. However, no significant impact on OS was observed; many patients recurred shortly after adjuvant imatinib cessation and they then received imatinib as a rescue therapy in the metastatic setting. This implies that adjuvant imatinib delays rather than prevents the relapse. Moreover, this trial enrolled many patients with low risk of recurrence according to current criteria. Substantial clinical benefit of adjuvant therapy was most obvious in the group of patients with high risk of relapse according to NCCN-AFIP criteria, with an improvement of 2-year recurrence-free survival (RFS) from 41% to 77% (P<.0001).[19,100] This raised interest in the assessment of a more long-term administration of adjuvant imatinib in high risk GIST.

Data from the SSGXVIII/AIO trial, comparing 12 versus 36 months of adjuvant imatinib treatment after resection of GIST with a high risk of recurrence, were initially presented in 2011 at the 47th Annual Meeting of the American Society of Clinical Oncology (ASCO).[96] The results showed significant improvement in the 36-month arm compared with the 12-month arm, both in RFS (5-year RFS: 65.6% vs 47.9%; P<.0001) and OS (5-year OS: 92.0% vs 81.7%; P = .01). The best results were obtained in GIST harboring KIT exon 11 mutations. Imatinib was generally well tolerated with anemia, periorbital edema, fatigue, nausea, diarrhea, leucopenia, and muscle cramps as the most common adverse events. More patients discontinued imatinib therapy in the 3-year arm in comparison with the 1-year arm (for reasons other than GIST recurrence) (26% vs 12%; P<.001).[20,32,96,101] Based on these data, the Food and Drug Administration and the European Medicines Agency, as well as ESMO and NCCN recommended 36 months of treatment with imatinib after surgery for adult patients with CD117-positive GIST considered at high risk of relapse.[50,51,102] Subsequent analyses confirmed the cost-effectiveness of prolonged adjuvant therapy in patients with GIST at high risk of disease recurrence.[103,104] The second, planned analysis of the SSGXVIII/AIO trial after a median follow-up time of 7.5 years confirmed the superior and sustained effect on RFS and OS of 3 years of adjuvant imatinib versus only 1 year of therapy.[105] Nevertheless, even after 3 years of adjuvant imatinib, a clear trend toward relapse occurs when imatinib is stopped. This implies an even further prolongation of adjuvant therapy in high-risk GIST and a very close follow-up after cessation of adjuvant therapy (especially in patients with higher mitotic index, who are especially susceptible for relapse).[94,105,106] The same observation was done for intermediate-risk and high-risk GIST in the EORTC 62024 trial,[97] suggesting that delaying relapse without a clear decrease in the relapse rate might actually exert a limited impact on survival. The highest impact is seen in the high-risk subgroup, probably with appropriate genotype profile. Recently reported interim results of an ongoing, nonrandomized phase II trial, evaluating the efficacy and safety of 5-year adjuvant imatinib in high-risk (based on modified NIH criteria) GIST after curative surgery, suggested a benefit of extended adjuvant imatinib therapy.[107] Currently, another nonrandomized phase II trial called PERSIST-5 (Post-resection Evaluation of Recurrence-free Survival for Gastrointestinal Stromal Tumors) is investigating 5 years of adjuvant imatinib therapy (400 mg daily) in patients with completely resected GIST (R0-resection) with significant risk of recurrence, with RFS as its primary endpoint.[108]

Characterizing the precise benefit of adjuvant imatinib in patients with moderate and high risk of recurrence by one of the new classifications, stratified by mutational subtype, is the next step in defining which patients should be treated. When using different risk-stratification schemes, such as the NCCN-AFIP, MSKCC (Memorial Sloan Kettering Cancer Center) nomogram, or the heat map, there is a consensus to treat all patients having at least 30% risk of recurrence, if their tumor carries a sensitive genotype.[30,34,37,50,51] Mutational status also has a predictive value for the clinical outcome after adjuvant treatment with imatinib and may help to tailor the treatment to patients with more sensitive mutations, such as KIT exon 11 mutants, or to exclude patients with imatinib-resistant mutations, such as PDGFRA D842V mutation. The data from randomized clinical trials ACOSOG Z9001 and SSGXVIII/AIO clearly demonstrated

744   Rutkowski & Hompes

Table 3
The most important clinical trials of adjuvant therapy with imatinib in primary GIST

Trial	Imatinib Dose and Duration	Inclusion Criteria	Efficacy Results	
			Primary Endpoints	Secondary Endpoints
ACOSOG Z9001[94] Randomized, phase III, placebo-controlled	400 mg daily (n = 359) vs placebo (n = 354) for 1 y	• KIT + primary GIST • Tumor size ≥3 cm • R0-resection • Low, intermediate or high risk of recurrence	1-y RFS: 98% with imatinib vs 83% placebo (83%) median FU: 19.7 mo HR 0.35, P<.0001	No significant difference in 1-y OS median FU: 19.7 mo HR 0.66, P = .47
ACOSOG Z9000[95] One-arm, open-label, phase II	400 mg daily (n = 107) for 1 y	• KIT + primary GIST • R0-resection • High risk of relapse ○ Tumor size ≥10 cm OR ○ Tumor rupture OR ○ Peritoneal metastases <5	1-y OS: 99% 2-y OS: 97% 3-y OS: 97% Median FU: 4 y	1-y RFS: 94% 2-y RFS: 73% 3-y RFS: 61% Median FU: 4 y
SSGXVIII/AIO[96] Randomized, open-label, phase III	400 mg daily for 1 y (n = 200) vs 3 y (n = 200)	• KIT + primary GIST • High risk of recurrence[b]: ○ Tumor size >10 cm OR ○ Mitotic rate >10/50 HPFs OR ○ Mitotic rate >5/50 and tumor size >5 cm OR ○ Tumor rupture	5-y RFS: 65.6% after 3 y vs 47.9% after 1 y of imatinib (71.1% vs 52.3% in Intention-to-treat population) Median FU: 54 mo HR 0.46, 95% CI 0.32–0.65; P<.0001	5-y OS: 92% after 3 y vs 81.7% after 1 y of imatinib Median 54-mo FU HR 0.45, 95% CI 0.22–0.89; P = .019
EORTC 62024[97] Two-arms, open-label, randomized, phase III	400 mg daily vs observation (n = 908) for 2 y	• KIT + primary GIST • R0-resection • Intermediate or high risk of relapse[a]: ○ Tumor size> 5 cm AND/OR ○ Mitotic index >5/50 HPF	5-y imatinib failure-free survival (IFFS): 84% with imatinib arm vs 84% in control arm HR = 0.80, P = .23 5-y IFFS in high-risk GIST: 89% vs 73%; P = .11	RFS (at 3 y): 84% after 2 y vs 66% in control arm Median FU: 4.7 y HR 0.45, 95% CI 0.22–0.89; P = .019 OS: no significant difference

Study	Treatment	Inclusion criteria	RFS	OS
Kang et al[98] Single-arm, prospective, phase II	400 mg daily (n = 47) for 2 y	• Primary GIST with KIT exon 11 mutation • R0-resection • High risk of recurrence: ○ Tumor size ≥10 cm OR ○ Mitotic rate ≥10/50 HPFs OR ○ Tumor size ≥5 cm and mitotic rate ≥5/50 HPFs	1-y RFS: 97.7% 2-y RFS: 92.7% Median FU: 26.9 mo	—
Li et al[99] Open-label, nonrandomized, phase II	400 mg daily (n = 56) vs no treatment (n = 49) for 3 y	• KIT + primary GIST • R0-resection • Intermediate or high risk of recurrence[a]: ○ Tumor size >5 cm and/or ○ Mitotic rate >5/50 HPFs	RFS with imatinib vs no treatment: 1-y RFS: 100% vs 90% 2-y RFS: 96% vs 57% 3-y RFS: 89% vs 48% Median FU: 45 mo HR 0.188, 95% CI 0.085–0.417; $P<.001$	Significantly reduced risk of death with imatinib vs no treatment Median FU: 45 mo HR 0.254, 95% CI 0.070–0.931; $P = .025$

Abbreviations: ACOSOG, American College of Surgeons Oncology Group; AE, adverse event; AIG, Arbeitsgemeinschaft Interistisch Onkologie; CI, confidence interval; EORTC, European Organisation for Research and Treatment of Cancer; FU, follow-up; GIST, gastrointestinal stromal tumors; Gr, Grade; HPF, high-power microscope field; HR, hazard ratio; NIH, National Institutes of Health; OS, overall survival; RFS, recurrence-free survival; RTOG, Radiation Therapy Oncology Group; SSG, Scandinavian Sarcoma Group.

[a] NIH classification.
[b] Modified NIH classification.

that patients with GIST with KIT exon 11 mutation benefited mostly from adjuvant therapy.[94,96,101] Although controversial in the adjuvant setting, patients with metastatic GIST harboring mutations in *KIT* exon 9 may benefit from an increase of the imatinib dose up to 800 mg daily. Thus, *KIT* and *PDGFRA* genotyping in GIST should be mandatory also in the adjuvant setting.[109,110] In our centers, we routinely use tumor mutation analysis as a predictive tool in the adjuvant setting. There is also a consensus not to treat patients having 10% or less risk of recurrence, even if their tumor carries a sensitive genotype. Although the concept that only high-risk patients derive benefit from adjuvant imatinib has not been prospectively validated, based on these data, it would seem reasonable to offer adjuvant therapy to all patients who fall into a "high-risk" category, regardless of the risk-stratification model used.

The EORTC 62024 trial, which compared 2-year adjuvant treatment with imatinib versus observation only, provided some data on imatinib resistance on rechallenge after disease relapse in the patients with intermediate-risk and high-risk GIST who had undergone resection of the primary tumor. In the high-risk subgroup, a non–statistically significant trend in favor of the adjuvant arm was observed in terms of imatinib failure-free survival. This implies that adjuvant therapy does not lead to the development of secondary imatinib resistance.[97,111] This observation confirms observations from a subgroup analysis of the SGXVIII/AIO trial, which demonstrated that most patients who received prior adjuvant imatinib treatment do respond to a rechallenge with imatinib to treat recurrence.[112] Thus, a rechallenge with imatinib is indicated in case of disease recurrence after adjuvant imatinib. In rare cases of disease progression on imatinib, second-line therapy with sunitinib should be used.[113]

RECURRENT/METASTATIC GASTROINTESTINAL STROMAL TUMORS

Imatinib mesylate at initial dose of 400 mg daily is the first-line standard treatment of patients with metastatic, recurrent, and/or inoperable GIST.[9,114] Approximately two-thirds of patients with GIST achieve an objective response during imatinib treatment with a standard dose of 400 mg daily, and further 20% of patients show durable disease stabilization[4,9,10]; however, complete remissions are rare. A recently emerging issue is the surgical removal of disease remnants during imatinib therapy, which may lead to complete remission in selected patients with GIST after the achievement of a partial response (PR). This policy appears attractive, because the excision of the tumor would be performed before the development of imatinib resistance, thus reducing the risk of resistant clone selection, which theoretically might prolong durable remission. The dramatic efficacy of imatinib is time-limited, with a common persistence of viable GIST cells after imatinib therapy and the probability of developing resistant clones of GIST cells is proportional to the tumor mass.[61,115]

The optimal time for the implementation of surgical treatment is probably the moment of disease stabilization; that is, the radiological observation of maximal remission. Usually, this point is reached after a time interval of 6 to 18 months from the onset of imatinib therapy.[61] Several series of patients treated surgically during imatinib therapy have been published, although randomized trials to formally confirm a survival benefit did not prove feasible. Therefore, the ESMO consensus guidelines advise that for metastatic disease the surgical option during imatinib treatment should be individualized after sharing the decision with the patient in cases of uncertainty.[50]

Systemic therapy should be continued indefinitely, as its interruption is followed by relatively rapid tumor progression in virtually all cases, even after successful metastasectomy.[61,116,117] Two trials, 1 in Europe (EORTC 62023) and 1 in China, attempted to address the question of which patients with metastatic or recurrent GIST might benefit from resection after upfront response to imatinib, but both were stopped prematurely due to poor accrual. The Chinese randomized trial reported data on 41 patients of 210 planned and showed a 2-year PFS of 88.4% in the surgery arm versus 57.7% in imatinib-alone arm (P = .08; median follow-up: 23 months).[118]

Despite the absence of randomized controlled trials, some general conclusions might still be drawn from the results of some single-institution retrospective studies examining disease control after resection in selected patients with limited metastatic disease (**Table 4**).[61,62,113,117,119–121] Generally, the conclusions of these studies were consistent. They demonstrated that complete excision of residual metastatic lesions was associated with improved prognosis, but outcome remained dependent on satisfactory responses to imatinib. Recently, the Spanish Group for Research in Sarcomas analyzed 2 cohorts of patients with advanced GIST: treated (n = 27) or not treated (n = 144) with surgery after PR or stable disease (SD) by imatinib. With a median follow-up time of 56.6 months, they concluded that median OS was strikingly superior in the group treated surgically during imatinib therapy (87.6 months) compared with 59.9 months in the imatinib-only group (P = .022). The 5-year OS rates were 79% and 50%, respectively. The effect of surgery remained significant in multivariate analysis. Median PFS differences were also superior for surgically treated patients: 73.4 months versus 44.6 months.[122] Researchers from Korea studied the role of surgery in patients with metastatic/recurrent GIST, who had at least 6 months of SD or response under imatinib. At a median follow-up of 58.9 months, median OS was not reached in patients who underwent surgery (n = 42), compared with 88.8 months in those who did not undergo surgery (n = 92) (P = .001). PFS was 87.7 and 42.8 months, respectively (P = .001). Surgery remained an independent factor for better PFS and OS in multivariate analysis.[123] Similarly, a data analysis from the Polish Clinical GIST Registry of 430 consecutive patients with inoperable/metastatic/recurrent GIST initially treated with imatinib showed that surgery of residual disease (n = 94) was an independent prognostic factor associated with longer OS and PFS. Eight-year OS and PFS rates were 67.4% and 50.4%, respectively, for patients undergoing resection of residual disease during imatinib therapy.[114] Systematic review of surgery and imatinib mesylate in treatment of advanced GIST also concluded that patients with stable or responding disease tend to have better PFS and OS after surgery when compared with those patients who have focal or generalized preoperative disease progression.[124] This was also supported by data from the prospective phase II RTOG 0132 trial for patients who underwent surgical debulking in the context of perioperative tyrosine kinase inhibitor (TKI) therapy.[81] The EORTC STBSG performed a cross-matched comparison of patients who underwent surgical resection at disease response (complete response, PR, or SD) with patients who were in response at the same time interval from imatinib start, but did not undergo surgery.[125] Fifty-eight patients were available for postsurgery survival analysis: 29 patients underwent resection of their metastatic disease while in response and they were matched with 29 nonoperated patients. Patients who underwent surgery for residual disease had a better survival after surgery than those who did not, especially during the first 3 years. Two-year postsurgery survival was 95.5% (95% confidence interval [CI] 87.2–100.0) versus 82.5% (95% CI 74.4–90.6) and 5-year postsurgery survival was 63.9% (95% CI 52.4–75.3) versus 56.0% (95% CI 43.3–68), respectively. A similar result was seen for postsurgery PFS, during the first year after surgery.[125]

Bauer and colleagues[120] analyzed the largest series of 239 consecutive patients with GIST who had undergone surgery for metastatic GIST in 4 large institutions from EORTC STBSG. In 79% of patients, R0/R1 resection was performed. OS data of patients in whom macroscopically complete resection could be achieved (R0/R1

Table 4
Series of patients with unresectable/metastatic GIST treated with surgery during imatinib therapy

	Number of Cases, Clinical Indications	Key Results
Raut et al,[62] 2006	n = 69 • Group I: Surgery at stable disease • Group II: Surgery at limited progression • Group III: Surgery at generalized progression	• Group I: 1-y PFS: 80%, 1-y OS: 95% • Group II: 1-y PFS: 33%, 1-y OS: 86% • Group III: 1-y PFS: 0%, 1-y OS: 0%
Rutkowski et al,[61] 2006	n = 141 unresectable/metastatic GIST treated initially with imatinib: • Group I (n = 24, 17%): resection of residual disease after complete/partial response or lack of further response to imatinib • Group II (n = 8, 6%): surgery as salvage therapy for progression after initially successful imatinib therapy	• Group I: 5 patients: imatinib not continued after surgery → 4 recurrences, 19 patients: imatinib continued after surgery → 1 recurrence 89.6% alive at last follow-up • Group II: 5/8 patients progressed Median follow-up time 12 mo
Gronchi et al,[117] 2007	n = 159 advanced/metastatic GIST treated initially with imatinib: • Group I (n = 27): surgery at response • Group II (n = 8): surgery at progression	• Group I: postsurgery PFS 96% at 12 mo and 69% at 24 mo; 100% alive at 12 mo • Group II: postsurgery PFS 0% at 12 mo, 60% alive at 12 mo (secondary progression: mainly related to postsurgical imatinib discontinuation, irrespective of pathologic or molecular variables)
DeMatteo et al,[119] 2007	n = 40 metastatic GIST treated with tyrosine kinase inhibitors • Group I (n = 20): response • Group II (n = 13): surgery at focal progression • Group III (n = 7): surgery at multifocal progression	• Group I: 2-y PFS of 61% and 2-y OS of 100% • Group II: 2-y PFS: 24% and the 2-y OS: 36%, median TTP: 12 mo • Group III: 1-y OS: 36%, median TTP: 3 mo Median follow-up 15 mo
Mussi et al,[113] 2010	n = 80 metastatic GIST after imatinib therapy: • Group A (n = 49): surgery at best response • Group B (n = 31): surgery at focal progression	• Group A: 2-y PFS: 64.4% and 5-y DSS: 82.9%, median PFS and DSS were not reached • Group B: 2-y PFS: 9.7%, median PFS: 8 mo and 5-y DSS: 67.6%, median DSS was not reached Morbidity: n = 13 patients (16.3%)
Bauer et al,[120] 2014	239 patients with GIST undergoing surgery for metastatic GIST • Group I (n = 177): Complete resection (R0/R1) • Group II: incomplete resection (R2)	• Group I: Median OS: 8.7 y, median OS was not reached when surgery was performed at remission, median TTP was not reached. • Group II: Median OS: 5.3 y, median OS was 5.1 y when surgery was performed at remission, median TTP: 1.9 y when surgery was performed at response. • Group I & II: No difference in median PFS was seen in patients progressing at time of surgery
Tielen et al,[121] 2012	n = 55 advanced/metastatic GIST after imatinib: • Group I (n = 35): responders • Group II (n = 20): nonresponders	• Group I: 48% recurrence/progression, Median PFS and OS were not reached 5-y OS: 78%. • Group II: 85% recurrence/progression, median PFS: 4 mo, median OS: 25 mo, 3-y OS: 26%.

Abbreviations: GIST, gastrointestinal stromal tumor; n, number of patients; OS, overall survival; PFS, progression-free survival; TTP, time to progression.

group, 79% of patients) were compared with those with residual tumor after resection (R2). Median OS was 8.7 years in the R0/R1 group versus 5.3 years in the R2 group ($P = .0001$). When patients with progressing disease (focal or general progression) at time of surgery were excluded, median OS was not reached in the R0/R1 group and it was 5.1 years in the R2 group ($P = .0001$). Female gender, short interval of imatinib to surgery, resection status (R0/R1), remission at time of surgery (ie, non–progressive disease [PD]), and liver site were identified as positive prognostic factors. Median survival was not reached in R0/R1 patients with hepatic-only metastases compared with 8.7 and 5.9 years in patients with peritoneal ($P = .064$) versus peritoneal and hepatic metastases ($P = .001$ and $P = .024$). Similarly, when patients with PD at time of surgery were excluded, the median PFS was not reached for those patients with complete resection (R0/R1) versus 3.9 years in those in whom surgery resulted in incomplete resection (R2).[120]

Generally, the data mentioned previously support the role of surgery for residual metastatic disease in patients with GIST responding to imatinib, but it has never been clearly demonstrated prospectively whether this is due to the surgery itself or to patient selection. Nevertheless, as the available data point to surgery of residual disease in the absence of disease progression as the most independent prognostic factor for better outcomes in advanced GIST, a real impact on the natural course of the disease can be expected from this treatment strategy. Surgery for residual disease, based on individual decisions within a multidisciplinary tumor board, is estimated to be an option in approximately 20% of patients responding to systemic therapy.[61,117,126] It also should be mentioned that cytoreduction before treatment with imatinib does not seem to improve the prognosis.[127] Therefore, surgery should not be the first treatment step for first recurrence, with the exception of emergency indications. Elective surgery should be considered only as a treatment option after imatinib therapy has been initiated. Data from several series have shown surgery after tyrosine kinase inhibitors to be a feasible and safe procedure.[57,61,62,117,119,126] Under elective circumstances, overall complication rates varied from 12% to 33%, with bleeding, prolonged ileus, anastomotic leakage, and fistulae as the most frequently reported postoperative complications. Nevertheless, the need for reintervention due to postoperative complications remains low and no postoperative mortality was reported in these series. In case of surgery for emergency complications during tyrosine kinase inhibitors therapy, on the other hand, complication rates may increase to up to 50% and postoperative mortality has been reported.[57,62] Furthermore, emergency surgery for GIST seems to increase the chances of obtaining an R2-resection.[57] Mutilating surgery in metastatic GIST should be avoided, as systemic therapy is the mainstay of treatment in this setting and surgery is only adjunctive to tyrosine kinase inhibitors therapy. As mentioned earlier, continuation of imatinib after surgery is crucial.[61,116,117] **Fig. 2** illustrates an example of a carefully selected patient with oligometastatic disease confined to the liver, who derived long-term benefit from surgery on imatinib.

Another field for surgery in advanced GIST during treatment with tyrosine kinase inhibitors comprises the resection of focally PD to delay resistance to systemic therapy. In patients who develop limited resistance to imatinib, surgery might be considered, although the benefit is unknown. In cases of generalized progression, currently available data do not support a clinical benefit of surgery.[61,119] Raut and colleagues[62] reported that the 1-year PFS was 80%, 33%, and 0% for patients with SD, limited progression, and generalized progression, respectively. Similarly, we found that patients with responsive or SD had significantly improved RFS and OS when compared with patients with PD.[61] Surgery for focally progressive lesions on imatinib results is a median time to secondary progression of 6 to 14 months,[61,128] which in some cases

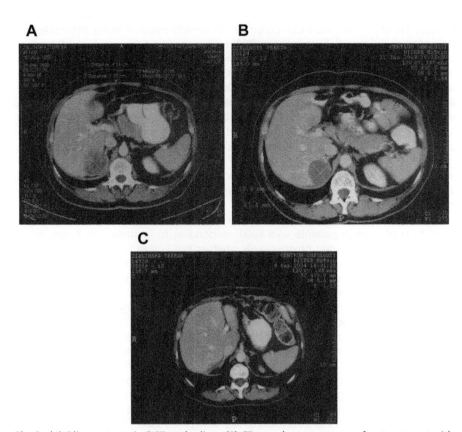

Fig. 2. (*A*) Oligometastatic GIST to the liver. (*B*) CT scan shows response after treatment with imatinib; metastasectomy was performed after response to imatinib. (*C*) Patient continues imatinib and remains in CR 11 years after surgery.

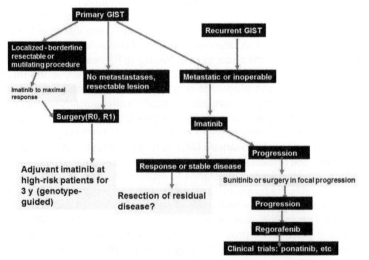

Fig. 3. The current algorithm of therapy in GIST, boxes with light background indicate the fields for combined therapy for surgery and tyrosine kinase inhibitors.

may delay a switch to treatment with sunitinib. Nevertheless, the final impact of this strategy on survival as well as the time of implementation of surgery is still controversial. Generally, the role of elective surgical therapy of advanced GIST during further lines of systemic treatment beyond imatinib is very limited and should be carefully individualized. Only few data are available on this matter.[129,130]

SUMMARY

Fig. 3 summarizes the current algorithm for the treatment of GIST.

REFERENCES

1. Joensuu H. Gastrointestinal stromal tumor (GIST). Ann Oncol 2006;17(Suppl 10):x280–6.
2. Miettinen M, Lasota J. Gastrointestinal stromal tumors–definition, clinical, histological, immunohistochemical, and molecular genetic features and differential diagnosis. Virchows Arch 2001;438(1):1–12.
3. DeMatteo RP, Lewis JJ, Leung D, et al. Two hundred gastrointestinal stromal tumors: recurrence patterns and prognostic factors for survival. Ann Surg 2000; 231(1):51–8.
4. Rutkowski P, Nowecki ZI, Michej W, et al. Risk criteria and prognostic factors for predicting recurrences after resection of primary gastrointestinal stromal tumors (GISTs). Ann Surg Oncol 2007;14:2018–27.
5. Nilsson B, Bumming P, Meis-Kindblom JM, et al. Gastrointestinal stromal tumors: the incidence, prevalence, clinical course, and prognostication in the preimatinib mesylate era–a population-based study in western Sweden. Cancer 2005; 103(4):821–9.
6. Corless CL, Fletcher JA, Heinrich MC. Biology of gastrointestinal stromal tumors. J Clin Oncol 2004;22(18):3813–25.
7. Lasota J, Miettinen M. KIT and PDGFRA mutations in gastrointestinal stromal tumors (GISTs). Semin Diagn Pathol 2006;23(2):91–102.
8. Rutkowski P, Debiec-Rychter M, Ruka W. Gastrointestinal stromal tumors: key to diagnosis and choice of therapy. Mol Diagn Ther 2008;12:131–43.
9. Demetri GD, von Mehren M, Blanke CD, et al. Efficacy and safety of imatinib mesylate in advanced gastrointestinal stromal tumors. N Engl J Med 2002;347(7): 472–80.
10. Verweij J, Casali PG, Zalcberg J, et al. Progression-free survival in gastrointestinal stromal tumours with high-dose imatinib: randomised trial. Lancet 2004; 364(9440):1127–34.
11. Blanke CD, Rankin C, Demetri GD, et al. Phase III randomized, intergroup trial assessing imatinib mesylate at two dose levels in patients with unresectable or metastatic gastrointestinal stromal tumors expressing the kit receptor tyrosine kinase: S0033. J Clin Oncol 2008;26(4):626–32.
12. Rutkowski P, Nowecki ZI, Debiec-Rychter M, et al. Predictive factors for long-term effects of imatinib therapy in patients with inoperable/metastatic CD117(+) gastrointestinal stromal tumors (GISTs). J Cancer Res Clin Oncol 2007;133(9):589–97.
13. Blanke CD, Demetri GD, von Mehren M, et al. Long-term results from a randomized phase II trial of standard- versus higher-dose imatinib mesylate for patients with unresectable or metastatic gastrointestinal stromal tumors expressing KIT. J Clin Oncol 2008;26(4):620–5.

14. Vincenzi B, Nannini M, Fumagalli E, et al. Imatinib dose escalation versus sunitinib as a second line treatment in KIT exon 11 mutated GIST: a retrospective analysis. Oncotarget 2015. [Epub ahead of print].
15. Patel S. Managing progressive disease in patients with GIST: factors to consider besides acquired secondary tyrosine kinase inhibitor resistance. Cancer Treat Rev 2012;38(5):467–72.
16. Zalcberg J, Desai J. Dose optimization of tyrosine kinase inhibitors to improve outcomes in GIST. Asia Pac J Clin Oncol 2012;8(1):43–52.
17. Yoo C, Ryu MH, Ryoo BY, et al. Efficacy, safety, and pharmacokinetics of imatinib dose escalation to 800 mg/day in patients with advanced gastrointestinal stromal tumors. Invest New Drugs 2013;31(5):1367–74.
18. Patel S, Zalcberg JR. Optimizing the dose of imatinib for treatment of gastrointestinal stromal tumours: lessons from the phase 3 trials. Eur J Cancer 2008;44:501–9.
19. DeMatteo R, Ballman KV, Antonescu CR, et al, American College of Surgeons Oncology Group (ACOSOG) Intergroup Adjuvant GIST Study Team. Adjuvant imatinib mesylate after resection of localised, primary gastrointestinal stromal tumour: a randomised, double-blind, placebo-controlled trial. Lancet 2009;373(9669):1079–104.
20. Joensuu H, Eriksson M, Sundby Hall K, et al. One vs three years of adjuvant imatinib for operable gastrointestinal stromal tumor: a randomized trial. JAMA 2012;307(12):1265–72.
21. Miettinen M, Lasota J. Gastrointestinal stromal tumors: pathology and prognosis at different sites. Semin Diagn Pathol 2006;23:70–83.
22. Fletcher C, Berman JJ, Corless C, et al. Diagnosis of gastrointestinal stromal tumors: a consensus approach. Hum Pathol 2002;33:459–65.
23. Wozniak A, Sciot R, Guillou L, et al. Array CGH analysis in primary gastrointestinal stromal tumors: cytogenetic profile correlates with anatomic site and tumor aggressiveness, irrespective of mutational status. Genes Chromosomes Cancer 2007;46:261–76.
24. Wozniak A, Rutkowski P, Schöffski P, et al. Tumor genotype is an independent prognostic factor in primary gastrointestinal stromal tumors of gastric origin: a European multicenter analysis based on ConticaGIST. Clin Cancer Res 2014;20(23):6105–16.
25. Miettinen M, Furlong M, Sarlomo-Rikala M, et al. Gastrointestinal stromal tumors, intramural leiomyomas, and leiomyosarcomas in the rectum and anus: a clinicopathologic, immunohistochemical, and molecular genetic study of 144 cases. Am J Surg Pathol 2001;25:1121–33.
26. Miettinen M, Kopczynski J, Makhlouf HR, et al. Gastrointestinal stromal tumors, intramural leiomyomas, and leiomyosarcomas in the duodenum: a clinicopathologic, immunohistochemical, and molecular genetic study of 167 cases. Am J Surg Pathol 2003;27:625–41.
27. Miettinen M, Sobin LH, Lasota J. Gastrointestinal stromal tumors of the stomach: a clinicopathologic, immunohistochemical, and molecular genetic study of 1765 cases with long-term follow-up. Am J Surg Pathol 2005;29:52–68.
28. Miettinen M, Makhlouf H, Sobin LH, et al. Gastrointestinal stromal tumors of the jejunum and ileum: a clinicopathologic, immunohistochemical, and molecular genetic study of 906 cases before imatinib with long-term follow-up. Am J Surg Pathol 2006;30:477–89.
29. Edge SB, Byrd DR, Compton CC, et al, editors. American Joint Committee on cancer staging manual. 7th edition. New York: Springer; 2009.

30. Rutkowski P, Wozniak A, Dębiec-Rychter M, et al. Clinical utility of the new American Joint Committee on cancer staging system for gastrointestinal stromal tumors: current overall survival after primary tumor resection. Cancer 2011; 117(21):4916–24.

31. Hohenberger P, Ronellenfitsch U, Oladeji O, et al. Pattern of recurrence in patients with ruptured primary gastrointestinal stromal tumour. Br J Surg 2010; 97(12):1854–9.

32. Joensuu H, Vehtari A, Riihimäki J, et al. Risk of recurrence of gastrointestinal stromal tumour after surgery: an analysis of pooled population-based cohorts. Lancet Oncol 2012;13(3):265–74.

33. Joensuu H. Risk stratification of patients diagnosed with gastrointestinal stromal tumor. Hum Pathol 2008;39:1411–9.

34. Rutkowski P, Bylina E, Wozniak A, et al. Validation of the Joensuu risk criteria for primary resectable gastrointestinal stromal tumour—the impact of tumour rupture on patient outcomes. Eur J Surg Oncol 2011;37:890–6.

35. Bumming P, Ahlman H, Andersson J, et al. Population-based study of the diagnosis and treatment of gastrointestinal stromal tumours. Br J Surg 2006;93: 836–43.

36. Pierie JP, Choudry U, Muzikansky A, et al. The effect of surgery and grade on outcome of gastrointestinal stromal tumors. Arch Surg 2001;136:383–9.

37. Gold JS, Gonen M, Gutierrez A, et al. Development and validation of a prognostic nomogram for recurrence-free survival after complete surgical resection of localised primary gastrointestinal stromal tumour: a retrospective analysis. Lancet Oncol 2009;10(11):1045–52.

38. Rossi S, Miceli R, Messerini L, et al. Natural history of imatinib-naive GISTs: a retrospective analysis of 929 cases with long-term follow-up and development of a survival nomogram based on mitotic index and size as continuous variables. Am J Surg Pathol 2011;35(11):1646–56.

39. Bischof DA, Kim Y, Behman R, et al. A nomogram to predict disease-free survival after surgical resection of GIST. J Gastrointest Surg 2014;18(12):2123–9.

40. Lasota J, Jasinski M, Sarlomo-Rikala M, et al. Mutations in exon 11 of c-Kit occur preferentially in malignant versus benign gastrointestinal stromal tumors and do not occur in leiomyomas or leiomyosarcomas. Am J Pathol 1999;154:53–60.

41. Lasota J, Dansonka-Mieszkowska A, Sobin LH, et al. A great majority of GISTs with PDGFRA mutations represent gastric tumors of low or no malignant potential. Lab Invest 2004;84:874–83.

42. Wardelmann E, Losen I, Hans V, et al. Deletion of Trp-557 and Lys-558 in the juxtamembrane domain of the c-kit protooncogene is associated with metastatic behavior of gastrointestinal stromal tumors. Int J Cancer 2003;106:887–95.

43. Lasota J, Dansonka-Mieszkowska A, Stachura T, et al. Gastrointestinal stromal tumours with internal tandem duplications in 3' end of KIT juxtamembrane domain occur predominantly in stomach and generally seem to have a favorable course. Mod Pathol 2003;16:1257–64.

44. Andersson J, Bümming P, Meis-Kindblom JM, et al. Gastrointestinal stromal tumors with KIT exon 11 deletions are associated with poor prognosis. Gastroenterology 2006;130:1573–81.

45. Martin J, Poveda A, Llombart-Bosch A, et al. Deletions affecting codons 557–558 of the c-KIT gene indicate a poor prognosis in patients with completely resected gastrointestinal stromal tumors: a study by the Spanish Group for Sarcoma Research (GEIS). J Clin Oncol 2005;23(25):6190–8.

46. Wozniak A, Rutkowski P, Piskorz A, et al, on behalf of Polish GIST Registry. Prognostic value of KIT/PDGFRA mutations in gastrointestinal stromal tumours (GIST): Polish Clinical GIST Registry experience. Ann Oncol 2012;23:353–60.

47. Rossi S, Gasparotto D, Miceli R, et al. KIT, PDGFRA, and BRAF mutational spectrum impacts on the natural history of imatinib-naive localized GIST: a population-based study. Am J Surg Pathol 2015;39(7):922–30.

48. Joensuu H, Rutkowski P, Nishida T, et al. KIT and PDGFRA mutations and the risk of GI stromal tumor recurrence. J Clin Oncol 2015;33(6):634–42.

49. Lartigue L, Neuville A, Lagarde P, et al. Genomic index predicts clinical outcome of intermediate-risk gastrointestinal stromal tumours, providing a new inclusion criterion for imatinib adjuvant therapy. Eur J Cancer 2015;51(1):75–83.

50. The ESMO/European Sarcoma Network Working Group. Gastrointestinal stromal tumors: ESMO clinical practice guidelines for diagnosis, treatment and follow-up. Ann Oncol 2012;23(Suppl 7):vii49–55.

51. NCCN clinical practice guidelines in oncology. Soft tissue sarcoma. Version 2.2012.

52. Pandey R, Kochar R. Management of gastrointestinal stromal tumors: looking beyond the knife. An update on the role of adjuvant and neoadjuvant imatinib therapy. J Gastrointest Can 2012;43:547–52.

53. Rutkowski P, Gronchi A, Hohenberger P, et al. Neoadjuvant imatinib in locally advanced gastrointestinal stromal tumors (GIST): the EORTC STBSG experience. Ann Surg Oncol 2013;20(9):2937–43.

54. Hohenberger P, Eisenberg B. Role of surgery combined with kinase inhibition in the management of gastrointestinal stromal tumor (GIST). Ann Surg Oncol 2010; 17(10):2585–600.

55. Gronchi A, Raut CP. The combination of surgery and imatinib in GIST: a reality for localized tumors at high risk, an open issue for metastatic ones. Ann Surg Oncol 2012;19(4):1051–5.

56. LeCesne A, Van Glabbeke M, Verweij J, et al. Absence of progression as assessed by response evaluation criteria in solid tumors predicts survival in advanced GI stromal tumors treated with imatinib mesylate: the intergroup EORTC-ISG-AGITG phase III trial. J Clin Oncol 2009;27(24):3969–74.

57. Bonvalot S, Eldweny H, Péchoux CL, et al. Impact of surgery on advanced gastrointestinal stromal tumors (GIST) in the imatinib era. Ann Surg Oncol 2006;13(12):1596–603.

58. Haller F, Detken S, Schulten HJ, et al. Surgical management after neoadjuvant imatinib therapy in gastrointestinal stromal tumours (GISTs) with respect to imatinib resistance caused by secondary KIT mutations. Ann Surg Oncol 2007;14: 526–32.

59. Tirumani SH, Shinagare AB, Jagannathan JP, et al. Radiologic assessment of earliest, best, and plateau response of gastrointestinal stromal tumors to neoadjuvant imatinib prior to successful surgical resection. Eur J Surg Oncol 2014; 40(4):420–8.

60. Blesius A, Cassier PA, Bertucci F, et al. Neoadjuvant imatinib in patients with locally advanced non metastatic GIST in the prospective BFR14 trial. BMC Cancer 2011;11:72.

61. Rutkowski P, Nowecki ZI, Nyckowski P, et al. Surgical treatment of patients with initially inoperable and/or metastatic gastrointestinal stromal tumors (GIST) during therapy with imatinib mesylate. J Surg Oncol 2006;4:304–11.

62. Raut CP, Posner M, Desai J, et al. Surgical management of advanced gastrointestinal stromal tumors after treatment with targeted systemic therapy using kinase inhibitors. J Clin Oncol 2006;24(15):2325–31.

63. Sicklick JK, Lopez NE. Optimizing surgical and imatinib therapy for the treatment of gastrointestinal stromal tumors. J Gastrointest Surg 2013;17(11): 1997–2006.

64. Bumming P, Andersson J, Meis-Kindblom JM, et al. Neoadjuvant, adjuvant and palliative treatment of gastrointestinal stromal tumours (GIST) with imatinib: a centre-based study of 17 patients. Br J Cancer 2003;89(3):460–4.

65. de Vos tot Nederveen Cappel RJ, van Hillegersberg R, Rodenhuis S, et al. Downstaging of an advanced gastrointestinal stromal tumor by neoadjuvant imatinib. Dig Surg 2004;21(1):77–9.

66. Lo SS, Papachristou GI, Finkelstein SD, et al. Neoadjuvant imatinib in gastrointestinal stromal tumor of the rectum: report of a case. Dis Colon Rectum 2005; 48:1316–9.

67. Loughrey MB, Mitchell C, Mann GB, et al. Gastrointestinal stromal tumour treated with neoadjuvant imatinib. J Clin Pathol 2005;58:779–81.

68. Shah JN, Sun W, Seethala RR, et al. Neoadjuvant therapy with imatinib mesylate for locally advanced GI stromal tumor. Gastrointest Endosc 2005;61:625–7.

69. Goh BK, Chow PK, Chuah KL, et al. Pathologic, radiologic and PET scan response of gastrointestinal stromal tumors after neoadjuvant treatment with imatinib mesylate. Eur J Surg Oncol 2006;32:961–3.

70. Salazar M, Barata A, Andre S, et al. First report of a complete pathological response of a pelvic GIST treated with imatinib as neoadjuvant therapy. Gut 2006;55:585–6.

71. Andtbacka RH, Ng CS, Scaife CL, et al. Surgical resection of gastrointestinal stromal tumors after treatment with imatinib. Ann Surg Oncol 2007;14(1):14–24.

72. Fiore M, Palassini E, Fumagalli E, et al. Preoperative imatinib mesylate for unresectable or locally advanced primary gastrointestinal stromal tumors (GIST). Eur J Surg Oncol 2009;35(7):739–45.

73. Yoon KJ, Kim NK, Lee KY, et al. Efficacy of imatinib mesylate neoadjuvant treatment for a locally advanced rectal gastrointestinal stromal tumor. J Korean Soc Coloproctol 2011;27(3):147–52.

74. Li SX, Li ZY, Zhang LH, et al. Application of perioperative imatinib mesylate therapy in initial resectable primary local advanced gastrointestinal stromal tumor at intermediate or high risk. Zhonghua Wei Chang Wai Ke Za Zhi 2013;16(3): 226–9.

75. Katz D, Segal A, Alberton Y, et al. Neoadjuvant imatinib for unresectable gastrointestinal stromal tumor. Anticancer Drugs 2004;15:599–602.

76. Koontz MZ, Visser BM, Kunz PL. Neoadjuvant imatinib for borderline resectable GIST. J Natl Compr Canc Netw 2012;10:1477–82.

77. Xu J, Ling TL, Wang M, et al. Preoperative imatinib treatment in patients with advanced gastrointestinal stromal tumors: patient experiences and systematic review of 563 patients. Int Surg 2015;100(5):860–9.

78. Tielen R, Verhoef C, van Coevorden F, et al. Surgical treatment of locally advanced, non-metastatic, gastrointestinal stromal tumours after treatment with imatinib. Eur J Surg Oncol 2013;39(2):150–5.

79. Berney CR. Laparoscopic resection of locally advanced gastrointestinal stromal tumour (GIST) of the stomach following neoadjuvant imatinib chemoreduction. Int J Surg Case Rep 2015;8C:103–6.

80. Neofytou K, Costa Neves M, Giakoustidis A, et al. Effective downsizing of a large oesophageal gastrointestinal stromal tumour with neoadjuvant imatinib enabling an uncomplicated and without Tumour Rupture Laparoscopic-Assisted Ivor-Lewis Oesophagectomy. Case Rep Oncol Med 2015;2015: 165736.

81. Eisenberg BL, Harris J, Blanke CD, et al. Phase II trial of neoadjuvant/adjuvant imatinib mesylate (IM) for advanced primary and metastatic/recurrent operable gastrointestinal stromal tumor (GIST): early results of RTOG 0132/ACRIN 6665. J Surg Oncol 2009;99:42–7.

82. Wang D, Zhang Q, Blanke CD, et al. Phase II trial of neoadjuvant/adjuvant imatinib mesylate for advanced primary and metastatic/recurrent operable gastrointestinal stromal tumors: long-term follow-up results of Radiation Therapy Oncology Group 0132. Ann Surg Oncol 2012;19(4):1074–80.

83. Hohenberger P, Langer C, Wendtner CM, et al. Neoadjuvant treatment of locally advanced GIST: results of APOLLON, a prospective, open label phase II study in KIT- or PDGFRA-positive tumors. J Clin Oncol 2012;30(Suppl) [abstract: 10031].

84. Hohenberger P, Langer C, Pistorius S, et al. Indication and results of surgery following imatinib treatment of locally advanced or metastatic GI stromal tumors (GIST) [meeting abstracts]. J Clin Oncol 2006;24:9500.

85. McAuliffe JC, Hunt KK, Lazar AJ, et al. A randomized, phase II study of preoperative plus postoperative imatinib in GIST: evidence of rapid radiographic response and temporal induction of tumor cell apoptosis. Ann Surg Oncol 2009;16:910–9.

86. Rink L, Skorobogatko Y, Kossenkov AV, et al. Gene expression signatures and response to imatinib mesylate in gastrointestinal stromal tumor. Mol Cancer Ther 2009;8(8):2172–82.

87. Doyon C, Sidéris L, Leblanc G, et al. Prolonged therapy with imatinib mesylate before surgery for advanced gastrointestinal stromal tumor results of a phase II trial. Int J Surg Oncol 2012;2012:761576.

88. Tielen R, Verhoef C, van Coevorden F, et al. Surgical management of rectal gastrointestinal stromal tumors. J Surg Oncol 2013;107(4):320–3.

89. Heinrich MC, Corless CL, Demetri GD, et al. Kinase mutations and imatinib response in patients with metastatic gastrointestinal stromal tumor. J Clin Oncol 2003;21(23):4342–9.

90. Heinrich MC, Shoemaker JS, Corless CL, et al. Correlation of target kinase genotype with clinical activity of imatinib mesylate (IM) in patients with metastatic GI stromal tumors (GISTs) expressing KIT (KIT+) [meeting abstracts]. J Clin Oncol 2005;23(Suppl 16):7.

91. Debiec-Rychter M, Sciot R, Le Cesne A, et al. KIT mutations and dose selection for imatinib in patients with advanced gastrointestinal stromal tumours. Eur J Cancer 2006;42(8):1093–103.

92. Gastrointestinal Stromal Tumor Meta-Analysis Group (MetaGIST). Comparison of two doses of imatinib for the treatment of unresectable or metastatic gastrointestinal stromal tumors: a meta-analysis of 1,640 patients. J Clin Oncol 2010; 28(7):1247–53.

93. Debiec-Rychter M, Dumez H, Judson I, et al. Use of c-KIT/PDGFRA mutational analysis to predict the clinical response to imatinib in patients with advanced gastrointestinal stromal tumours entered on phase I and II studies of the EORTC Soft Tissue and Bone Sarcoma Group. Eur J Cancer 2004;40(5):689–95.

94. Corless CL, Ballman KV, Antonescu CR, et al. Pathologic and molecular features correlate with long-term outcome after adjuvant therapy of resected primary GI stromal tumor: the ACOSOG Z9001 trial. J Clin Oncol 2014;32(15):1563–70.
95. DeMatteo RP, Ballman KV, Antonescu CR, et al, American College of Surgeons Oncology Group (ACOSOG) Intergroup Adjuvant GIST Study Team for the Alliance for Clinical Trials in Oncology. Long-term results of adjuvant imatinib mesylate in localized, high-risk, primary gastrointestinal stromal tumor: ACOSOG Z9000 (Alliance) intergroup phase 2 trial. Ann Surg 2013;258(3):422–9.
96. Joensuu H, Eriksson M, Hartmann J, et al. Twelve versus 36 months of adjuvant imatinib (IM) as treatment of operable GIST with a high risk of recurrence: final results of a randomized trial (SSGXVIII/AIO). J Clin Oncol 2011;29:aLBA1.
97. Casali PG, Le Cesne A, Poveda Velasco A, et al. Time to definitive failure to the first tyrosine kinase inhibitor in localized gastrointestinal stromal tumors (GIST) treated with imatinib as an adjuvant: a randomized trial from the EORTC Soft Tissue and Bone Sarcoma Group (STBSG), Australasian Gastrointestinal Tumor Study Group (AGITG), UNICANCER, Italian Sarcoma Group (ISG), Spanish Group for Research on Sarcomas (GEIS). J Clin Oncol 2015;33(36):4276–83.
98. Kang B, Lee J, Ryu M, et al. A phase II study of imatinib mesylate as adjuvant treatment for curatively resected high-risk localized gastrointestinal stromal tumors. J Clin Oncol 2009;27 [abstract: e21515].
99. Li J, Gong JF, Wu AW, et al. Post-operative imatinib in patients with intermediate or high risk gastrointestinal stromal tumor. Eur J Surg Oncol 2011;37(4):319–24.
100. Blackstein ME, Corless CL, Ballman KV, et al, American College of Surgeons Oncology Group (ACOSOG) Intergroup. Risk assessment for tumor recurrence after surgical resection of localized primary gastrointestinal stromal tumor (GIST): North American Intergroup phase III trial ACOSOG Z9001. ASCO; 2010. Gastrointestinal Cancers Symposium. [abstract: 6].
101. Joensuu H. Adjuvant treatment of GIST: patient selection and treatment strategies. Nat Rev Clin Oncol 2012;9(6):351–8.
102. Rutkowski P, Przybyl J, Zdzienicki M. Extended adjuvant therapy with imatinib in patients with gastrointestinal stromal tumors. Mol Diagn Ther 2013;17(1):9–19.
103. Majer IM, Gelderblom H, van den Hout WB, et al. Cost-effectiveness of 3-year vs 1-year adjuvant therapy with imatinib in patients with high risk of gastrointestinal stromal tumour recurrence in the Netherlands; a modelling study alongside the SSGXVIII/AIO trial. J Med Econ 2013;16(9):1106–19.
104. Rutkowski P, Gronchi A. Efficacy and economic value of adjuvant imatinib for gastrointestinal stromal tumors. Oncologist 2013;18(6):689–96.
105. Joensuu H, Eriksson M, Sundby Hall K, et al. Three vs. 1 year of adjuvant imatinib (IM) for operable high-risk GIST: the second planned analysis of the randomized SSGXVIII/AIO trial. J Clin Oncol 2015;33(Suppl):2015 [abstract: 10505].
106. Joensuu H, Martin-Broto J, Nishida T, et al. Follow-up strategies for patients with gastrointestinal stromal tumour treated with or without adjuvant imatinib after surgery. Eur J Cancer 2015;51(12):1611–7.
107. Jiang WZ, Guan GX, Lu HS, et al. Adjuvant imatinib treatment after R0 resection for patients with high-risk gastrointestinal stromal tumors: a median follow-up of 44 months. J Surg Oncol 2011;104(7):760–4.
108. PERSIST 5.
109. Corless CL, Ballman KV, Antonescu C, et al. American College of Surgeons Oncology Group; relation of tumor pathologic and molecular features to outcome after surgical resection of localized primary gastrointestinal stromal

tumor (GIST): results of the intergroup phase III trial ACOSOG Z9001. J Clin Oncol 2010;28(15s) [abstract: 10006].

110. Casali PG, Blay JY. ESMO/CONTICANET/EUROBONET consensus panel of experts gastrointestinal stromal tumours: ESMO clinical practice guidelines for diagnosis, treatment and follow-up. Ann Oncol 2010;21(Suppl 5):v98–102.

111. Casali PG, Le Cesne A, Poveda Velasco A, et al. Imatinib failure-free survival (IFS) in patients with localized gastrointestinal stromal tumors (GIST) treated with adjuvant imatinib (IM): The EORTC/AGITG/FSG/GEIS/ISG randomized controlled phase III trial. J Clin Oncol 2013;31(Suppl) [abstract: 10500].

112. Reichardt P, Hartmann J, Sundby Hall K, et al. Response to imatinib rechallenge of GIST that recurs following completion of adjuvant imatinib treatment: the first analysis in the SSGXVIII/AIO trial patient population. European Multidisciplinary Cancer Congress 2011. Stockholm (Sweden), September 23–27, 2011.

113. Reichardt P, Blay JY, Boukovinas I, et al. Adjuvant therapy in primary GIST: state-of-the-art. Ann Oncol 2012;23(11):2776–81.

114. Rutkowski P, Andrzejuk J, Bylina E, et al. What are the current outcomes of advanced gastrointestinal stromal tumors: who are the long-term survivors treated initially with imatinib? Med Oncol 2013;30(4):765.

115. Mussi C, Ronellenfitsch U, Jakob J, et al. Post-imatinib surgery in advanced/metastatic GIST: is it worthwhile in all patients? Ann Oncol 2010;21(2):403–8.

116. Le Cesne A, Ray-Coquard I, Bui BN, et al. Discontinuation of imatinib in patients with advanced gastrointestinal stromal tumors after 3 years of treatment: an open-label multicentre randomised phase 3 trial. Lancet Oncol 2010;11(10):942–9.

117. Gronchi A, Fiore M, Miselli F, et al. Surgery of residual disease following molecular-targeted therapy with imatinib mesylate in advanced/metastatic GIST. Ann Surg 2007;245(3):341–6.

118. Du CY, Zhou Y, Song C, et al. Is there a role of surgery in patients with recurrent or metastatic gastrointestinal stromal tumours responding to imatinib: a prospective randomised trial in China. Eur J Cancer 2014;50:1772–8.

119. DeMatteo RP, Maki RG, Singer S, et al. Results of tyrosine kinase inhibitor therapy followed by surgical resection for metastatic gastrointestinal stromal tumor. Ann Surg 2007;245(3):347–52.

120. Bauer S, Rutkowski P, Hohenberger P, et al. Long-term follow-up of patients with GIST undergoing metastasectomy in the era of imatinib–analysis of prognostic factors (EORTC-STBSG collaborative study). Eur J Surg Oncol 2014;40(4):412–9.

121. Tielen R, Verhoef C, van Coevorden F, et al. Surgery after treatment with imatinib and/or sunitinib in patients with metastasized gastrointestinal stromal tumors: is it worthwhile? World J Surg Oncol 2012;10:111.

122. Rubió-Casadevall J, Martinez-Trufero J, Garcia-Albeniz X, et al. Spanish group for research on sarcoma (GEIS). Role of surgery in patients with recurrent, metastatic, or unresectable locally advanced gastrointestinal stromal tumors sensitive to imatinib: a retrospective analysis of the Spanish group for research on sarcoma (GEIS). Ann Surg Oncol 2015;22(9):2948–57.

123. Park SJ, Ryu MH, Ryoo BY, et al. The role of surgical resection following imatinib treatment in patients with recurrent or metastatic gastrointestinal stromal tumors: results of propensity score analyses. Ann Surg Oncol 2014;21(13):4211–7.

124. Cirocchi R, Farinella E, La Mura F, et al. Efficacy of surgery and imatinib mesylate in the treatment of advanced gastrointestinal stromal tumor: a systematic review. Tumori 2010;96(3):392–9.

125. Hohenberger P, Bonvalot S, Litiere S, et al. Surgical resection of metastatic GIST on imatinib delays recurrence and death: results of a cross-match comparison in the EORTC Intergroup 62005 study. CTOS; 2014.
126. Sym SJ, Ryu MH, Lee JL, et al. Surgical intervention following imatinib treatment in patients with advanced gastrointestinal stromal tumors (GISTs). J Surg Oncol 2008;98:27–33.
127. An HJ, Ryu MH, Ryoo BY, et al. The effects of surgical cytoreduction prior to imatinib therapy on the prognosis of patients with advanced GIST. Ann Surg Oncol 2013;20(13):4212–8.
128. Tse GH, Wong EH, O'Dwyer PJ. Resection of focally progressive gastrointestinal stromal tumours resistant to imatinib therapy. Surgeon 2012;10(6):309–13.
129. Raut CP, Wang Q, Manola J, et al. Cytoreductive surgery in patients with metastatic gastrointestinal stromal tumor treated with sunitinib malate. Ann Surg Oncol 2010;17(2):407–15.
130. Ruka W, Rutkowski P, Szawłowski A, et al. Surgical resection of residual disease in initially inoperable imatinib-resistant/intolerant gastrointestinal stromal tumor treated with sunitinib. Eur J Surg Oncol 2009;35(1):87–91.

Liposarcoma

Multimodality Management and Future Targeted Therapies

Aimee M. Crago, MD, PhD[a,b,c],*, Mark A. Dickson, MD[a,d,e]

KEYWORDS

- Sarcoma • Liposarcoma • Myxoid liposarcoma • Pleomorphic liposarcoma • CDK4
- MDM2 • FUS-CHOP • Trabectedin

KEY POINTS

- Common genomic events define 3 biological groups of liposarcoma (LPS) – amplification of 12q13–15 in well-differentiated LPS (WDLS) and dedifferentiated LPS (DDLS), FUS-DDIT3 translocation in myxoid LPS (MLS)/round cell LPS (RCLS), and complex genomic changes in pleomorphic LPS.
- Surgery is the gold standard for cure of LPS, but grade, histology, and tumor site (retroperitoneal vs extremity) determine prognosis and pattern of recurrence.
- Retroperitoneal LPSs are almost always well-differentiated and dedifferentiated tumors that recur locally even after complete surgical resection, so active research focuses on optimizing surgical protocols and defining the role of radiation in multimodality therapy.
- WDLS and DDLS are relatively chemoresistant; however, MLS/RCLS and pleomorphic LPSs respond well to cytotoxic therapies, and MLS/RCLS is particularly radiosensitive.
- Among targeted therapies, CDK4 inhibitors are effective in WDLS and DDLS, and trabectedin, which prevents FUS-DDIT3 binding to DNA, is effective in MLS/RCLS.

INTRODUCTION

LPS is one of the most common histologies of soft tissue sarcoma (STS), representing 50% of retroperitoneal and 25% of extremity STS.[1] There are 3 separate biologic groups of LPS encompassing 5 histologic subtypes. Each group is characterized by

The authors have nothing to disclose.
[a] Sarcoma Disease Management Team, Memorial Sloan Kettering Cancer Center, 1275 York Avenue, New York, NY 10065, USA; [b] Gastric and Mixed Tumor Service, Department of Surgery, Memorial Sloan Kettering Cancer Center, 1275 York Avenue, H1220, New York, NY 10065, USA; [c] Department of Surgery, Weill Cornell Medical College, 1300 York Avenue, New York, NY, USA; [d] Sarcoma Oncology Service, Department of Medicine, Memorial Sloan Kettering Cancer Center, 300 East 66th Street, New York, NY 10065, USA; [e] Department of Medicine, Weill Cornell Medical College, 1300 York Avenue, New York, NY 10065, USA
* Corresponding author. Gastric and Mixed Tumor Service, Department of Surgery, 1275 York Avenue, H1220, New York, NY 10065.
E-mail address: cragoa@mskcc.org

Surg Oncol Clin N Am 25 (2016) 761–773
http://dx.doi.org/10.1016/j.soc.2016.05.007
1055-3207/16/$ – see front matter © 2016 Elsevier Inc. All rights reserved.

surgonc.theclinics.com

specific genetic alterations presumed to drive tumor initiation (**Table 1**). WDLS and DDLS represent more than 60% of all LPS and are almost universally associated with amplification of chromosome segment 12q13–15, which carries the oncogenes *MDM2*, *CDK4*, and *HMGA2*.[2–6] More than 95% of MLS and RCLS carry a translocation of *FUS* and *DDIT3* (*CHOP*) genes.[7–9] Pleomorphic LPS has a complex karyotype often causing loss of tumor suppressors p53 and Rb.[5] This subtype, which is associated with a poor prognosis, is the rarest subtype of LPS, comprising approximately 5% of cases.[6]

Surgery remains the mainstay of treatment of LPS, but the 3 subgroups have highly variable response to systemic therapies, affecting recommendations regarding adjuvant therapy (**Table 2**). The different genomic underpinnings that define the groups mean that research has identified variable means of targeting these diseases using novel therapies. This article examines the data supporting current treatment strategies, including multimodality paradigms that integrate radiation and chemotherapy. Ongoing genomic and molecular studies elucidating novel methods for treating the diseases and results of clinical trials aimed at translating these findings into clinical practice are also examined.

WELL-DIFFERENTIATED LIPOSARCOMA AND DEDIFFERENTIATED LIPOSARCOMA

WDLS and DDLS are the most common histologic variants of LPS. DDLS represents progression of WDLS from an indolent, sometimes locally aggressive lesion to more rapidly growing disease with metastatic potential.[6,10,11] Five-year disease-specific survival in patients with DDLS is 44% compared with 93% in patients diagnosed with pure WDLS.[6] Genomic alterations are more complex in DDLS than in WDLS. In addition to amplification of 12q13–15, copy number alterations affecting segments of chromosome 11, 19, and 3, among others, are common in retroperitoneal DDLS and may affect genomic stability as well as prognosis.[12]

Management of Primary Well-differentiated Liposarcoma and Dedifferentiated Liposarcoma in the Extremity

Treatment strategies for WDLS/DDLS diagnosed in the extremity parallel those of STS in general[1]; however, diagnosis can often be made radiographically and not based on core biopsy. DDLS appears as an enhancing nodule in association with a lipomatous tumor (WDLS); the adipogenic component appears similar to fat on CT or MRI (**Fig. 1A**). High-grade DDLS is managed primarily with surgical resection. The tumor

---

Table 1
Genomic alterations in liposarcoma

Histologic Subtypes	Genomic Alterations	Affected Oncogenes	Clinical Correlation
Well-differentiated and dedifferentiated	12q13–15 amplification	MDM2 and CDK4	N/A
	3p14–21 loss	Unknown	Dedifferentiation
	11q23–24 loss	Unknown	Dedifferentiation, genomic instability
	19q13 loss	Unknown	Dedifferentiation, poor prognosis
Myxoid/round cell	FUS-DDIT3 translocation	Unknown	N/A
Pleomorphic	Rb/p53 loss	Rb and p53	N/A

Table 2
Clinical characteristics of liposarcoma histologic subtypes

Subtype	Local Recurrence Rate	Distal Recurrence Rate	Chemosensitivity	Radiosensitivity
Well-differentiated	Low	Low	Low	Moderate
Dedifferentiated	Moderate	Low	Low	Moderate
Myxoid	Low	Low	High	High
Round cell	Moderate	High	High	High
Pleomorphic	Moderate	High	High	Moderate

is removed with margins of 1 cm of normal tissue or a major fascial barrier circumferentially. Encasement of a major neurovascular structure may require resection with arterial reconstruction. When the tumor abuts the neurovascular bundle or bone, then the neurovascular sheath, perineurium, or periosteum can be resected as closest margin. Adjuvant radiation is used to reduce risk of local recurrence in cases of high-grade DDLS of the extremity that is greater than 5 cm in diameter or after R1 resection that cannot be improved without causing major morbidity. Radiation planned in the neoadjuvant setting is an indication for preoperative biopsy as opposed to clinical diagnosis. Because DDLS is relatively chemoresistant, systemic therapies are rarely used for localized DDLS.[13,14]

WDLS in the extremity is also termed atypical lipomatous tumor. As in the case of DDLS, diagnosis of WDLS can be suggested by preoperative imaging. WDLS appears as a lipomatous mass, with similar signal intensity as normal fat (**Fig. 1**B). The differential diagnosis for lipomatous mass in the extremity includes WDLS and lipoma. Final diagnosis is accurately determined only after pathologic evaluation of the surgically resected specimen, because core biopsy results are susceptible to sampling error, but WDLS may be suspected in deep lesions. WDLS tends to be larger than lipoma (>10 cm), diagnosed in older patients (≥55 years), and identified in the context of recurrence.[15] MRI may show enhancing septae in WDLS.[16] Outcomes for patients

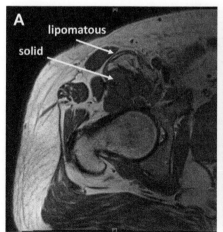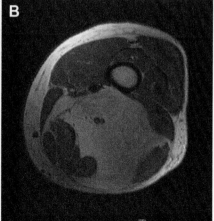

Fig. 1. MRI T1 images showing cross-sectional evaluation of (A) DDLS in the hip and (B) WDLS in the thigh. Arrows show lipomatous components representing a well-differentiated component of the dedifferentiated tumor and the nodular high-grade component.

with WDLS of the extremity are good, with 5-year and 10-year local recurrence-free survival rates of 100% and 78%, respectively; the tumors have no metastatic potential unless they have a dedifferentiated component.[17] The surgical approach can, therefore, be more conservative than that for DDLS. For example, WDLS that encases a neurovascular bundle may be bivalved to preserve the structures, and margins of less than 1 cm can be planned to optimize function and cosmesis. Similarly, radiation is generally deferred after resection of extremity WDLS, because even in the context of local recurrence, disease-related deaths are exceedingly rare.[17]

An algorithm for the treatment of localized WDLS/DDLS of the extremity (and other LPSs) is shown in **Fig. 2**.

Management of Primary Well-differentiated Liposarcoma and Dedifferentiated Liposarcoma of the Retroperitoneum

WDLS/DDLS is the most common type of STS in the retroperitoneum. Like extremity WDLS/DDLS, WDLS/DDLS of the retroperitoneum can often be diagnosed based on imaging studies. Highly suggestive of WDLS/DDLS is cross-sectional imaging demonstrating a lipomatous lesion with pushing borders and enhancing septae, with or without solid nodules. Surgery can be planned without biopsy when imaging is reviewed by an experienced diagnostician. The primary goal of surgery for retroperitoneal WDLS/DDLS should be complete gross resection of all disease. For retroperitoneal sarcoma, R2 resection is associated with significantly poorer outcomes than R0 or R1 resection, and, in most series, patients with gross residual disease have outcomes as poor as patients who did not undergo any surgery.[18] Whether R0 resections have better outcomes than R1 resections is unclear, because results have varied among the retrospective analyses of retroperitoneal sarcomas.[19,20] Therefore, there is no clear consensus regarding the importance of obtaining an R0 versus R1 resection.

This controversy regarding the role of R0 resection underlies ongoing debate on extended compartmental resection for patients with primary retroperitoneal disease, particularly because retroperitoneal WDLS/DDLS often recurs locally, and death is often caused by unresectable local recurrence that compresses visceral organs as opposed to distant metastases.[11] Retrospective series compared patients treated

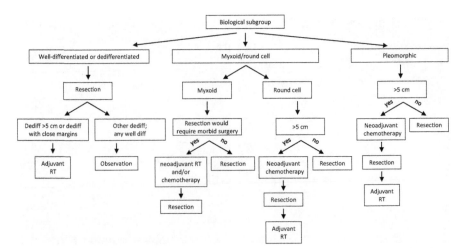

Fig. 2. Flow-diagram delineating basic treatment algorithm used for management of patients with localized LPS of the extremity. Dediff, dedifferentiated liposarcoma; RT, radiation therapy; Well diff, well-differentiated liposarcoma.

with excision of primary tumor, including surrounding fat and fascial planes (eg, kidney capsule) where feasible, with patients treated by extended compartmental resection, that is, removal of the tumor with surrounding organs where those organs would provide an additional 1-cm margin (eg, kidney, colon, pancreas, and spleen). Decreased rates of local recurrence were reported for the extended compartmental resection group, and, with longer follow-up, results suggested improvements in overall survival.[20–22] Many major sarcoma centers, however, have not adopted this practice, for reasons delineated in depth in multiple reviews.[23–25] Briefly, extended compartmental resection is criticized for high rates of postoperative morbidity and for the limited ability to optimize margins because most retroperitoneal lesions lie close to central vessels and unresectable organs (eg, liver and duodenum). Prior reports have also associated multivisceral organ resection with poorer outcomes for LPS, suggesting that the need for aggressive surgery to control disease may be a function of poor tumor biology.[11] More recent data suggest that rates of local recurrence (in the absence synchronous distant metastases) are highest in grade II (French or Fédération Nationale des Centres de Lutte Contre le Cancer [FNCLCC]) DDLS, so extended resections may be most appropriate for this subset.[26]

Most STS specialists agree on the need for complete gross resection of retroperitoneal WDLS/DDLS, and, as in the extremity, adjuvant systemic therapy is rarely considered. Given poor rates of response, systemic therapy is generally reserved for unresectable disease, in some instances preoperatively for marginally resectable disease, or in the context of metastatic disease. The role for radiation is debatable; radiation is considered at many institutions because of high rates of local recurrence. When given, it is generally as neoadjuvant to prevent injury to surrounding normal tissues. Adjuvant radiation causes, for example, small bowel enteritis in up to 60% of patients.[27] The efficacy of neoadjuvant radiation has been partially defined by 2 prospective series with a combined 72 patients, although only 40% of the patients had LPS and 25% had recurrent disease. Among the 54 radiation-treated patients who were able to undergo complete gross resection, 5-year local recurrence-free survival was 60% compared with nonirradiated historic controls, with 5-year local recurrence-free survivals of 30% to 60%.[28] The benefit was not clear-cut, however, and the role of neoadjuvant radiation in primary retroperitoneal sarcoma is currently being examined in a phase III, randomized European Organisation for Research and Treatment of Cancer trial.[29]

Management of Recurrent Disease

Local recurrence rates in the extremity are low, and follow-up can be performed with serial examinations or MRI yearly for WDLS (every 6 months for DDLS). Local recurrences of extremity disease are managed in much the same way as primary disease. If reoperation carries significant morbidity, WDLS recurrence can be observed with serial imaging, given its lack of metastatic potential. When surgery is required, all attempt is made to preserve the limb. Patients with DDLS should undergo chest imaging every 4 to 6 months, because distant recurrence of extremity DDLS is generally noted in the lung. Metastasectomy can be performed if technically favorable and if the patient has good prognostic indicators, such as a solitary site and long disease-free interval, with the caveat that these recommendations are generally based on studies covering a range of sarcoma histologies. For patients who had retroperitoneal WDLS/DDLS, distant recurrence is less often a problem although up to 22% of patients may develop metastatic disease in the lungs, but local recurrence is common. CT of the abdomen and pelvis is completed every 3 to 6 months in the first 2 years after surgery, then every 6 months for 2 years.[30] Chest imaging is indicated for patients treated for DDLS.

Because of the relative resistance of WDLS/DDLS to systemic therapy, surgical re-resection has been the standard management for recurrent disease. Resection of recurrent disease is associated, however, with increased rates of complications, so careful patient selection is essential in determining who may benefit from alternative treatments. Recurrent disease is rarely curable, and surgery should be seen as a temporizing measure and reserved for instances in which significant disease control is anticipated. Recurrence after re-resection is least frequent in patients who had a long disease-free interval and whose recurrence is small and not multifocal, so these characteristics identify ideal surgical candidates. In a multivariate analysis of 393 patients with primary or recurrent disease,[31] those with multifocal lesions had significantly poorer outcomes regardless of resectability. Patients with more than 7 lesions had 5-year overall survival of only 7%. This outcome was similar to that in patients undergoing incomplete gross resection.[31] Both disease-free interval and size of recurrence were examined in a study of 61 patients with retroperitoneal LPS undergoing resection of a first local recurrence. Patients with tumors that grew faster than 0.9 cm per month since the prior complete gross resection had median disease-specific survival of only 13 months.[32] Therefore, patients with rapid recurrence and multifocal disease are generally considered for systemic therapies, and operative intervention is reserved for palliation of symptoms.

Systemic Therapies for Well-differentiated Liposarcoma and Dedifferentiated Liposarcoma

Doxorubicin-based chemotherapy (either as a single agent or with ifosfamide) has been a standard treatment of recurrent STS for many years. In a retrospective review of 208 STS patients, the observed response rate to doxorubicin-based chemotherapy was 12%[33]; liposomal doxorubicin is also a reasonable option with comparable activity in STS.[34] Unfortunately, few patients with LPS were included in clinical trials, so histology-specific rates of response are unclear although it is considered a first-line treatment in most patients. Ifosfamide also has some single-agent activity in WDLS/DDLS.[35] Combination therapy with doxorubicin and ifosfamide in STS in general has been shown to improve response rates and progression-free survival (PFS) compared with doxorubicin alone but not to improve survival. Thus, single-agent therapy in the setting of recurrent disease is likely best for most patients unless the disease burden requires an urgent response to palliate symptoms. Dacarbazine shows some activity in second-line or third-line regimens, and the combination of gemcitabine and docetaxel is also widely used in advanced STS, although there are few data on response rates in WDLS/DDLS.[36] A subgroup analysis of a randomized phase II trial of gemcitabine versus gemcitabine and docetaxel showed 75% of patients with WDLS/DDLS had some stabilization of disease, although this was only durable (≥24 weeks) in 2 of 12 patients.[37]

Although a range of systemic options are available for patients with advanced WDLS/DDLS, they seem to have limited efficacy, at least compared with MLS and pleomorphic LPS. Therefore, significant effort has been made to identify targeted therapies for the disease by understanding the genetic events that drive tumorigenesis. As discussed previously, WDLS/DDLS almost universally has amplification of 12q13–15. A high-throughput small hairpin RNA screen of genes amplified on this chromosome identified more than 20 potential drivers of liposarcomagenesis. One of the most commonly amplified among these was CDK4, a cell-cycle regulator that promotes G1 to S phase transition by phosphorylating RB and inducing transcription of E2F targets.[5] Palbociclib, an inhibitor of CDK4, was recently Food and Drug Administration (FDA) approved for treatment in breast cancer, and an initial phase II trial of palbociclib in WDLS/DDLS has been reported.[38,39] In this report, examining 29 patients with unresectable WDLS/DDLS and disease progressing through prior treatments, PFS at 12 weeks was 66% and there was 1 partial response; median PFS was 4.7 months. Although these results do not approximate those for targeted therapy in other subtypes of STS (eg, imatinib in metastatic gastrointestinal stromal tumor), a small subset of patients had prolonged PFS of over a year.[39] Ongoing research is aimed at discovering predictive markers for response to palbociclib.[40]

Chromosome 12q13–15 also contains the *MDM2* gene. MDM2 promotes degradation of p53 to prevent apoptosis and/or cell-cycle arrest and may have p53-independent effects on alternative tumor suppressors, such as p21 and regulators of the epithelial-to-mesenchymal transition.[41–45] MDM2 inhibitors that prevent its binding to p53 (eg, Nutlin) have yielded promising results in vitro and in mouse xenografts.[46] In patient trials, however, MDM2 inhibitors have been associated with significant adverse events (up to 40% of patients), which have precluded their chronic administration.[47] Recent data suggest, however, that in vitro abrogation of MDM2 may exert cytostatic effects on the cell (senescence, an irreversible form of growth arrest) without altering cellular levels of p53.[40] Specific targeting of the p53-independent activities of MDM2 may have therapeutic potential and minimize toxicity, a hypothesis that warrants further study.

Some additional 12q13–15 amplicon genes, such as *YEATS4*, have been implicated in WDLS/DDLS, but research examining their oncogenic functions is limited, minimizing their impact on clinical therapeutics. Similarly, studies of dedifferentiation of WDLS have identified potential oncogenes and tumor suppressors that drive tumor progression, such as 11q23–25, 3p14–21, 3q29, and 19q13.[12] Although integrated copy number and gene expression data have implicated the loss of tumor suppressors, such as CEBP-α in dedifferentiation, mechanisms for inducing re-expression of such proteins have been elusive. One possible mechanism is targeting the epigenetic modification that contributes to down-regulation of these tumor suppressors. For example, methylation of the CEBP-α gene was identified in 10 of 42 DDLS samples (24%). Treatment of DDLS cell lines with demethylating agents induced cellular apoptosis in increased expression of CEBP-α.[48] Future studies are likely to examine these findings in greater depth as well as the findings of aberrant expression of receptor tyrosine kinases (eg, MET and AXL) and microRNAs (eg, mir-193b) in subsets of WDLS/DDLS.[48,49]

MYXOID LIPOSARCOMA AND ROUND CELL LIPOSARCOMA

MLS is identified primarily in the extremity and, unlike WDLS/DDLS, only rarely in the retroperitoneum. MLS uniformly has a translocation involving *FUS-DDIT3* or *EWSR1-DDIT3* fusion. Like most other translocation-associated STSs, MLS occurs in young patients (typically ages 35–55). Its histology spans a spectrum, with more small blue round cells or primitive round cells in the high-grade form (RCLS). Some debate exists regarding the percentage of round cells associated with poor prognosis, although the authors' institution uses a 5% cutpoint to define the high-grade RCLS as opposed to the low-grade MLS histology and generally considers diagnosis of the high-grade form a poor prognostic indicator.[6]

Multimodality Management of Primary Disease

Unlike in WDLS/DDLS, core biopsy is required to confirm diagnosis of MLS/RCLS and provide some insight into tumor grade. The surgical approach to MLS and RCLS of the extremity is, however, almost identical to that of WDLS/DDLS, with function-sparing procedures the standard of care.

The local recurrence risk of a low-grade MLS is exceedingly low. Based on a nomogram for extremity sarcomas, even a tumor over 5 cm in diameter with a microscopically positive margin has a risk of local recurrence of only approximately 15% 3 years postoperatively.[50] If margins are widely negative, this rate falls to less than 10%. This is concordant with a report that only 8% of patients with MLS experienced local recurrence at median follow-up of over 5 years.[51] Given this, the authors' practice has generally been to defer adjuvant radiation in patients with completely resected MLS, reserving radiation for patients with a significant round cell component. MLS/RCLS is most often in the thigh, and given the high morbidity associated with preoperative radiation in this region, the authors tend to prescribe radiation in the adjuvant setting unless a tumor were particularly close to the joint. Both MLS and RCLS are, however, more sensitive to radiation therapy than are other histologic subtypes; mean tumor volume of MLS on average is reduced by approximately 50% after neoadjuvant radiation.[52] Therefore, in rare cases of surgical resection expected to be morbid, neoadjuvant radiation can be considered, even for a low-grade lesion, to minimize the size of the surgical bed.

Both MLS and RCLS have metastatic potential. For MLS, metastasis is estimated to occur in approximately 10% of patients, whereas in RCLS the risk of developing distant disease leads to disease-specific survival of only approximately 60% of patients 10 years after complete resection.[6] The minimal risk associated with MLS means that adjuvant chemotherapy is not generally considered. In general, randomized trials have not shown benefit to adjuvant chemotherapy. Some experts have argued, however, that because most of these trials are performed on a cohort with mixed histologies, the treatment may still benefit patients with select histologies, and retrospective data support its use in patients with high-risk MLS/RCLS. In a retrospective cohort study, including 61 patients undergoing resection for MLS/RCLS, treatment with adjuvant or neoadjuvant ifosfamide-based chemotherapy was associated with a 22% improvement in disease-specific survival.[13] Up to 44% of patients with MLS/RCLS have objective responses to doxorubicin, suggesting that it is a uniquely chemosensitive subtype of STS.[53] The authors' practice has been to consider neoadjuvant doxorubicin and ifosfamide in high-risk lesions (RCLS >5 cm in largest diameter).

Management of Recurrent Disease

As discussed previously, MLS/RCLS has metastatic potential regardless of grade, unlike most STSs where low-grade lesions generally show little metastatic potential. The location of metastases also differs significantly from that of other STS. Although most STSs metastasize primarily to the lung, and NCCN guidelines suggest that regular imaging of the chest is sufficient to follow for evidence of distant disease, MLS/RCLS more commonly metastasizes to soft tissue sites, such as the retroperitoneal and axillary fat pads. MLS/RCLS can also metastasize to spine, so complete staging of a high-risk patient requires CT of the chest, abdomen and pelvis as well as MRI of the total spine.[54]

The relative chemosensitivity and radiosensitivity of MLS/RCLS means that, in many patients, metastases can be managed for years. Surgical resection of oligometastases is an option, and doxorubicin and ifosfamide yield at least partial responses in more than 40% of patients. Radiation yields 100% pathologic treatment response in a subset of radiated lesions, making palliative RT an important means of controlling disease as well.[52] An improved understanding of the biology of MLS/RCLS may also lead to novel therapeutics for advanced disease. Mutations in PI3 kinase and consequent Akt activation have been identified in almost 20% of MLS/RCLS, so PI3 kinase inhibitors have potential for select patients.[5]

More recently, results of clinical trials for trabectedin have been published and the FDA has approved its use for patients with metastatic LPS. The drug binds to the minor groove of DNA and causes the FUS-DDIT3 chimera to be displaced from promoters.[55] This promotes adipogenic differentiation in vitro. Trabectedin has been available in Europe since 2007 and was FDA approved in the United States in 2015 based on a randomized phase 3 trial. Patients with LPS (all subtypes) and leiomyosarcoma were eligible and the trial showed an improvement in PFS compared with treatment with dacarbazine.[56] The most substantial improvement in PFS was seen in patients with MLS/RCLS (median PFS 5.6 months with trabectedin vs 1.5 months with dacarbazine). A retrospective review of 51 patients with MLS/RCLS treated in Europe demonstrated a remarkable response rate of 51%.[57] Thus, although trabectedin is now available as a treatment in all patients with LPS, it is uniquely useful for the myxoid/round cell subtype.

The newest drug for LPS is eribulin, a novel microtubule inhibitor, which was approved by the FDA in 2016 based on a large phase 3 study comparing eribulin to dacarbazine.[58] Treatment with eribulin was associated with improved overall survival and PFS. Outcomes for the different LPS subtypes have not been reported. Thus, eribulin is a reasonable option for patients with all LPS subtypes, although trabectedin is preferred for MLS/RCLS. Another new drug for STS, pazopanib, has been tested in multiple subtypes of STS and ultimately was approved by the FDA in 2012. The phase 3 study, however, excluded patients with LPS because of low PFS rates observed in the earlier phase 2 study.[59] Thus, pazopanib is approved for STS but specifically not for LPS, and its use in LPS patients is considered off-label and supported by few data.

PLEOMORPHIC LIPOSARCOMA

Pleomorphic LPS is uniformly high grade and is the rarest subtype of LPS, representing only approximately 5% of cases. Surgical management and application of radiation parallel the management of other high-grade tumors (as discussed previously); all but the smallest tumors resected with wide margins are treated with adjuvant radiation. Outcomes for patients with pleomorphic LPS are poor. More than 50% of patients develop metastatic disease, and overall survival is poor.[6] Like RCLS, however, pleomorphic LPS responds to the doxorubicin and ifosfamide combination, and in retrospective studies neoadjuvant/adjuvant therapy has been associated with improved disease-specific survival.[13] Given this, the authors' practice has been to treat eligible patients and tumors greater than 5 cm in diameter with neoadjuvant chemotherapy before surgical resection.

Metastases generally occur in the lung, and serial pulmonary imaging is used to follow patients after complete resection. Doxorubicin and ifosfamide are used in the metastatic setting as in the adjuvant setting, although the tumors may also respond to gemcitabine-based therapies. As discussed previously, trabectedin and eribulin are also options for advanced disease. Significant work remains to be done to develop novel therapies for this disease. To date, most studies have failed to identify targetable aberrations and noted only consistent losses in p53 and Rb pathway proteins.[5] These genomic alterations are notoriously difficult to exploit for therapeutic benefit.

SUMMARY

LPS is one of the most common types of STS, although it includes 3 heterogeneous groups, WDLS/DDLS, MLS/RCLS, and pleomorphic LPS. Careful analyses have determined optimal surgical and adjuvant approaches to these diseases and delineated both commonalities between groups and variations in treatment response and genomic drivers. Surgery remains the gold standard to cure localized disease, but increased understanding of how each subtype of tumor responds to systemic and radiation therapies has improved the ability to manage these diseases (see **Fig. 2**). Similarly, an improved understanding of the genomic underpinnings of each disease is allowing rapidly identifying potential novel therapies. These therapies may have the ability to further alter treatment paradigms over the coming years.

ACKNOWLEDGMENTS

This work was supported by the Memorial Sloan-Kettering Cancer Center Core Grant (P30 CA008748) and the Kristen Ann Carr Fund. The authors thank Janet Novak for editorial assistance.

REFERENCES

1. Crago AM, Brennan MF. Principles in management of soft tissue sarcoma. Adv Surg 2015;49(1):107–22.
2. Mandahl N, Akerman M, Aman P, et al. Duplication of chromosome segment 12q15-24 is associated with atypical lipomatous tumors: a report of the CHAMP collaborative study group. CHromosomes and MorPhology. Int J Cancer 1996; 67(5):632–5.
3. Pedeutour F, Forus A, Coindre JM, et al. Structure of the supernumerary ring and giant rod chromosomes in adipose tissue tumors. Genes Chromosomes Cancer 1999;24(1):30–41.
4. Fletcher CD, Akerman M, Dal Cin P, et al. Correlation between clinicopathological features and karyotype in lipomatous tumors. A report of 178 cases from the Chromosomes and Morphology (CHAMP) Collaborative Study Group. Am J Pathol 1996;148(2):623–30.
5. Barretina J, Taylor BS, Banerji S, et al. Subtype-specific genomic alterations define new targets for soft-tissue sarcoma therapy. Nat Genet 2010;42(8):715–21.
6. Dalal KM, Kattan MW, Antonescu CR, et al. Subtype specific prognostic nomogram for patients with primary liposarcoma of the retroperitoneum, extremity, or trunk. Ann Surg 2006;244(3):381–91.
7. Knight JC, Renwick PJ, Dal Cin P, et al. Translocation t(12;16)(q13;p11) in myxoid liposarcoma and round cell liposarcoma: molecular and cytogenetic analysis. Cancer Res 1995;55(1):24–7.
8. Crozat A, Aman P, Mandahl N, et al. Fusion of CHOP to a novel RNA-binding protein in human myxoid liposarcoma. Nature 1993;363(6430):640–4.
9. Rabbitts TH, Forster A, Larson R, et al. Fusion of the dominant negative transcription regulator CHOP with a novel gene FUS by translocation t(12;16) in malignant liposarcoma. Nat Genet 1993;4(2):175–80.
10. McCormick D, Mentzel T, Beham A, et al. Dedifferentiated liposarcoma. Clinicopathologic analysis of 32 cases suggesting a better prognostic subgroup among pleomorphic sarcomas. Am J Surg Pathol 1994;18(12):1213–23.
11. Singer S, Antonescu CR, Riedel E, et al. Histologic subtype and margin of resection predict pattern of recurrence and survival for retroperitoneal liposarcoma. Ann Surg 2003;238(3):358–70 [discussion: 370–1].
12. Crago AM, Socci ND, Decarolis P, et al. Copy number losses define subgroups of dedifferentiated liposarcoma with poor prognosis and genomic instability. Clin Cancer Res 2012;18(5):1334–40.

13. Eilber FC, Eilber FR, Eckardt J, et al. The impact of chemotherapy on the survival of patients with high-grade primary extremity liposarcoma. Ann Surg 2004; 240(4):686–95 [discussion: 695–7].

14. Woll PJ, Reichardt P, Le Cesne A, et al. Adjuvant chemotherapy with doxorubicin, ifosfamide, and lenograstim for resected soft-tissue sarcoma (EORTC 62931): a multicentre randomised controlled trial. Lancet Oncol 2012;13(10):1045–54.

15. Fisher SB, Baxter KJ, Staley CA 3rd, et al. The General Surgeon's quandary: atypical lipomatous tumor vs lipoma, who needs a surgical oncologist? J Am Coll Surg 2013;217(5):881–8.

16. Jelinek JS, Kransdorf MJ, Shmookler BM, et al. Liposarcoma of the extremities: MR and CT findings in the histologic subtypes. Radiology 1993;186(2):455–9.

17. Kooby DA, Antonescu CR, Brennan MF, et al. Atypical lipomatous tumor/well-differentiated liposarcoma of the extremity and trunk wall: importance of histological subtype with treatment recommendations. Ann Surg Oncol 2004;11(1): 78–84.

18. Crago AM, Singer S. Clinical and molecular approaches to well differentiated and dedifferentiated liposarcoma. Curr Opin Oncol 2011;23(4):373–8.

19. Lewis JJ, Leung D, Woodruff JM, et al. Retroperitoneal soft-tissue sarcoma: analysis of 500 patients treated and followed at a single institution. Ann Surg 1998; 228(3):355–65.

20. Bonvalot S, Rivoire M, Castaing M, et al. Primary retroperitoneal sarcomas: a multivariate analysis of surgical factors associated with local control. J Clin Oncol 2009;27(1):31–7.

21. Bonvalot S, Miceli R, Berselli M, et al. Aggressive surgery in retroperitoneal soft tissue sarcoma carried out at high-volume centers is safe and is associated with improved local control. Ann Surg Oncol 2010;17(6):1507–14.

22. Gronchi A, Lo Vullo S, Fiore M, et al. Aggressive surgical policies in a retrospectively reviewed single-institution case series of retroperitoneal soft tissue sarcoma patients. J Clin Oncol 2009;27(1):24–30.

23. Pisters PW. Resection of some – but not all – clinically uninvolved adjacent viscera as part of surgery for retroperitoneal soft tissue sarcomas. J Clin Oncol 2009;27(1):6–8.

24. Gronchi A, Pollock R. Surgery in retroperitoneal soft tissue sarcoma: a call for a consensus between Europe and North America. Ann Surg Oncol 2011;18(8): 2107–10.

25. Crago AM. Extended surgical resection and histology in retroperitoneal sarcoma. Ann Surg Oncol 2015;22(5):1401–3.

26. Gronchi A, Miceli R, Allard MA, et al. Personalizing the approach to retroperitoneal soft tissue sarcoma: histology-specific patterns of failure and postrelapse outcome after primary extended resection. Ann Surg Oncol 2015;22(5):1447–54.

27. Ballo MT, Zagars GK, Pollock RE, et al. Retroperitoneal soft tissue sarcoma: an analysis of radiation and surgical treatment. Int J Radiat Oncol Biol Phys 2007; 67(1):158–63.

28. Pawlik TM, Pisters PW, Mikula L, et al. Long-term results of two prospective trials of preoperative external beam radiotherapy for localized intermediate- or high-grade retroperitoneal soft tissue sarcoma. Ann Surg Oncol 2006;13(4): 508–17.

29. EORTC. A phase III randomized study of preoperative radiotherapy plus surgery versus surgery alone for patients with Retroperitoneal sarcomas (RPS) - STRASS. Available at: http://www.eortc.be/clinicaltrials/Details.asp?Protocol=62092&T=. Accessed January 29, 2016.

30. Tirumani SH, Tirumani H, Jagannathan JP, et al. Metastasis in dedifferentiated liposarcoma: Predictors and outcome in 148 patients. Eur J Surg Oncol 2015; 41(7):899–904.

31. Anaya DA, Lahat G, Liu J, et al. Multifocality in retroperitoneal sarcoma: a prognostic factor critical to surgical decision-making. Ann Surg 2009;249(1):137–42.

32. Park JO, Qin LX, Prete FP, et al. Predicting outcome by growth rate of locally recurrent retroperitoneal liposarcoma: the one centimeter per month rule. Ann Surg 2009;250(6):977–82.

33. Italiano A, Cioffi A, Penel N, et al. Comparison of doxorubicin and weekly paclitaxel efficacy in metastatic angiosarcomas. Cancer 2012;118(13):3330–6.

34. Judson I, Radford JA, Harris M, et al. Randomised phase II trial of pegylated liposomal doxorubicin (DOXIL/CAELYX) versus doxorubicin in the treatment of advanced or metastatic soft tissue sarcoma: a study by the EORTC Soft Tissue and Bone Sarcoma Group. Eur J Cancer 2001;37(7):870–7.

35. Martin-Liberal J, Alam S, Constantinidou A, et al. Clinical activity and tolerability of a 14-day infusional Ifosfamide schedule in soft-tissue sarcoma. Sarcoma 2013; 2013:868973.

36. Garcia-Del-Muro X, Lopez-Pousa A, Maurel J, et al. Randomized phase II study comparing gemcitabine plus dacarbazine versus dacarbazine alone in patients with previously treated soft tissue sarcoma: a Spanish Group for Research on Sarcomas study. J Clin Oncol 2011;29(18):2528–33.

37. Maki RG, Wathen JK, Patel SR, et al. Randomized phase II study of gemcitabine and docetaxel compared with gemcitabine alone in patients with metastatic soft tissue sarcomas: results of sarcoma alliance for research through collaboration study 002 [corrected]. J Clin Oncol 2007;25(19):2755–63.

38. Beaver JA, Amiri-Kordestani L, Charlab R, et al. FDA approval: palbociclib for the treatment of postmenopausal patients with estrogen receptor-positive, HER2-negative metastatic breast cancer. Clin Cancer Res 2015;21(21):4760–6.

39. Dickson MA, Tap WD, Keohan ML, et al. Phase II trial of the CDK4 inhibitor PD0332991 in patients with advanced CDK4-amplified well-differentiated or dedifferentiated liposarcoma. J Clin Oncol 2013;31(16):2024–8.

40. Kovatcheva M, Liu DD, Dickson MA, et al. MDM2 turnover and expression of ATRX determine the choice between quiescence and senescence in response to CDK4 inhibition. Oncotarget 2015;6(10):8226–43.

41. Haupt Y, Maya R, Kazaz A, et al. Mdm2 promotes the rapid degradation of p53. Nature 1997;387(6630):296–9.

42. Kubbutat MH, Jones SN, Vousden KH. Regulation of p53 stability by Mdm2. Nature 1997;387(6630):299–303.

43. Jin Y, Lee H, Zeng SX, et al. MDM2 promotes p21waf1/cip1 proteasomal turnover independently of ubiquitylation. EMBO J 2003;22(23):6365–77.

44. Zhang Z, Wang H, Li M, et al. Stabilization of E2F1 protein by MDM2 through the E2F1 ubiquitination pathway. Oncogene 2005;24(48):7238–47.

45. Wang SP, Wang WL, Chang YL, et al. p53 controls cancer cell invasion by inducing the MDM2-mediated degradation of Slug. Nat Cell Biol 2009;11(6):694–704.

46. Singer S, Socci ND, Ambrosini G, et al. Gene expression profiling of liposarcoma identifies distinct biological types/subtypes and potential therapeutic targets in well-differentiated and dedifferentiated liposarcoma. Cancer Res 2007;67(14):6626–36.

47. Ray-Coquard I, Blay JY, Italiano A, et al. Effect of the MDM2 antagonist RG7112 on the P53 pathway in patients with MDM2-amplified, well-differentiated or

dedifferentiated liposarcoma: an exploratory proof-of-mechanism study. Lancet Oncol 2012;13(11):1133–40.

48. Taylor BS, DeCarolis PL, Angeles CV, et al. Frequent alterations and epigenetic silencing of differentiation pathway genes in structurally rearranged liposarcomas. Cancer Discov 2011;1(7):587–97.

49. Peng T, Zhang P, Liu J, et al. An experimental model for the study of well-differentiated and dedifferentiated liposarcoma; deregulation of targetable tyrosine kinase receptors. Lab Invest 2011;91(3):392–403.

50. Cahlon O, Brennan MF, Jia X, et al. A postoperative nomogram for local recurrence risk in extremity soft tissue sarcomas after limb-sparing surgery without adjuvant radiation. Ann Surg 2012;255(2):343–7.

51. Hoffman A, Ghadimi MP, Demicco EG, et al. Localized and metastatic myxoid/round cell liposarcoma: clinical and molecular observations. Cancer 2013; 119(10):1868–77.

52. Pitson G, Robinson P, Wilke D, et al. Radiation response: an additional unique signature of myxoid liposarcoma. Int J Radiat Oncol Biol Phys 2004;60(2):522–6.

53. Patel SR, Burgess MA, Plager C, et al. Myxoid liposarcoma. Experience with chemotherapy. Cancer 1994;74(4):1265–9.

54. Schwab JH, Boland PJ, Antonescu C, et al. Spinal metastases from myxoid liposarcoma warrant screening with magnetic resonance imaging. Cancer 2007;110(8):1815–22.

55. Di Giandomenico S, Frapolli R, Bello E, et al. Mode of action of trabectedin in myxoid liposarcomas. Oncogene 2014;33(44):5201–10.

56. Demetri GD, von Mehren M, Jones RL, et al. Efficacy and Safety of Trabectedin or Dacarbazine for Metastatic Liposarcoma or Leiomyosarcoma After Failure of Conventional Chemotherapy: Results of a Phase III Randomized Multicenter Clinical Trial. J Clin Oncol 2016;34(8):786–93.

57. Grosso F, Jones RL, Demetri GD, et al. Efficacy of trabectedin (ecteinascidin-743) in advanced pretreated myxoid liposarcomas: a retrospective study. Lancet Oncol 2007;8(7):595–602.

58. Schoffski P, Chawla S, Make RG, et al. Randomized, open-label, multicenter, phase III study of eribulin versus dacarbazine in patients (pts) with leiomyosarcoma (LMS) and adipocytic sarcoma (ADI). J Clin Oncol 2015;33(Suppl) [abstract: LBA10502].

59. Sleijfer S, Ray-Coquard I, Papai Z, et al. Pazopanib, a multikinase angiogenesis inhibitor, in patients with relapsed or refractory advanced soft tissue sarcoma: a phase II study from the European organisation for research and treatment of cancer-soft tissue and bone sarcoma group (EORTC study 62043). J Clin Oncol 2009;27(19):3126–32.

Myxofibrosarcoma

Christina L. Roland, MD[a],*, Wei-Lien Wang, MD[b],
Alexander J. Lazar, MD, PhD[b], Keila E. Torres, MD, PhD[a]

KEYWORDS

- Myxofibrosarcoma • Surgery • MRI • Recurrence

KEY POINTS

- Myxofibrosarcoma is a unique subtype of soft tissue sarcoma with a locally infiltrative behavior and a predilection for local recurrence.
- Histology reveals a highly myxoid neoplasm with a distinctly hypocellular appearance, although some lesions have more cellular areas and can be higher grade.
- Patients presenting with a diagnosis of myxofibrosarcoma should undergo high-quality T1- and T2-weighted MRI with pre- and postgadolinium imaging to accurately define the extent of the disease.
- Wide surgical resection with a 2 cm soft tissue margin encompassing the entire area of increased signal on T2-weighted MRI is required, which can require complex vascular and plastic surgery reconstruction.
- A subset of patients with higher-grade lesions will develop distant metastases.

INTRODUCTION: NATURE OF THE PROBLEM

Myxofibrosarcoma (MFS) is a unique subtype of soft tissue sarcoma often characterized by a diffusely infiltrative pattern. This represents approximately 5% of soft tissue sarcoma diagnoses (**Fig. 1**). With the introduction of more stringent morphologic and immunohistochemical criteria in 2002 and reaffirmed in 2013, the World Health Organization (WHO) renamed the myxoid variant of malignant fibrous histiocytoma (MFH) with a predominant myxoid component (>50%) myxofibrosarcoma.[1,2] Series of MFS and myxoid MFH studies describe these tumors as having a significant propensity for local recurrence, while exhibiting an overall better prognosis when compared with other complex karyotype sarcomas such as leiomyosarcoma.[3–5] Given its relatively recent recognition as a distinct pathologic entity, the clinical behavior and outcomes for patients with MFS are uncertain, and there are no randomized trials to guide treatment protocols.

Disclosure: The authors have nothing to disclose.
[a] Department of Surgical Oncology, University of Texas MD Anderson Cancer Center, 1400 Pressler Street, Unit 1484, Houston, TX 77030, USA; [b] Department of Pathology, University of Texas MD Anderson Cancer Center, 1515 Holcombe Boulevard, Unit 0085, Houston, TX 77030, USA
* Corresponding author.
E-mail address: clroland@mdanderson.org

Surg Oncol Clin N Am 25 (2016) 775–788
http://dx.doi.org/10.1016/j.soc.2016.05.008
surgonc.theclinics.com

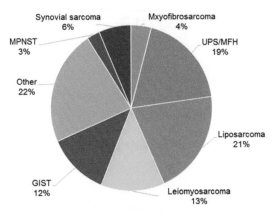

Fig. 1. Frequency by histology for patients with soft tissue sarcoma treated at MD Anderson Cancer Center (MDACC) between 2008 to 2013 (n = 3574). *UPS/MFH* undifferentiated pleomorphic sarcoma, *GIST* gastrointestinal stromal tumor, *MPNST* malignant peripheral nerve sheath tumor.

Therefore, treatment decisions and understanding of this disease are based on case–control and retrospective studies.

PATHOPHYSIOLOGY

Myxofibrosarcoma was first formally described in 1977.[6] Diagnostic terminology has evolved over the years and thus merits some further discussion. In the original 1977 description in the journal *Cancer*, Enzinger and Weiss used the terminology "myxoid variant of malignant fibrous histiocytoma." They noted that the myxoid variant of MFH had extensive, distinct myxoid features and exhibited less aggressive behavior than storiform or pleomorphic MFH.[6] Use of the term myxofibrosarcoma extends back to at least 1951.[7] However, it was only in the late 1970s that this terminology was applied to this specific entity.[8] In the 1990s, MFH attracted attention as a potentially problematic and possibly nonspecific diagnostic category likely contaminated with multiple entities.[9–11] Among the multiple histologic types of MFH, attempts were made to help better distinguish myxofibrosarcoma as a separate diagnostic category.[10] Malignant fibrous histiocytoma (MFH) was renamed undifferentiated pleomorphic sarcoma (UPS) and was defined as a diagnosis of exclusion in both the 2002 and 2013 WHO Classification of Tumors of Soft Tissue and Bone.[1,2] Given the use of modern methods including immunohistochemistry and molecular studies, UPS is now better defined and much less likely to be contaminated by mimics such as poorly differentiated carcinoma or spindle cell melanoma. Under the current WHO classification, the preferred diagnostic terminology for tumors formerly referred as myxoid malignant fibrous histiocytoma is myxofibrosarcoma.

Not surprisingly, given the alterations in diagnostic terminology, the diagnostic criteria for myxofibrosarcoma have also evolved over the years. The original 1977 description detailed a grossly multilobular tumor with mucoid features on cut surface (**Fig. 2**). Histology reveals a highly myxoid neoplasm with a distinctly hypocellular appearance (**Fig. 3**A). The myxoid areas are sparsely populated spindle cells or sometimes pleomorphic cells embedded in a matrix of the acid mucopolysaccharides (**Fig. 3**B, C). Due to the myxoid features, the vasculature is distinct. Areas of more diffuse cellularity are often present (**Fig. 3**D), and these areas often have conspicuous

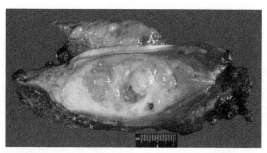

Fig. 2. Gross appearance of myxofibrosarcoma. The tumor is composed of lobulated areas of myxoid and nonmyxoid areas.

mitotic activity that is not usually a feature of the highly myxoid areas. Sometimes pseudo-lipoblasts (multivacuolated cells filled with mucin rather than lipid, see inset **Fig. 3**E) are apparent in myxoid areas. It was recognized early on that areas of this myxofibrosarcoma may show much higher degrees of cellularity that were indistinguishable from malignant fibrous histiocytoma or what is now called undifferentiated pleomorphic sarcoma.[6,12,13] The original 1997 article demonstrated that the degree of hypercellularity was related to the ultimate metastatic potential of these neoplasms.[6] Rarely, myxofibrosarcoma can show epithelioid cellularity rather than spindle cells admixed within the myxoid areas or growing as a diffusely cellular proliferation (**Fig. 4**). These epithelioid myxofibrosarcomas appear to behave more aggressively than their traditional spindle cell counterparts.[14]

Although the hypocellular myxoid component of myxofibrosarcoma is relatively easy to recognize, there has been debate in the field over how much of the neoplasm must be comprised of this hypocellular myxoid component in order to diagnose this entity. Opinions vary widely, with requirements of as much as 75% to as little as 5% hypercellular myxoid content.[3,6,8,13,15,16] Furthermore, myxofibrosarcoma can progress to a completely cellular neoplasm devoid of a myxoid component that is indistinguishable from UPS (see **Fig. 3**D). There is a tendency for myxofibrosarcomas to become more cellular over time and with local recurrence, suggesting this is a form of tumor progression in at least some cases. Neoplasms composed mainly of the hypocellular myxoid component tend to show local recurrence rather than distant metastasis.[3] A recent paper by Singer and colleagues indicates that even a minimal hypocellular myxoid component of at least 5% confers a better prognosis for myxofibrosarcoma relative to undifferentiated pleomorphic sarcoma lacking this myxoid component.[15] They thus suggest defining myxofibrosarcoma as having at least a 5% hypocellular myxoid component, while anything with less than 5% myxoid is best considered as undifferentiated pleomorphic sarcoma. Given the virtually complete morphologic overlap of the hypercellular and generally nonmyxoid portions of myxofibrosarcoma with undifferentiated pleomorphic sarcoma, distinguishing these 2 entities can be challenging when only a minimal myxoid component is present. At the authors' institution, a cut-off of roughly 20% characteristic myxoid component is used for the diagnosis of myxofibrosarcoma.

Myxofibrosarcoma can be graded under the FNCLCC (Fédération Nationale des Centres de Lutte Contre le Cancer) system.[17] Hypocellular cases tend have low mitotic activity and no necrosis and are thus considered low-grade when the entire lesion is composed of this characteristic component. Areas of increased cellularity

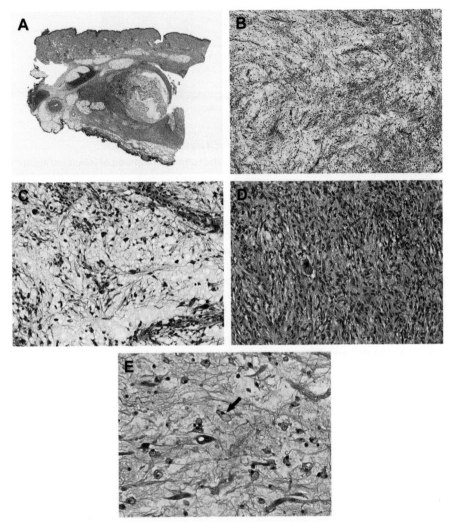

Fig. 3. Histologic appearance of myxofibrosarcoma. (*A*) Low power reveals lobular architecture with myxoid areas and less myxoid, more cellular areas. (*B, C*) Higher-power examination of myxoid areas reveals the prominent myxoid stroma, spindle cells with mild-to-moderate atypia, thin-walled vessels; mitotic activity is generally very low. (*D*) More cellular areas have less myxoid stroma, often composed of more atypical spindled-to-pleomorphic cells. These areas are reminiscent of undifferentiated pleomorphic sarcoma and often demonstrate prominent mitotic activity. (*E*) Scattered pseudolipoblasts are sometimes encountered in the myxoid areas (*arrow*). These cells have a vacuolated appearance but are filled with mucin and not lipids and should not be interpreted as evidence of lipogenic differentiation.

with mitotic activity result in designation of a higher grade. Many of these neoplasms turn out to be intermediate- rather than high-grade, as the tumor differentiation score for myxofibrosarcoma is 2, in contrast to undifferentiated pleomorphic sarcoma, which is assigned a differentiation score of 3. Thus, myxofibrosarcoma must exhibit both high mitotic rate and necrosis to achieve a designation of high-grade under the FNCLCC system. However, many institutions and the American Joint Committee

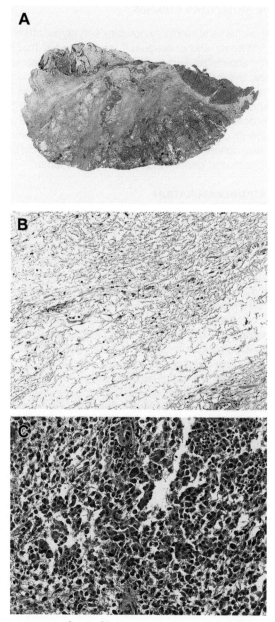

Fig. 4. Histologic appearance of myxofibrosarcoma with epithelioid features. (*A*) Low power reveals myxoid and more cellular areas. (*B*) Myxoid areas can be prominent and relatively devoid of atypical cellularity. (*C*) More cellular areas contain epithelioid cells that can become diffuse.

on Cancer (AJCC), group intermediate- and high-grade tumors into 1 category for purposes of staging given that intermediate sarcomas have some potential for distant metastasis.[18] Given the challenges and debate in the literature regarding the diagnostic criteria and grading, management approaches vary for the more cellular and higher-grade myxofibrosarcomas.

CYTOGENETICS AND MOLECULAR FINDINGS

Most cases of MFS demonstrate a highly complex karyotype, often with tripoid or tetrapoid alterations.[6] Willems and colleagues[19] demonstrated that most cases have complex cytogenetic anomalies, and such alterations were observed in tumors of all grades. Furthermore, this group observed that the tumors that locally recurred had more complex cytogenetic aberrations when compared with those that did not recur. Based on this observation, the authors proposed the concept of MFS progression as a multistep genetic process that is lead by genetic instability. MFS is among the sarcoma subtypes currently being characterized by The Cancer Genome Atlas (TCGA) for sarcoma, and this collaborative project should provide additional insights into the relatively uncharacterized genomic landscape of this tumor.

CLINICAL PRESENTATION/EXAMINATION

MFS usually affects older patients (**Table 1**).[6,13,16] Although the age range is broad, most patients are in their fifth to seventh decades of life, and men are affected slightly more often than women. The most common sites of presentation are the extremities (77%), with a predilection for the lower extremities (**Fig. 5**A). MFS tumors can also be located on the trunk (12%) and head and neck region (3%), but to a lesser extent.[13] MFS is uncommon in the abdominal cavity and retroperitoneum. It has been reported in the skin, breast, heart, and paratesticular region.

The tumor most commonly arises as a slowly enlarging, painless mass. It may present as a predominantly deep or subcutaneous multinodular growth (**Fig. 5**B). Mentzel and colleagues[16] classified MFS into 2 groups: superficial (dermal/subcutaneous) and deep (intramuscular/mainly subfascial). The superficial group tends to infiltrate through the fascia, whereas the deep lesions tend to form a single discrete mass. The superficial lesions may involve the dermal layer and present as a cutaneous lesion as well. Deep-seated lesions tend to be less nodular and can demonstrate an infiltrative growth pattern. Usually, they are larger than their superficial counterparts.

DIAGNOSTIC PROCEDURES

One of the major challenges of myxofibrosarcoma is to define the boundaries of the tumor. As with other soft tissue sarcomas of the extremity, MRI is the diagnostic modality of choice. MFS has low attenuation on computed tomography (CT) and shows low-to-intermediate signal on T1-weighted MRI (**Fig. 6**A). The solid and myxomatous components both show high signal on T2-weighted MRI, with the myxoid component showing higher signal intensity similar to that of fluid (**Figs. 6**B–D). Nodular and peripheral enhancement is often seen in the solid components.

MFS often show abnormal signal infiltration along the facial plan on MRI that correspond to an infiltrative growth pattern histologically, named the "tail sign (**Figs. 6**B and D)."[5,20] One of the first groups to evaluate the diagnostic value of the tail sign in

Table 1 Clinical features of myxofibrosarcoma	
Features	**Low-Grade Myxofibrosarcoma**
Peak age	Elderly
Depth	Subcutaneous tissue
Stroma	Usually uniformly myxoid
Atypia	Present

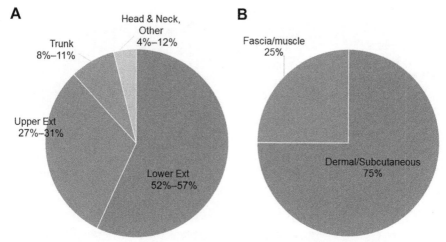

Fig. 5. Distribution of myxofibrosarcoma tumors by (*A*) site and (*B*) tumor depth. (*Data from* Refs.[3,13,16])

a large number of patients with MFS was Kaya and colleagues.[20] Eighty-one percent of MFS tumors had a multidirectional signal spreading along the facial plane (tail sign) on T2-weighted MRI. Interestingly, the authors found histologic infiltrative growth pattern on patients with focal growth pattern on MRI. The discrepancy may be due to the use of T2-weighted images instead of gadolinium-enhanced images that can depict tumor infiltration more accurately. Lefkowitz and colleagues[21] sought to determine whether the tail sign is helpful in distinguishing myxofibrosarcoma from other myxoid-containing neoplasms. In a group of 44 MFS, the tail sign was observed by 3 radiologists, with a sensitivity of 64% to 77% and a specificity of 79% to 90% among myxoid-predominant lesions. In addition, this group also found that the lesions demonstrated an infiltrative growth pattern histologically regardless of the MRI characteristics, emphasizing the importance of clearly defining the extent of disease with imaging prior to resection. Yoo and colleagues[22] observed that tumors that had a focal growth pattern on T2-weighted images would also demonstrate a tail sign on postcontrast images. Tails at MRI are not unique to MFS; they are also observed in other soft tissue tumors such as unclassified sarcomas.[22] Waters and colleagues[5] evaluated the features of recurrent low-grade myxofibrosarcoma lesions on CT and MRI imaging and found the tail sign was present in recurrent disease as well.

The infiltrative growth pattern of low-grade myxofibrosarcoma can result in anatomically deceptive boundaries at surgery because of microscopic extension into the dermis and skeletal muscles.[5,23] A completely infiltrative growth pattern along facial planes without the formation of a discrete nodular lesion has been described in some cases. Given the various clinical and histopathologic appearances of this tumor, the potential for diagnostic and staging errors highlights the importance of multidisciplinary, preoperative planning. As part of the preoperative imaging, it is critical that patients presenting with a diagnosis of MFS undergo high-quality T1- and T2-weighted MRI with pre-and postgadolinium imaging.

THERAPEUTIC OPTIONS/SURGICAL TECHNIQUE

Margin-negative surgical resection is the cornerstone of treatment for patients with soft tissue sarcoma, including MFS. In the 1970s, half of patients presenting with

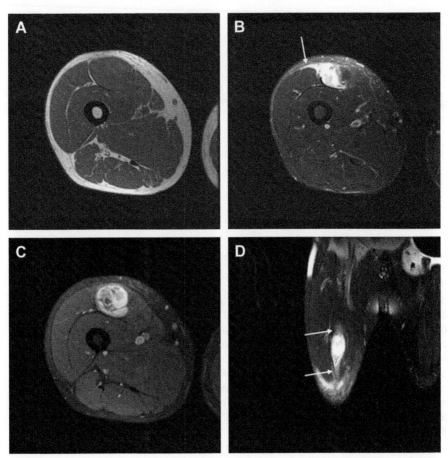

Fig. 6. A 54-year-old man with 7.3 cm myxofibrosarcoma of the right thigh. (*A–C*) Axial views. (*D*) Coronal view demonstrates a fusiform intramuscular soft tissue tumor in the rectus femoris muscle in the right midthigh. The lobulated intramuscular tumor is isointense on T1 (*A*), heterogeneously hyperintense on T2 (*B*), and shows nonhomogeneous enhancement on the postcontrast images (*C*). On T2-weighted images with fat suppression (*B, D*), the tail sign can be seen extending along the facial planes (*white arrows*).

extremity sarcomas were treated with amputation for local control of their tumors. Radical resection was defined as complete removal of an entire anatomic compartment, including nerves, vessels, and any involved bone. Often, amputation was the only possible procedure for adequate compartmental resection. Disappointingly, it was noted that although local recurrence rates were less than 10% following radical surgery, a significant proportion of patients continued to die from metastatic disease.[24] This realization led to the establishment of limb salvage surgery combined with radiation therapy. However, for patients whose tumor cannot be grossly resected with a limb-sparing procedure that leaves a functional extremity (rare, at < 5%), amputation remains the treatment of choice.[25]

MFS presents a unique challenge due multidirectional spread along the facial planes. Therefore, obtaining negative margins may be challenging despite careful preoperative planning (**Fig. 7**).[20] As described previously, a high-quality T1- and

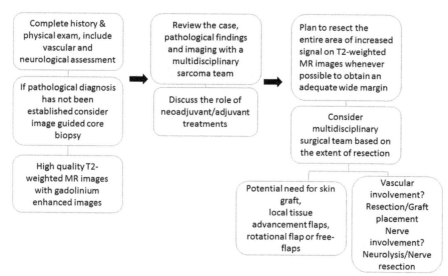

Fig. 7. Preoperative planning algorithm for patients with myxofibrosarcoma.

T2-weighted MRI with pre-and postgadolinium imaging is part of the preoperative planning for a patient with a diagnosis of MFS. Clinical, pathologic, and radiographic data should be reviewed by an experienced multidisciplinary team in a specialized referral center. The input of an experienced sarcoma multidisciplinary team (surgical oncologist, radiation oncologist, medical oncologist, sarcoma pathologist, and radiologist) is critical to the planning and implementation of these complex resections. Wide resection should include a 2 cm margin of soft tissue surrounding the tumor, with planned resection of the entire area on increased signal on T2-weighted images. The biopsy tract or incision should be removed en bloc with the resection specimen.

Although evidence of major vascular, bony, or nerve involvement may be indications for amputation, en bloc resection of the tumor with vascular structures, bone, or segments of nerve can be performed with reconstruction and interposition grafting. Often, the superficial and infiltrative nature of MFS results in large surgical resection beds that require complex reconstruction for wound closure. Consultation with plastic surgeons for local tissue advancement flaps, rotational flap, and free-flaps are sometimes necessary. The complexity of this type of excision may require a multidisciplinary surgical team including a vascular surgeon, neurosurgeon, and a reconstructive plastic surgeon in addition to a sarcoma surgical oncologist. The authors highly recommend for the patient to have the opportunity to meet and discuss the surgical plan with each of the surgical specialties involved in the case and understand and be prepared for the resection and the necessary vascular and/or reconstructive procedures.

Intraoperative margin assessment with frozen section is notoriously difficult and unreliable.

CLINICAL OUTCOMES

Overall survival for patients with localized MFS ranges from 61% to 77% at 5-year **(Table 2)**.[3,26] Resection margin status at initial operation remains the most important factor associated with survival.[3,27,28]

MFS are locally aggressive tumors that have a propensity for local recurrence (LR) **(Table 3)**. LR rates range from 16% to 57%, with a significant proportion of

Table 2
Disease-specific and overall survival rates for myxofibrosarcoma

Reference, Study Year	Number of Patients	5-y Disease-Specific Survival (%)	5-y Overall Survival (%)
Lin et al,[27] 2006	61	73	—
Huang et al,[28] 2010	49	96	—
Sanfilippo et al,[3] 2011	158	—	77
Lee et al,[15] 2016	197	51	—
Look Hong et al,[26] 2013	69	—	61
Haglund et al,[30] 2012	36	—	65 (4 y)

patients developing multiple recurrences (25%–52%).[3,15,26–30] Median time to LR is approximately 8 to 27 months but can occur up to 8 years after initial treatment.[3] Margin status at initial resection is the most important predictor of LR, as patients with a microscopically negative margin are less likely to recur than those with microscopically positive margins.[3,30] Further, Haglund and colleagues[30] demonstrated reduced local recurrence rates for patients with wider microscopic margins. Among patients with negative margins, 6 of 15 patients with less than 1 cm margin had an LR, whereas none of the patients with a margins of at least 1 cm had an LR.

Tumor grade has also been evaluated in relationship to LR.[8,13,16,31] As discussed previously, various grading systems have been used, making it difficult to compare between studies (**Table 4**). However, the risk of recurrence ranged from approximately 48% for low-grade tumors to 62% for high-grade tumors.

Interestingly, Huang and colleagues[31] found that when low-grade tumors recur, they often recur at a higher grade, demonstrating evidence of tumor progression. Furthermore, of those who demonstrated tumor progression, up to 50% of patients developed distant metastases compared with only 17% of patients who did not have histologic progression.

The tendency for local recurrences makes limb salvage difficult. MFS amputation rates are as high 17% to 41%,[30,32] as compared with approximately 5% for all other soft tissue sarcoma histologies, highlighting the importance of optimal, multimodal therapy at initial presentation.

Table 3
Local recurrence rates for myxofibrosarcoma

Reference, Study Year	Number of Patients	Local Recurrence Rate Number	Multiple Recurrences Number	5 Year RFS
Lin et al,[27] 2006	61	27 (44%)	13 (48%)	30%
Huang et al,[28] 2010	49	28 (57%)	7/28 (25%)	40%
Sanfilippo et al,[3] 2011	158	20 (17%)	14/27 (52%)	82%
Haglund et al,[30] 2012	36	11 (31%)	4/11 (45%)	60% (4 y)
Lee et al,[15] 2016	197	54 (27%)	—	25%
Dewan et al,[29] 2012	172	27 (17%)	—	—
Look Hong et al,[26] 2013	69	11 (16%)	4/11 (36%)	72%
		16%–57%	25%–52%	25%–82%

Table 4
Relationship between histologic grade and local recurrence for myxofibrosarcoma

Study, Year	Grade 1	Grade 2	Grade 3	Grade 4
Mentzel et al,[16] 1996	6/12 (50%)	9/13 (69%)	18/33 (55%)	—
Angervall et al,[8] 1977	0/2	2/7 (29%)	6/10 (60%)	7/11 (64%)
Merck et al,[13] 1983	3/8 (38%)	13/27 (48%)	21/41 (51%)	17/28 (61%)
Huang et al,[31] 2004	28/49 (57%)	—	—	—
	~48%	~49%	55%	62%

Like other soft tissue sarcomas, a proportion of patients with initially localized disease will develop distant metastases (**Tables 5** and **6**). Overall 5-year metastasis-free survival is 47% to 90% and varies by tumor grade (**Table 7**).[8,13,15,16,31]

ROLE OF RADIATION

Given that local recurrence is a critical problem in patients with MFS, the potential for adjuvant therapies is appealing to reduce potential local and distant recurrences. Based on randomized trials including a multitude of sarcoma subtypes, there is assumed to be an improvement in local control with radiation therapy in the treatment of MFS.[33,34] However, there are no randomized data specific to MFS evaluating the role of radiation therapy (XRT). Several retrospective cohort studies[3,26,32] have evaluated the association of XRT and recurrence (see **Table 7**). Unfortunately, these studies are small and likely underpowered to demonstrate a significant difference. Currently, the use of XRT for patients with MFS varies by institution and should be based on an individualized patient basis.

ROLE OF CHEMOTHERAPY

The role of chemotherapy in the treatment of MFS is less clear. There are no randomized clinical trials evaluating chemotherapy in the treatment of MFS. Several cohort studies[3,26,32] have evaluated overall survival of patients with primary resected MFS, some of whom were treated with chemotherapy (**Table 8**). None of these studies demonstrated a benefit in distant metastases or overall survival with the use of chemotherapy. Therefore, the use of chemotherapy should be used in the setting of a clinical trial.

Table 5
Relation between histologic grade and rate of metastasis for myxofibrosarcoma

Reference, Study Year	Grade 1	Grade 2	Grade 3	Grade 4
Mentzel et al,[16] 1996	0/12	5/13 (38%)	10/33 (29%)	—
Angervall et al,[8] 1977	0/2	2/7 (29%)	2/11 (18%)	3/11 (27%)
Merck et al,[13] 1983	0/8	6/27 (21%)	21/45 (47%)	11/29 (38%)
Huang et al,[31] 2004	—	7/49 (14%)	—	—
		26%	31%	33%

Table 6
Impact of radiation therapy on local recurrence in myxofibrosarcoma

Reference, Study Year	# Patients	Radiation Tx (%)	Local Recurrence HR (95% CI)
Sanfilippo et al,[3] 2011	158	35% (RT) 14% CRT	1.1 (0.5–2.6)[b]
Look Hong et al,[26] 2013	69	77%	0.43 (0.12–1.51)[a]
Mutter et al,[32] 2012	114	80%	0.6 (0.29–1.27)[a]

Abbreviations: CRT, chemoradiation therapy; RT, radiation therapy.
[a] Univariate analysis.
[b] Multivariable analysis.

Table 7
Five-year metastasis-free-survival for myxofibrosarcomas

Reference, Study Year	Number of Patients	5-Year Metastasis-Free Survival (%)
Lin et al,[27] 2006	61	60
Huang et al,[28] 2010	49	90
Sanfilippo et al,[3] 2011	158	85
Lee et al,[15] 2016	197	47
Look Hong et al,[26] 2013	69	82
		47–90

Table 8
Impact of chemotherapy on overall survival in myxofibrosarcoma

Reference, Study Year	Number of Patients	Chemo Tx (%)	Overall Survival HR (95% Confidence Interval)
Sanfilippo et al,[3] 2011	158	14% CRT	0.8 (0.3–2.2)[b]
Look Hong et al,[26] 2013	69	12% CRT 18% CTx	0.92 (0.27–3.14)[a]
Mutter et al,[32] 2012	114	11%	1.31 (0.71–2.4)[a]

Abbreviations: CRT, chemoradiation therapy; CTx, chemotherapy only.
[a] Univariate analysis.
[b] Multivariable analysis.

SUMMARY

Myxofibrosarcoma is a unique subtype of soft tissue sarcoma with a locally infiltrative behavior. High-quality MRI imaging is critical for preoperative planning. Wide surgical resection with 2 cm soft tissue margin is the mainstay of treatment and can require complex vascular and plastic surgery reconstruction. Local recurrence is common, and a subset of patients with high-grade lesions will develop distant metastases. Radiation may be beneficial in reducing local recurrence

REFERENCES

1. Fletcher CD, Bridge JA, Hogendoorn PC, et al. WHO classification of tumours of soft tissue and bone. 4th edition. Lyon (France): IARC Press; 2013.

2. Fletcher C, Unni K, Mertens F. Pathology and genetics of tumours of soft tissue and bone. 3rd edition. Lyon (France): IARC Press; 2002.

3. Sanfilippo R, Miceli R, Grosso F, et al. Myxofibrosarcoma: prognostic factors and survival in a series of patients treated at a single institution. Ann Surg Oncol 2011; 18(3):720–5.

4. Gronchi A, Lo Vullo S, Colombo C, et al. Extremity soft tissue sarcoma in a series of patients treated at a single institution: local control directly impacts survival. Ann Surg 2010;251(3):506–11.

5. Waters B, Panicek DM, Lefkowitz RA, et al. Low-grade myxofibrosarcoma: CT and MRI patterns in recurrent disease. AJR Am J Roentgenol 2007;188(2):W193–8.

6. Weiss SW, Enzinger FM. Myxoid variant of malignant fibrous histiocytoma. Cancer 1977;39(4):1672–85.

7. Von Leden H. Myxofibrosarcoma of the external auditory canal. Ann Otol Rhinol Laryngol 1951;60(1):258–9.

8. Angervall L, Kindblom LG, Merck C. Myxofibrosarcoma. A study of 30 cases. Acta Pathol Microbiol Scand A 1977;85A(2):127–40.

9. Fletcher CD. Pleomorphic malignant fibrous histiocytoma: fact or fiction? A critical reappraisal based on 159 tumors diagnosed as pleomorphic sarcoma. Am J Surg Pathol 1992;16(3):213–28.

10. Hollowood K, Fletcher CD. Malignant fibrous histiocytoma: morphologic pattern or pathologic entity? Semin Diagn Pathol 1995;12(3):210–20.

11. Fletcher CD, Gustafson P, Rydholm A, et al. Clinicopathologic re-evaluation of 100 malignant fibrous histiocytomas: prognostic relevance of subclassification. J Clin Oncol 2001;19(12):3045–50.

12. Bakhalova NV. Effect of methylergometrine on the secretory function of the breasts. Zdravookhr Kirg 1977;(1):10–5 [in Russian].

13. Merck C, Angervall L, Kindblom LG, et al. Myxofibrosarcoma. A malignant soft tissue tumor of fibroblastic-histiocytic origin. A clinicopathologic and prognostic study of 110 cases using multivariate analysis. Acta Pathol Microbiol Immunol Scand Suppl 1983;282:1–40.

14. Nascimento AF, Bertoni F, Fletcher CD. Epithelioid variant of myxofibrosarcoma: expanding the clinicomorphologic spectrum of myxofibrosarcoma in a series of 17 cases. Am J Surg Pathol 2007;31(1):99–105.

15. Lee AY, Agaram NP, Qin LX, et al. Optimal percent myxoid component to predict outcome in high-grade myxofibrosarcoma and undifferentiated pleomorphic sarcoma. Ann Surg Oncol 2016;23(3):818–25.

16. Mentzel T, Calonje E, Wadden C, et al. Myxofibrosarcoma. Clinicopathologic analysis of 75 cases with emphasis on the low-grade variant. Am J Surg Pathol 1996;20(4):391–405.

17. Neuville A, Chibon F, Coindre JM. Grading of soft tissue sarcomas: from histological to molecular assessment. Pathology 2014;46(2):113–20.

18. Edge SB, American Joint Committee on Cancer. AJCC cancer staging manual. 7th edition. New York: Springer; 2010.

19. Willems SM, Debiec-Rychter M, Szuhai K, et al. Local recurrence of myxofibrosarcoma is associated with increase in tumour grade and cytogenetic aberrations, suggesting a multistep tumour progression model. Mod Pathol 2006;19(3): 407–16.

20. Kaya M, Wada T, Nagoya S, et al. MRI and histological evaluation of the infiltrative growth pattern of myxofibrosarcoma. Skeletal Radiol 2008;37(12):1085–90.

21. Lefkowitz RA, Landa J, Hwang S, et al. Myxofibrosarcoma: prevalence and diagnostic value of the "tail sign" on magnetic resonance imaging. Skeletal Radiol 2013;42(6):809–18.
22. Yoo HJ, Hong SH, Kang Y, et al. MR imaging of myxofibrosarcoma and undifferentiated sarcoma with emphasis on tail sign; diagnostic and prognostic value. Eur Radiol 2014;24(8):1749–57.
23. Wada T, Hasegawa T, Nagoya S, et al. Myxofibrosarcoma with an infiltrative growth pattern: a case report. Jpn J Clin Oncol 2000;30(10):458–62.
24. Shiu MH, Castro EB, Hajdu SI, et al. Surgical treatment of 297 soft tissue sarcomas of the lower extremity. Ann Surg 1975;182(5):597–602.
25. Brennan MF, Casper ES, Harrison LB, et al. The role of multimodality therapy in soft-tissue sarcoma. Ann Surg 1991;214(3):328–36 [discussion: 336–8].
26. Look Hong NJ, Hornicek FJ, Raskin KA, et al. Prognostic factors and outcomes of patients with myxofibrosarcoma. Ann Surg Oncol 2013;20(1):80–6.
27. Lin CN, Chou SC, Li CF, et al. Prognostic factors of myxofibrosarcomas: implications of margin status, tumor necrosis, and mitotic rate on survival. J Surg Oncol 2006;93(4):294–303.
28. Huang HY, Li CF, Fang FM, et al. Prognostic implication of ezrin overexpression in myxofibrosarcomas. Ann Surg Oncol 2010;17(12):3212–9.
29. Dewan V, Darbyshire A, Sumathi V, et al. Prognostic and survival factors in myxofibrosarcomas. Sarcoma 2012;2012:830879.
30. Haglund KE, Raut CP, Nascimento AF, et al. Recurrence patterns and survival for patients with intermediate- and high-grade myxofibrosarcoma. Int J Radiat Oncol Biol Phys 2012;82(1):361–7.
31. Huang H. Low-grade myxofibrosarcoma: a clinicopathologic analysis of 49 cases treated at a single institution with simultaneous assessment of the efficacy of 3-tier and 4-tier grading systems. Hum Pathol 2004;35(5):612–21.
32. Mutter RW, Singer S, Zhang Z, et al. The enigma of myxofibrosarcoma of the extremity. Cancer 2012;118(2):518–27.
33. Yang JC, Chang AE, Baker AR, et al. Randomized prospective study of the benefit of adjuvant radiation therapy in the treatment of soft tissue sarcomas of the extremity. J Clin Oncol 1998;16(1):197–203.
34. Beane JD, Yang JC, White D, et al. Efficacy of adjuvant radiation therapy in the treatment of soft tissue sarcoma of the extremity: 20-year follow-up of a randomized prospective trial. Ann Surg Oncol 2014;21(8):2484–9.

Malignant Peripheral Nerve Sheath Tumor

Aaron W. James, MD[a], Elizabeth Shurell, MD[b], Arun Singh, MD[c],
Sarah M. Dry, MD[d], Fritz C. Eilber, MD[e],*

KEYWORDS

- Neurofibroma • Atypical neurofibroma • Malignant peripheral nerve sheath tumor
- Neurofibromatosis • NF1

KEY POINTS

- Malignant peripheral nerve sheath tumor (MPNST) is the sixth most common soft tissue sarcoma, often arises from a neurofibroma, and in half of cases occurs in a patient with neurofibromatosis type I.
- The most accurate radiographic evaluation of MPNST uses a combination of PET along with CT or MRI.
- The pathologic diagnoses of peripheral nerve sheath tumors with atypia represent a histologic continuum, and include neurofibroma with atypical features, low-grade MPNST, and high-grade MPNST.
- Management and prognosis significantly differ between low-grade MPNST and high-grade MPNST.

INTRODUCTION TO MALIGNANT PERIPHERAL NERVE SHEATH TUMOR

MPNST is the sixth most common type of soft-tissue sarcoma, accounting for approximately 5% to 10% of cases.[1–3] Although its exact cellular origins remain unclear, most MPNSTs arise in association with a peripheral nerve and are hypothesized to be of neural crest origin.[4] Approximately 50% of all MPNST cases arise sporadically, whereas the other 50% of cases are observed in patients with neurofibromatosis

Disclosure Statement: The authors have nothing to disclose.
[a] Department of Pathology, Johns Hopkins University, 600 North Wolfe Street, Baltimore, MD 21287-6417, USA; [b] Memorial Sloan Kettering Cancer Center, 1275 York Avenue, New York, NY 10065, USA; [c] Sarcoma Service, Division of Hematology/Oncology, University of California, Los Angeles, 2825 Santa Monica Boulevard, Suite 213 TORL, Santa Monica, CA 90404, USA; [d] Department of Pathology & Laboratory Medicine, University of California, Los Angeles, Box 951732, 13-145D CHS, Los Angeles, CA 90095-1732, USA; [e] Division of Surgical Oncology, University of California, Los Angeles, 10833 LeConte Avenue, Room 54-140 CHS, Los Angeles, CA 90095-1782, USA
* Corresponding author.
E-mail address: fceilber@mednet.ucla.edu

type 1 (NF1).[5,6] NF1 (also termed von Recklinghausen disease) is an autosomal-dominant genetic disorder with high penetrance that is characterized by mutations in the *Neurofibromin 1* gene, in which patients develop both superficial and deep neurofibromas, among other tumor types.[7,8] Guidelines for the diagnosis of NF1 are summarized in **Box 1**. NF1 patients carry an estimated 8% to 13% lifetime risk of developing MPNST, and 30% of NF1-associated MPNSTs progress from a deeply situated neurofibroma.[8,9] The incidence of MPNST among NF1 patients is 1:3,500, in comparison to the incidence among the general population of 1:100,000.[6] NF1 patients are also predisposed to developing astrocytic brain tumors, pheochromocytoma, and myeloid leukemia, among a diverse array of other benign and malignant tumors.[10,11] Another main risk factor for the development of MPNST is radiation exposure. An estimated 3% to 10% of all MPNST patients have a clinical history of prior radiation exposure.[5] The latency period for radiation-associated MPNST is typically more than 15 years.[12] The median age at diagnosis among sporadic MPNST patients is 41 years of age, whereas NF1-associated MPNST patients are generally younger (mean age of 28 years).[13] Although infrequent, NF1-associated MPNSTs in childhood do occur.[14] The incidence of sporadic MPNST is approximately equal among men and women,[15] whereas NF1-associated MPNST is somewhat more common in men.[5]

In general, the clinical presentation of MPNST is typical of a soft tissue sarcoma. MPNST presents as an enlarging mass for several months. The location is most commonly near nerve roots and bundles of the extremities and the pelvis, including the sciatic nerve, brachial plexus, and sacral plexus.[15] Therefore, a majority of MPNST occur in the proximal portions of the upper and lower extremities. Symptoms include pain, paresthesia, and neurologic deficits.[16] New-onset pain in an existing neurofibroma, especially in an NF1 patient, should prompt evaluation for MPNST. Currently, the clinical standard of care for localized high-grade MPNST is surgical resection and adjuvant radiation. An estimated 40% to 65% of MPNST patients experience local recurrence and 30% to 60% develop metastasis, with the most common site primarily located in the lungs.[17–20] Although chemotherapy is administered to systemically manage metastatic MPNST, survival rates remain low.[21,22] In general, a diagnosis of MPNST carries a poor prognosis. For all patients with high-grade MPNST, overall 5-year survival rate ranges from 20% to 50% and a mortality rate of up to 75%.[1,4] Although it was previously believed that patients with NF1-associated tumors have a worse prognosis,[9] this has been disproved across multiple studies.

Box 1
Diagnostic criteria for neurofibromatosis type 1

Two or more of the following signs or factors

Six or more café au lait macules

Two or more neurofibromas or one plexiform neurofibroma

Axillary or inguinal region freckling

Optic glioma

Two or more iris hamartomas (Lisch nodules)

First-degree relative with NF1

Adapted from NIH consensus development conference statement of neurofibromatosis. Bethesda (MD): US Department of Health and Human Services; 1987.

MOLECULAR PATHOGENESIS OF MALIGNANT PERIPHERAL NERVE SHEATH TUMOR

MPNSTs exhibit many different genetic aberrations that lead to the dysregulation of crucial signaling pathways that modulate cellular proliferation, growth, and apoptosis. Specifically, proteins that have been implicated in MPNST pathogenesis include neurofibromin 1, phosphatase and tensin homolog (PTEN), insulinlike growth factor 1 receptor (IGF1R), epidermal growth factor receptor (EGFR), and mitogen-activated protein kinases (MAPKs). As such, targeting these signal transduction pathways is an active area of research.

Neurofibromin 1

Mutations in the neurofibromin 1 tumor suppressor gene responsible for NF1 have been examined in research into the molecular pathogenesis of MPNST. In 1 study, Cichowski and Jacks[11] found that the neurofibromin 1 gene is closely linked to the tumor suppressor gene *p53* on chromosome 11 in mice. Specifically, mice carrying null mutations of both genes developed MPNST at high frequencies, indicating that concomitant loss of these tumor suppressors enables tumor cells to avoid growth arrest and apoptosis.[23]

Phosphatase and Tensin Homolog

The tumor suppressor PTEN is a central negative regulator of the PI3K/AKT/mTOR signaling cascade, which controls cell growth, proliferation, and survival.[24] PTEN is the most commonly altered component of the PI3K pathway in human malignancies, including MPNST.[24] Specifically, the reduction or deletion of PTEN is associated with the malignant transformation of neurofibroma to MPNST in humans and animal models.[6,25,26]

For example, Keng and colleagues[26] created transgenic mice lacking both the *Pten* and *Nf1* in Schwann cells and their precursors to elucidate the role of these 2 tumor suppressor genes in vivo. When coupled with *Nf1* loss, both the decrease and loss of *Pten* resulted in MPNST development from neurofibromas and seemed to accelerate the progression from low-grade to high-grade MPNST.[26] Additionally, genetic analysis of human MPNST exhibited down-regulation of *PTEN* expression, suggesting that *PTEN*-regulated pathways play key roles as tumor suppressors to inhibit the progression of benign neurofibroma to MPNST.[26]

Likewise, Gregorian and colleagues[25] found that concomitant activation of the *K-ras* oncogene along with single allelic deletion of *Pten* led to 100% development of NF1 lesions and subsequent progression to MPNST in mice.[25] In the same study, they observed loss of PTEN expression in human NF1-associated MPNST lesions, because less than 20% of the tumor cells were PTEN positive.

In a similar study, Bradtmoller and colleagues[6] discovered significantly reduced PTEN expression in human MPNST samples (5%) compared with benign neurofibromas (30%). Furthermore, a significantly higher methylation frequency in MPNST was observed compared with benign peripheral nerve sheath tumor (PNST), including neurofibroma.[6] These findings indicated that the methylation of CpG island 3' as one mechanism that down-regulates PTEN in MPNST.[6]

In summary, deletion of the tumor suppressor PTEN in the cell-cycle regulatory PI3K/AKT/mTOR pathway plays a critical role in the malignant transformation of neurofibroma to MPNST. For a more detailed review on the role of PTEN in neoplastic growth, please refer to the article by Chow and Baker.[24]

Insulinlike Growth Factor 1 Receptor and Epidermal Growth Factor Receptor

Genetic alterations of the IGF1R pathway have been correlated to MPNST progression. For example, Yang and colleagues[27] observed *IGF1R* amplification and increased IGF1R protein expression, respectively, in 24% and 82% of human MPNST samples. Higher IGF1R protein expression correlated with worse tumor-free survival and increased risk of tumor progression.[27] Moreover, activation of IGF1R induces MPNST cell proliferation, migration, and invasion via up-regulation of the PI3K/AKT/mTOR pathway.[27] Specifically, inhibition of IGF1R in ST88 to 14 MPNST cells via small interfering RNA or the IGF1R inhibitor MK-0646 significantly decreased cell proliferation, invasion, and migration due to attenuation of the PI3K/AKT/mTOR pathway.[27]

Likewise, up-regulation of EGFR has also been implicated in the progression of MPNST. DeClue and colleagues[28] found significantly increased EGFR expression in the Schwann cells of MPNST compared with benign neurofibromas. Additionally, proliferation of cultured primary cells from human MPNST was inhibited by the EGFR antagonists mAb225, A-25, and AG-1478.[28]

Mitogen-Activated Protein Kinase

MAPK has also been found overexpressed in MPNST.[16,29,30] This signaling cascade, which includes rapidly accelerated fibrosarcoma (RAF), extracellular signal-regulated kinase (ERK), and MAPK/ERK kinase [MEK]), is responsible for cell-cycle progression from the G1 phase to the S phase.[16] Thus, dysregulation of the MAPK pathway leads to uncontrolled growth in cancer. For example, Zou and colleagues[30] observed that 91% of MPNST samples stained positive for phosphorylated MEK compared with only 21% of benign neurofibromas. See **Table 1** for a brief summary of main molecular pathways dysregulated in MPNST.

RADIOGRAPHIC DIAGNOSIS OF MALIGNANT PERIPHERAL NERVE SHEATH TUMOR

The detection of MPNST and its differentiation from benign neurofibromas remains a clinical challenge, because the symptomology of these 2 conditions, including tumor size, pain, and neurologic deficits, exhibits considerable overlap. Currently, the imaging modalities that are used to evaluate and diagnose MPNST include CT, MRI, and PET. Each is discussed.

Both CT and MRI are used to define the anatomic tumor size and local invasiveness of PNST. For example, Benz and colleagues[31] used CT imaging and observed that MPNSTs are larger than their benign counterparts. Specifically, the mean tumor size for malignant and benign PSNT were 7.4 cm $\pm$ 4.1 cm and mean 4.8 cm $\pm$ 2.7 cm, respectively.[31] Due to the clear overlap between the size ranges of benign and

Table 1
Dysregulation of molecular pathways in malignant peripheral nerve sheath tumor

Molecular Pathway	Normal Role	Change in Malignant Peripheral Nerve Sheath Tumor
NF1	Tumor suppressor	Down-regulation
PTEN	Tumor suppressor Negative regulator of PI3K/AKT/mTOR signaling cascade	Down-regulation
IGF1R	Positive regulator of PI3K/AKT/mTOR signaling cascade	Up-regulation
EGFR	Positive regulator of PI3K/AKT/mTOR signaling cascade	Up-regulation
MAPK	Phosphorylation of RAF/MEK/ERK signaling cascade	Up-regulation

malignant PNST, however, CT-based evaluation of tumor size is limited when used as the sole imaging modality to diagnose MPNST.

Several studies have established diagnostic criteria for distinguishing benign PNST and MPNST using MRI (**Table 2**). Mautner and colleagues,[32] however, evaluated the efficacy of MRI in the diagnosis of MPNST and concluded that MRI when used alone can likewise not reliably distinguish between malignant and benign PNST, especially when tumors are inhomogeneous. Overall, the central limitation of both CT and MRI is that they cannot effectively confirm malignant transformation of lesions.[31,33,34]

To improve on anatomic imaging, various studies have used quantitative fludeoxy-glucose F 18 (FDG) PET imaging to distinguish between benign PNST and MPNST based on a tumor's metabolic activity.[31,33,34] In these studies, the maximum standardized uptake value (SUVmax) is used to measure tumor glucose utilization; in summary, lower tumor FDG uptake is correlated with benign peripheral nerve sheath tumors, whereas higher tumor FDG uptake is correlated with MPNST.[31,33,34]

Benz and colleagues[31] determined that the mean SUVmax for MPNSTs (12.0 g/mL ± 7.1 g/mL) was significantly higher than that of benign peripheral nerve sheath tumors (3.4 g/mL ± 1.8 g/mL). In addition, they determined that the optimum threshold for separating MPNSTs from their benign counterparts was an SUVmax of 6.1 g/mL, with sensitivity and specificity of 94% and 91%, respectively.[31] In a similarly conducted study, Ferner and colleagues[40] determined that lesions in NF1 patients with an SUVmax of 3.5 g/mL should be resected to prevent progression towards MPNST, with sensitivity and specificity of 89% and 95%, respectively.

In summary, the definitive radiographic distinction of benign PNST and MPNST is a challenge. Currently, quantitative FDG-PET imaging used in conjunction with CT or MRI offers the best ability to distinguish benign PNST from MPNST. The authors think that these data should be combined with the clinical assessment of patients to identify patients undergoing and who have undergone malignant transformation. Radiographic imaging and clinical features of PNST/MPNST have not supplanted histopathologic examination as the gold standard for the diagnosis of MPNST.

HISTOPATHOLOGIC DIAGNOSIS OF MALIGNANT PERIPHERAL NERVE SHEATH TUMOR

The diagnosis of MPNST may be suspected prior to biopsy, based on a variety of factors, including known diagnosis of NF1, changes in the tempo of clinical symptoms, relationship to a peripheral nerve, relationship to preexisting neurofibroma, or imaging characteristics, including rapidly growing tumors and highly FDG-avid lesions. The typical histology of MPNST is that of a proliferation of spindle cells showing a

Table 2
Diagnostic criteria for malignant peripheral nerve sheath tumor using MRI

Parameter	Malignant Peripheral Nerve Sheath Tumor	Benign Peripheral Nerve Sheath Tumor
Tumor size (mm)	74–100	43–69
Intratumoral lobulation (%)	50–63	12–17
Intratumoral heterogeneity (%)	51–90	30–52
Irregular or peripheral contrast enhancement (%)	34–75	5–33
Intratumoral cystic changes (%)	21–39	10–17
Peritumoral edema (%)	29–66	0–23

Data from Refs.[35–39]

fascicular growth pattern, often with a branching hemangiopericytoma-like vascular pattern, as well as alternating hypercellular and hypocellular areas. The histologic appearance of MPNST may vary significantly — from tumors appearing similar to neurofibroma ranging to those more resembling a fibrosarcoma. From a biological perspective, this variation in appearance may reflect different elements within the native peripheral nerve sheath, including Schwann cells, perineural cells, and fibroblasts. Given this spectrum of findings and the lack of definitive markers for MPNST, it is important to recognize that there is still a lack of widely accepted diagnostic criteria for MPNST.

Typical cytologic features of MPNST include nuclei that are wavy, buckled or comma-shaped.[41] Other less common histologic features of MPNST that may be present include epithelioid or pleomorphic cytomorphology, heterologous elements, glandular differentiation, and melanin pigment. Heterologous elements are more common in MPNST compared with other tumor types and most commonly include mature islands of cartilage and bone (seen in up to 15% of MPNST).[42] Glandular differentiation is rare[43] and most commonly brings up the diagnostic alternative of biphasic synovial sarcoma.[41] Epithelioid MPNST constitutes less than 5% of MPNST and is distinctive for diffuse S100 immunoreactivity in a majority of tumors[44] as well as loss of INI1 in approximately half of cases.[45] A more comprehensive discussion of the histopathologic variation with MPNST can be found within the following reference.[41]

Immunohistochemistry (IHC) is of some help in the diagnosis of MPSNT, including the exclusion of competing diagnostic possibilities. All IHC markers, however, have limited sensitivity or specificity, so a single diagnostic marker for MPNST is not currently available. S100 protein expression is the most commonly used in the evaluation of MPNST. When present (estimated at anywhere from 50% to 90% frequency[46,47]), S100 immunostaining is usually focal. Diffuse S100 expression is more consistent with a cellular schwannoma, melanoma, or clear cell sarcoma. The exception to this is epithelioid MPNST, which often shows diffuse S100 immunostaining.[44] SOX10 may show improved sensitivity and specificity over S100 protein for MPNST.[48] Melanocytic markers are negative, whereas keratins may be positive (either in epithelioid MPNST or glandular MPNST). TLE1 expression is usually focal and weak in MPNST, rather than strong and diffuse, as seen in synovial sarcoma.[49]

Two diagnostic dilemmas that may face pathologists when considering the diagnosis of MPNST are discussed briefly. The first is distinguishing low-grade MPNST from neurofibroma and neurofibroma with atypical features. When neural differentiation is clearly identified, the next step is histopathologic subcategorization. The differentiation of atypical neurofibroma from low-grade MPNST is challenging and not entirely agreed on by experts in the field, because these lesions likely represent a histologic continuum.[41] For example, some investigators maintain that both hypercellularity and nuclear atypia, with or without mitoses, are consistent with low-grade MPNST.[50–52] Other experts add that if mitotic activity is not present, low-grade MPNST may be diagnosed if the cellularity and atypia are marked and the architectural pattern is fascicular.[41] Other experts accept any mitotic activity in a cellular or atypical neurofibroma, particularly in a patient with NF1, as evidence for malignant transformation.[53] In contrast, the current World Health Organization classification maintains that "hypercellularity of otherwise unremarkable neurofibroma cells, atypical tumour cells with hyperchromatic smudgy nuclei, or mitotic activity, alone or together, do not indicate malignant change."[54] This debate over the hematoxylin-eosin diagnosis is compounded by the fact that current molecular or immunohistochemical assays do not distinguish between these diagnostic categories. Current guidelines that the authors use in practice for the light microscopic diagnosis of neurofibroma are shown in **Box 2**, adapted from Goldblum and colleagues.[41]

The second potential diagnostic dilemma is distinguishing high-grade MPNST from other high-grade malignancies. Based on the hematoxylin-eosin appearance, high-grade MPNST has overlapping appearance with a diverse array of high-grade sarcomas and other malignancies. Other sarcomas with overlapping spindle cell morphology include monophasic synovial sarcoma, fibrosarcoma, leiomyosarcoma, malignant solitary fibrous tumor, dedifferentiated liposarcoma, dedifferentiated dermatofibrosarcoma protuberans, and high-grade spindle cell sarcoma not otherwise specified. In the case of a pleomorphic/anaplastic MPNST, other sarcomas with pleomorphic features must be considered, including, for example, high-grade myxofibrosarcoma, pleomorphic leiomyosarcoma, or high-grade pleomorphic sarcoma not otherwise specified. In the case of suspected anaplastic MPNST, a careful search for more typical areas of high-grade MPNST should be undertaken. As well, melanoma, in particular desmoplastic melanoma, must always be excluded; as discussed previously, IHC stains for S100, SOX-10, and melanoma-specific markers (such as HMB45 or MART-1) are helpful in this regard. Finally, poorly differentiated or sarcomatoid carcinomas may also mimic MPNST histologically. A careful hunt for distinguishing cytologic features as well as initial panel of immunohistochemical stains aid in the diagnosis. A potential list of immunohistochemical stains for the evaluation of suspected high-grade MPNST is in **Box 3**.

SURGICAL MANAGEMENT OF MALIGNANT PERIPHERAL NERVE SHEATH TUMOR

Complete surgical resection with wide negative margins is the current standard of care for localized high-grade MPNST and is a strong predictor of survival.[5,7,55] Specifically, it is recommended that tumors should be excised with wide margins.[7]

The location of MPNST affects tumor accessibility and consequently affects the rate at which negative surgical margins are successfully achieved. For example, Wong and

---

Box 2
Histologic criteria for distinguishing neurofibroma from low-grade malignant peripheral nerve sheath tumor

Neurofibroma

- Nuclear atypia (may be focal or diffuse)
- No diffuse cellularity
- No mitotic activity

Neurofibroma with atypical features

A combination of nuclear atypia, cellularity, and/or mitotic activity that falls short of the criteria for low-grade MPNST

Low-grade MPNST

All of the following 3 attributes must be present (In the absence of mitotic activity, atypia and cellularity must be marked):
- Generalized nuclear atypia
- Diffuse cellularity
- Low levels of mitotic activity

Adapted from Goldblum JR, Folpe AL, Weiss SW, et al. Enzinger and Weiss's soft tissue tumors. 6th edition. Philadelphia: Saunders/Elsevier; 2014. p. xiv, 1155.

Box 3
Potential immunohistochemical stains in the evaluation of high-grade malignant peripheral nerve sheath tumor

Pan cytokeratin

High-molecular-weight cytokeratin

S100

SOX10

HMB45/MelanA/MART1

CD34

SMA

Desmin

TLE1

STAT6

---

colleagues[18] observed large differences in the frequency of positive surgical margins dependent on anatomic site (reproduced in **Table 3**).

Various studies have indicated that the surgical margin status is a significant prognostic factor for high-grade MPNST.[18,56,57] Wong and colleagues[18] observed that MPNST patients with positive margins exhibited 3-year and 5-year overall survival rates of 47% and 22%, respectively, whereas those with negative margins exhibited higher rates of 74% and 67% respectively. Likewise, Porter and colleagues[57] found that only 6% of MPNST patients with negative surgical margins experienced local recurrence compared with 30% of patient with positive surgical margins. Additionally, the rate of 10-year distant metastases is higher for MPNST patients with positive margins (27%–31%) compared with those with negative margins (21%–27%).[15,58] Moreover, MPNST patients with positive resection margins exhibited a 1.8-fold risk of disease-specific mortality.[15] Follow-up guidelines regarding the management of MPNST after surgical resection have not been definitively established.

Importantly, the surgical management of low-grade MPNST versus high-grade MPNST may be different. Bernthal and colleagues[59] determined that surgical margins did not have a significant effect on the clinical outcome of patients with low-grade MPNST or atypical neurofibroma. Of the 23 patients studied, 78% exhibited positive surgical margins; strikingly, these patients also demonstrated a 0% occurrence of

---

Table 3
Frequency of positive margins in malignant peripheral nerve sheath tumor based on anatomic site

Anatomic Site	Frequency of Positive Margins in Malignant Peripheral Nerve Sheath Tumor (%)
Pelvis	42
Chest	32
Abdomen	27
Head/neck	22
Extremities	6

pulmonary metastasis and a 100% rate of disease-specific survival at 4 years.[59] Although local recurrence of disease occurred in 16.7% of patients with positive surgical margins, none of them developed metastatic disease or died of the disease itself. Therefore, this study suggests that obtaining wide resections with negative surgical margins in low-grade MPNST or atypical neurofibroma patients is not as critical compared with high-grade MPNST. The absolute requirement and timing for re-resection in low-grade MPNST with positive margins is not yet clear.

RADIATION THERAPY AND MALIGNANT PERIPHERAL NERVE SHEATH TUMOR

Both neoadjuvant and postoperative adjuvant radiation therapy have been used to locally control MPNST. For example, Kahn and colleagues[60] examined the clinical outcomes of adjuvant radiation therapy in both sporadic and NF1-associated MPNST patients. Tumors were located in the extremities (58%), trunk (36%), and the head/neck region (6%).[60] The various modalities of administered radiation therapy included external beam radiation, brachytherapy, proton therapy, and a combination of external beam radiation and brachytherapy.[60] The median total doses of sporadic and NF1-associated tumors were 58.5 Gy and 59.4 Gy, respectively.[55] Additionally, the local control rate at 5 years for NF1-associated tumors was 51%, and the rates of pulmonary metastasis in sporadic and NF1-associated tumors were 47% and 28%, respectively.[55] The median survival of all patients was 46.5 months, with a 43.7%% overall 5-year survival.[60] Strikingly, the median overall survival of NF1-associated MPNST patients treated with radiation was 33.1 months, whereas the median survival among those not treated with radiation was 17.4 months.[60] Thus, Kahn and colleagues[60] determined that adjuvant radiation therapy is effective in achieving local control and improving overall survival among patients with MPNST.

Various other studies have also recommended the use of intraoperative or postoperative adjuvant radiation therapy to treat MPNST.[55,61] For example, Wong and colleagues[18] found that the 3-year and 5-year overall survival rates for patients receiving either brachytherapy or intraoperative electron irradiation were 84% and 72%, respectively, compared with 61% and 50% among patients who did not receive the treatment.

Similarly, Kar and colleagues[55] concluded that postoperative adjuvant radiotherapy increased both 5-year disease-free and overall survival of MPNST patients. Adjuvant radiotherapy ranging in dosage from 54 Gy to 62 Gy was administered to patients who exhibited deep-seated, high-grade tumors that were larger than 5 cm.[55] Specifically, the 5-year disease-free survival rates among patients who did and did not receive postoperative radiotherapy were 42% and 0% respectively.[55] Likewise, the 5-year overall survival rates for patients who did and did not receive radiotherapy were 65% and 38%, respectively.[55]

Additionally, a group of clinicians and scientists specializing in MPNST reached an international consensus that recommended the use of postoperative radiation therapy to combat local recurrence of disease.[7] Moreover, Stucky and colleagues[61] recommended the use of postoperative therapy for tumors with the following characteristics: greater than or equal to 5 cm, high grade, and R1 (microscopically positive; closest margin within 2 mm of inked surface) or R2 (macroscopically positive) margin status.

SYSTEMIC THERAPY AND MALIGNANT PERIPHERAL NERVE SHEATH TUMOR

In contrast to surgical resection and radiation therapy, chemotherapy is usually limited to the management of metastatic MPNST or in patients with unresectable tumors.[7,21]

Treatment regimens typically consist of either single-agent doxorubicin or a combination of doxorubicin and ifosfamide.[7,21] In one study, Kroep and colleagues[21] observed a response rate, progression-free survival, and median overall survival of 21%, 17 weeks, and 48 weeks, respectively, among MPNST patients who underwent chemotherapy. The combination of ifosfamide and doxorubicin has a higher response rate than single-agent doxorubicin in MPNST and in most soft tissue sarcomas. In the recently completed EORTC 62012 trial, however, although the combination improves progression-free survival, it was not associated with improved overall survival in locally advanced/metastatic soft tissue sarcomas.[62]

At the authors' institution, neoadjuvant chemotherapy/radiation therapy is used in selected cases of MPNST in an effort to downstage borderline unresectable tumors and to determine the in vivo chemosensitivity of patients who have a high risk of disseminated disease. In these cases, doxorubicin plus ifosfamide is used due to the higher response rate. Furthermore, tumors with greater than 90% necrosis have been shown to have improve disease-specific survival.[33] This retrospective observation needs to be tested in prospective randomized trials.

CURRENT AND COMPLETED CLINICAL TRIALS OF TARGETED AGENTS

Recent advances in therapy have focused on targeting the various molecular pathways implicated in MPNST, such as the Ras-MAPK, PI3K/AKT/mTOR, Hsp90, and EGFR signaling cascades.[16,29] Although anecdotal reports have implicated the targeting of driving mutations, for the most part, a common driving genetic event has not been targeted in this disease. A summary of recently completed trials was reviewed by Farid and colleagues.[29] Information regarding recent clinical trials involving MPNST patients is in **Table 4**.

OUTCOMES OF MALIGNANT PERIPHERAL NERVE SHEATH TUMOR

A majority of MPNST are high-grade sarcomas, with a high probability of local recurrence and distant metastasis. As discussed previously, 40% to 65% of MPNST patients experience local recurrence and 30% to 60% develop metastasis.[15,17–20,30,63] Factors that predict local recurrence among high-grade MPNST include anatomic site, tumor size (greater than 10 cm), and positive margins.[15,30,63] Factors that predict metastasis include tumor size greater than 10 cm or tumors that are American Joint Committee on Cancer stage III.[15,30,63] Although it was previously believed that patients with NF1-associated tumors have a worse prognosis, this has later been disproved across multiple studies. Approximately 65% of metastases are to the lungs, whereas other sites of disease spread include the liver, brain, bone, and adrenal gland.[41] Regional lymph node involvement is uncommon, and for this reason lymph node dissection should not be routinely performed.

Table 4
Recent clinical trials offered to malignant peripheral nerve sheath tumor patients

Study Number	Clinical Trial Phase	Interventional Drug Under Investigation	Mechanism	Status
NCT02584647	I/II	PLX3397/sirolimus	mTOR inhibitor	Recruiting
NCT02008877	I/II	Ganetespib/sirolimus	mTOR inhibitor	Recruiting
NCT01661283	II	Everolimus/bevacizumab	mTOR inhibitor	Ongoing
NCT00068367	II	Erlotinib hydrochloride	EGFR inhibitor	Completed

SUMMARY

In summary, MPNST is a common high-grade soft tissue sarcoma. Its diagnosis and management is complex – and a team approach in an experienced sarcoma center is best for patients. Team members should include surgical oncologists, radiation oncologists, and medical oncologists as well as radiologists and pathologists with specialization in sarcoma. From a diagnostic perspective, there are many histologic mimics of MPNST and re-review of all outside slides is a critical step in the management of patients. From a therapeutic perspective, it is important to recognize the differences in management between low-grade MPNST and high-grade MPNST. Potential differences include the need for adjuvant radiation therapy and the prognostic importance of positive margins.

ACKNOWLEDGMENTS

The authors thank Ms Vi Nguyen for her excellent technical assistance.

REFERENCES

1. Eilber FC, Brennan MF, Eilber FR, et al. Validation of the postoperative nomogram for 12-year sarcoma-specific mortality. Cancer 2004;101(10):2270–5.
2. Grobmyer SR, Reith JD, Shahlaee A, et al. Malignant Peripheral Nerve Sheath Tumor: molecular pathogenesis and current management considerations. J Surg Oncol 2008;97(4):340–9.
3. Fuchs B, Spinner RJ, Rock MG. Malignant peripheral nerve sheath tumors: an update. J Surg Orthop Adv 2005;14(4):168–74.
4. Lin CT, Huang TW, Nieh S, et al. Treatment of a malignant peripheral nerve sheath tumor. Onkologie 2009;32(8–9):503–5.
5. Ducatman BS, Scheithauer BW, Piepgras DG, et al. Malignant peripheral nerve sheath tumors. A clinicopathologic study of 120 cases. Cancer 1986;57(10): 2006–21.
6. Bradtmoller M, Hartmann C, Zietsch J, et al. Impaired Pten expression in human malignant peripheral nerve sheath tumours. PLoS One 2012;7(11):e47595.
7. Ferner RE, Gutmann DH. International consensus statement on malignant peripheral nerve sheath tumors in neurofibromatosis. Cancer Res 2002;62(5):1573–7.
8. Tucker T, Wolkenstein P, Revuz J, et al. Association between benign and malignant peripheral nerve sheath tumors in NF1. Neurology 2005;65(2):205–11.
9. Evans DG, Baser ME, McGaughran J, et al. Malignant peripheral nerve sheath tumours in neurofibromatosis 1. J Med Genet 2002;39(5):311–4.
10. Bader JL. Neurofibromatosis and cancer. Ann N Y Acad Sci 1986;486:57–65.
11. Cichowski K, Jacks T. NF1 tumor suppressor gene function: narrowing the GAP. Cell 2001;104(4):593–604.
12. Ducatman BS, Scheithauer BW. Postirradiation neurofibrosarcoma. Cancer 1983; 51(6):1028–33.
13. Shurell E, Tran LM, Nakashima J, et al. Gender dimorphism and age of onset in malignant peripheral nerve sheath tumor preclinical models and human patients. BMC Cancer 2014;14:827.
14. Carli M, Ferrari A, Mattke A, et al. Pediatric malignant peripheral nerve sheath tumor: the Italian and German soft tissue sarcoma cooperative group. J Clin Oncol 2005;23(33):8422–30.

15. Anghileri M, Miceli R, Fiore M, et al. Malignant peripheral nerve sheath tumors: prognostic factors and survival in a series of patients treated at a single institution. Cancer 2006;107(5):1065–74.
16. Katz D, Lazar A, Lev D. Malignant peripheral nerve sheath tumour (MPNST): the clinical implications of cellular signalling pathways. Expert Rev Mol Med 2009;11:e30.
17. Goertz O, Langer S, Uthoff D, et al. Diagnosis, treatment and survival of 65 patients with malignant peripheral nerve sheath tumors. Anticancer Res 2014; 34(2):777–83.
18. Wong WW, Hirose T, Scheithauer BW, et al. Malignant peripheral nerve sheath tumor: analysis of treatment outcome. Int J Radiat Oncol Biol Phys 1998;42(2): 351–60.
19. Hruban RH, Shiu MH, Senie RT, et al. Malignant peripheral nerve sheath tumors of the buttock and lower extremity. A study of 43 cases. Cancer 1990;66(6): 1253–65.
20. Kourea HP, Bilsky MH, Leung DH, et al. Subdiaphragmatic and intrathoracic paraspinal malignant peripheral nerve sheath tumors: a clinicopathologic study of 25 patients and 26 tumors. Cancer 1998;82(11):2191–203.
21. Kroep JR, Ouali M, Gelderblom H, et al. First-line chemotherapy for malignant peripheral nerve sheath tumor (MPNST) versus other histological soft tissue sarcoma subtypes and as a prognostic factor for MPNST: an EORTC soft tissue and bone sarcoma group study. Ann Oncol 2011;22(1):207–14.
22. Zehou O, Fabre E, Zelek L, et al. Chemotherapy for the treatment of malignant peripheral nerve sheath tumors in neurofibromatosis 1: a 10-year institutional review. Orphanet J Rare Dis 2013;8:127.
23. Cichowski K, Shih TS, Schmitt E, et al. Mouse models of tumor development in neurofibromatosis type 1. Science 1999;286(5447):2172–6.
24. Chow LM, Baker SJ. PTEN function in normal and neoplastic growth. Cancer Lett 2006;241(2):184–96.
25. Gregorian C, Nakashima J, Dry SM, et al. PTEN dosage is essential for neurofibroma development and malignant transformation. Proc Natl Acad Sci U S A 2009;106(46):19479–84.
26. Keng VW, Rahrmann EP, Watson AL, et al. PTEN and NF1 inactivation in Schwann cells produces a severe phenotype in the peripheral nervous system that promotes the development and malignant progression of peripheral nerve sheath tumors. Cancer Res 2012;72(13):3405–13.
27. Yang J, Ylipaa A, Sun Y, et al. Genomic and molecular characterization of malignant peripheral nerve sheath tumor identifies the IGF1R pathway as a primary target for treatment. Clin Cancer Res 2011;17(24):7563–73.
28. DeClue JE, Heffelfinger S, Benvenuto G, et al. Epidermal growth factor receptor expression in neurofibromatosis type 1-related tumors and NF1 animal models. J Clin Invest 2000;105(9):1233–41.
29. Farid M, Demicco EG, Garcia R, et al. Malignant peripheral nerve sheath tumors. Oncologist 2014;19(2):193–201.
30. Zou C, Smith KD, Liu J, et al. Clinical, pathological, and molecular variables predictive of malignant peripheral nerve sheath tumor outcome. Ann Surg 2009; 249(6):1014–22.
31. Benz MR, Czernin J, Dry SM, et al. Quantitative F18-fluorodeoxyglucose positron emission tomography accurately characterizes peripheral nerve sheath tumors as malignant or benign. Cancer 2010;116(2):451–8.

32. Mautner VF, Friedrich RE, von Deimling A, et al. Malignant peripheral nerve sheath tumours in neurofibromatosis type 1: MRI supports the diagnosis of malignant plexiform neurofibroma. Neuroradiology 2003;45(9):618–25.

33. Shurell E, Eilber FC. Peripheral nerve sheath tumors: diagnosis using quantitative FDG-PET. In: Hayat MA, editor. Tumors of the central nervous system. New York: Springer; 2012. p. 161–6.

34. Benz MR, Tchekmedyian N, Eilber FC, et al. Utilization of positron emission tomography in the management of patients with sarcoma. Curr Opin Oncol 2009; 21(4):345–51.

35. Salamon J, Mautner VF, Adam G, et al. Multimodal imaging in neurofibromatosis type 1-associated nerve sheath tumors. Rofo 2015;187(12):1084–92.

36. Matsumine A, Kusuzaki K, Nakamura T, et al. Differentiation between neurofibromas and malignant peripheral nerve sheath tumors in neurofibromatosis 1 evaluated by MRI. J Cancer Res Clin Oncol 2009;135(7):891–900.

37. Wasa J, Nishida Y, Tsukushi S, et al. MRI features in the differentiation of malignant peripheral nerve sheath tumors and neurofibromas. AJR Am J Roentgenol 2010;194(6):1568–74.

38. Derlin T, Tornquist K, Munster S, et al. Comparative effectiveness of 18F-FDG PET/CT versus whole-body MRI for detection of malignant peripheral nerve sheath tumors in neurofibromatosis type 1. Clin Nucl Med 2013;38(1):e19–25.

39. Demehri S, Belzberg A, Blakeley J, et al. Conventional and functional MR imaging of peripheral nerve sheath tumors: initial experience. AJNR Am J Neuroradiol 2014;35(8):1615–20.

40. Ferner RE, Lucas JD, O'Doherty MJ, et al. Evaluation of (18)fluorodeoxyglucose positron emission tomography ((18)FDG PET) in the detection of malignant peripheral nerve sheath tumours arising from within plexiform neurofibromas in neurofibromatosis 1. J Neurol Neurosurg Psychiatry 2000;68(3):353–7.

41. Goldblum JR, Folpe AL, Weiss SW, et al. Enzinger and Weiss's soft tissue tumors. 6th edition. Philadelphia: Saunders/Elsevier; 2014. p. xiv, 1155.

42. deCou JM, Rao BN, Parham DM, et al. Malignant peripheral nerve sheath tumors: the St. Jude Children's Research Hospital experience. Ann Surg Oncol 1995;2(6): 524–9.

43. Cross PA, Clarke NW. Malignant nerve sheath tumour with epithelial elements. Histopathology 1988;12(5):547–9.

44. Laskin WB, Weiss SW, Bratthauer GL. Epithelioid variant of malignant peripheral nerve sheath tumor (malignant epithelioid schwannoma). Am J Surg Pathol 1991; 15(12):1136–45.

45. Hollmann TJ, Hornick JL. INI1-deficient tumors: diagnostic features and molecular genetics. Am J Surg Pathol 2011;35(10):e47–63.

46. Matsunou H, Shimoda T, Kakimoto S, et al. Histopathologic and immunohistochemical study of malignant tumors of peripheral nerve sheath (malignant schwannoma). Cancer 1985;56(9):2269–79.

47. Weiss SW, Langloss JM, Enzinger FM. Value of S-100 protein in the diagnosis of soft tissue tumors with particular reference to benign and malignant Schwann cell tumors. Lab Invest 1983;49(3):299–308.

48. Nonaka D, Chiriboga L, Rubin BP. Sox10: a pan-schwannian and melanocytic marker. Am J Surg Pathol 2008;32(9):1291–8.

49. Foo WC, Cruise MW, Wick MR, et al. Immunohistochemical staining for TLE1 distinguishes synovial sarcoma from histologic mimics. Am J Clin Pathol 2011; 135(6):839–44.

50. Woodruff JM. Pathology of tumors of the peripheral nerve sheath in type 1 neuro-fibromatosis. Am J Med Genet 1999;89(1):23–30.

51. Swanson PE, Scheithauer BW, Wick MR. Peripheral nerve sheath neoplasms. Clinicopathologic and immunochemical observations. Pathol Annu 1995;30(Pt 2):1–82.

52. Rodriguez FJ, Scheithauer BW, Abell-Aleff PC, et al. Low grade malignant peripheral nerve sheath tumor with smooth muscle differentiation. Acta Neuropathol 2007;113(6):705–9.

53. Liapis H, Dehner LP, Gutmann DH. Neurofibroma and cellular neurofibroma with atypia: a report of 14 tumors. Am J Surg Pathol 1999;23(9):1156–8.

54. Fletcher CDM, World Health Organization, International Agency for Research on Cancer. WHO classification of tumours of soft tissue and bone. 4th edition. Lyon (France): IARC Press; 2013.

55. Kar M, Deo SV, Shukla NK, et al. Malignant peripheral nerve sheath tumors (MPNST)–clinicopathological study and treatment outcome of twenty-four cases. World J Surg Oncol 2006;4:55.

56. Longhi A, Errani C, Magagnoli G, et al. High grade malignant peripheral nerve sheath tumors: outcome of 62 patients with localized disease and review of the literature. J Chemother 2010;22(6):413–8.

57. Porter DE, Prasad V, Foster L, et al. Survival in malignant peripheral nerve sheath tumours: a comparison between sporadic and neurofibromatosis type 1-associated tumours. Sarcoma 2009;2009:756395.

58. Gronchi A, Casali PG, Mariani L, et al. Status of surgical margins and prognosis in adult soft tissue sarcomas of the extremities: a series of patients treated at a single institution. J Clin Oncol 2005;23(1):96–104.

59. Bernthal NM, Putnam A, Jones KB, et al. The effect of surgical margins on outcomes for low grade MPNSTs and atypical neurofibroma. J Surg Oncol 2014; 110(7):813–6.

60. Kahn J, Gillespie A, Tsokos M, et al. Radiation therapy in management of sporadic and neurofibromatosis type 1-associated malignant peripheral nerve sheath tumors. Front Oncol 2014;4:324.

61. Stucky CC, Johnson KN, Gray RJ, et al. Malignant peripheral nerve sheath tumors (MPNST): the Mayo Clinic experience. Ann Surg Oncol 2012;19(3):878–85.

62. Judson I, Verweij J, Gelderblom H, et al, European Organisation and Treatment of Cancer Soft Tissue and Bone Sarcoma Group. Doxorubicin alone versus intensified doxorubicin plus ifosfamide for first-line treatment of advanced or metastatic soft-tissue sarcoma: a randomised controlled phase 3 trial. Lancet Oncol 2014; 15(4):415–23.

63. Okada K, Hasegawa T, Tajino T, et al. Clinical relevance of pathological grades of malignant peripheral nerve sheath tumor: a multi-institution TMTS study of 56 cases in Northern Japan. Ann Surg Oncol 2007;14(2):597–604.

Desmoid-Type Fibromatosis

Evolving Treatment Standards

Marco Fiore, MD[a],*, Andrea MacNeill, MD[a,b], Alessandro Gronchi, MD[a], Chiara Colombo, MD[a]

KEYWORDS

- Desmoid tumor • Desmoid-type fibromatosis • Aggressive fibromatosis
- Wait and see • Observation • Surgery • Chemotherapy • Radiotherapy

KEY POINTS

- Desmoid-type fibromatosis is a clonal proliferation without metastatic potential; mutations of the *CTNNB1* gene are documented in sporadic disease.
- Historically surgery has been the standard of care, but resultant functional impairment and high local recurrence rates have contributed to a paradigm shift toward more conservative management.
- Multiple pharmacologic therapies have been shown to be effective, including chemotherapy, hormone therapy, targeted therapies, and nonsteroidal anti-inflammatory drugs.
- Other therapeutic modalities, such as radiation therapy, cryoablation, and isolated limb perfusion can be considered in select cases.
- The natural history of desmoid-type fibromatosis is unpredictable and can include periods of prolonged stability or spontaneous regression.

INTRODUCTION
Definition

Desmoid-type fibromatosis (DF) is a rare benign fibroblastic/myofibroblastic proliferation that can occur in almost any anatomic location. Although the histologic appearance is consistent with fibrosis or reactive proliferation, the neoplastic nature of this disease was suggested by the discovery of a clonality in DF cells.[1,2] DF lacks metastatic

The authors have nothing to disclose.
Support was received by the Desmoid Tumor Research Foundation (to C. Colombo), Ministero della Salute - Ricerca Finalizzata 2009 (to A. Gronchi) and Associazione Italiana per la Ricerca sul Cancro (AIRC) (to C. Colombo).
[a] Sarcoma Service, Department of Surgery, Fondazione IRCCS Istituto Nazionale dei Tumori, Via Venezian, 1, Milan 20133, Italy; [b] Department of Surgical Oncology, Mount Sinai Hospital and Princess Margaret Cancer Centre, and Department of Surgery, University of Toronto, 600 University Avenue, Toronto, Ontario M5G 1X5, Canada
* Corresponding author.
E-mail address: marco.fiore@istitutotumori.mi.it

potential, but its propensity for local recurrence can entail considerable morbidity. In the latest edition of the World Health Organization's classification of tumors of bone and soft tissue, DF is defined as an intermediate/locally aggressive tumor.[3]

PATHOPHYSIOLOGY AND EMERGING BIOLOGICAL INSIGHTS
Adenomatous Poliposis Coli Gene

The earliest insight into the biology of DF stemmed from the observation of a high prevalence of desmoids in patients with familial adenomatous polyposis (FAP/Gardner syndrome). FAP is driven by mutations in the *Adenomatous Poliposis Coli (APC)* gene and is characterized by innumerable polyps in the gastrointestinal tract (primarily the colon) that can evolve to adenocarcinoma. FAP is also associated with frequent DF, arising mainly in the abdominal cavity (mesenteric DF) or in the abdominal wall within previous surgical scars.[4] As a general rule, FAP-related DF should be distinguished from sporadic DF, as the two exhibit different clinical behavior and necessitate different treatment strategies. *APC* is involved in controlling the level of β-catenin in the cytoplasm. When *APC* is mutated, β-catenin cannot be degraded and it translocates to the nucleus where it affects gene transcription.[5]

β-Catenin

β-catenin is a dual-function protein encoded by the *CTNNB1* gene, regulating the coordination of cell-cell adhesion in the cytoplasm as well as gene transcription in the nucleus. β-catenin is a subunit of the cadherin protein complex and acts as an intracellular signal transducer in the Wnt signaling pathway.[6]

Generally, cytoplasmic β-catenin levels are kept in equilibrium via continuous ubiquitin-proteasome–mediated degradation, a process that is regulated by a multiprotein complex containing axin, APC, GSK3β, and CK1α. β-catenin phosphorylation allows recognition by ubiquitin ligase, which targets the protein for destruction in the proteosome.[7] Unphosphorylated β-catenin is stable and can translocate to the nucleus to interact with the TCF family of transcription factors to activate downstream genes (**Fig. 1**).

APC mutations do not in fact underlie most sporadic DF; rather *CTNNB1* mutations were found in 85% to 88% of sporadic DF in historical published series.[2,8,9] With modern genome sequencing techniques, the frequency of *CTNBB1* mutations has been shown to be even higher, providing compelling evidence that alterations in the Wnt/APC/β-catenin pathway underlie the development and progression of this disease.[10,11] Most of the β-catenin mutations occur in the region encoding the phosphorylation domain on exon 3. Three main point mutations have been described in codons 41 and 45, which represent targets for phosphorylation by GSK3β and CK1, respectively (**Fig. 2**). The most common *CTNNB1* mutation in sporadic DF is T41A, accounting for around 50% of cases. S45F accounts for approximately 30% and S45P for 7%.[8] Rare mutations in exon 3, such as T40A[11] and small in-frame deletions have been reported.[9] Other genetic events, such as APC loss, chromosome 6 loss, or BMI I mutation, have been recently published.[11]

Target genes of the transcriptional complex β-catenin/TCF3 in DF are largely unknown, as few studies have evaluated potential desmoid-associated gene expression deregulation.[12–19] Available data on gene expression show some common deregulated genes between different published series, but the comparability of studies is limited by differences in tumor types and study technique. Despite the crucial role of β-catenin in the pathogenesis of DF, additional players must be involved as β-catenin is mutated and overexpressed in other tumors types, including hepatocellular carcinoma, colorectal, lung, breast, ovarian, and endometrial cancers.[20,21]

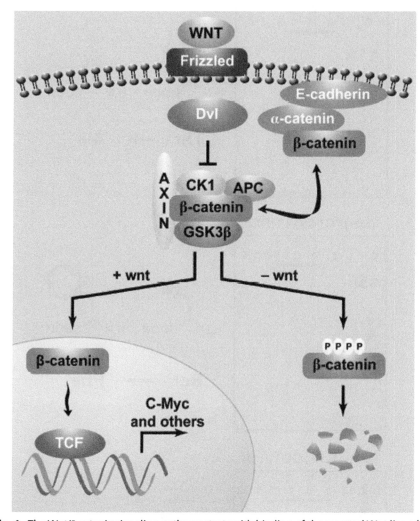

Fig. 1. The Wnt/β-catenin signaling pathway starts with binding of the secreted Wnt ligand to its cell surface receptors (Fz-Frizzled/LRP); such binding results in phosphorylation of the cytoplasmic disheveled (dvl) protein. Phosphorylated dvl prevents phosphorylation of β-catenin by the APC/axin/CK1/GSK3β. Phosphorylated β-catenin is destroyed in the proteosome complex. Unphosphorylated β-catenin is stable and can translocate to the nucleus to interact with cotranscriptional factors belonging to the TCF family to activate downstream genes (c-MYC, Cyclin D1, and so forth). (*From* Kotiligam D, Lazar AJ, Pollock RE, et al. Desmoid tumor: a disease opportune for molecular insight. Histol Histopathol 2008;23:121; with permission.)

β-Catenin Mutations and Beyond

The role of specific β-catenin mutations in DF is not yet fully understood. In surgically treated series, patients harboring a *CTNNB1* S45F mutation had more aggressive disease with higher rates of local recurrence compared with *CTNNB1* T41A mutants.[8] In an international multicenter study the 3- and 5-year recurrence-free survival (RFS) rates were 49% and 45% for those with a *CTNNB1* S45F mutation, 91% and 91% for wild-type (WT) genes, and 70% and 66% for all other mutations, including

806

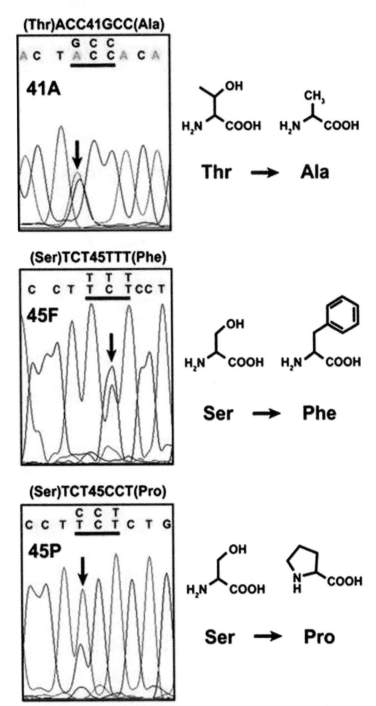

Fig. 2. Examples of Sanger sequencing for each mutational type encountered. A single amino acid substitution generates different mutation: ACC to GCC in codon 41 (41A; replacement of threonine by alanine); TCT to TTT in codon 45 (45F; replacement of serine by phenylalanine); and TCT to CCT in codon 45 (45P; replacement of serine with proline). (*From* Lazar AJ, Tuvin D, Hajibashi S, et al. Specific mutations in the beta-catenin gene [CTNNB1] correlate with local recurrence in sporadic desmoid tumors. Am J Pathol 2008;173(5):1521; with permission.)

T41A and S45P (P<.001).[22] In a recent series, van Broekhoven and colleagues[23] confirmed that an S45F mutation entailed worse RFS in patients treated surgically (5-year cumulative risk of recurrence of 63.8%); it remained an independent risk factor in multivariable analysis.

The biological effect of different β-catenin mutations is an area of ongoing active investigation, with the objective of eventually predicting disease behavior and response to treatment based on gene expression or miRNA signature. Two European trials of patients with DF being managed with a watchful-waiting strategy seek to elucidate the prognostic value of specific β-catenin mutations with respect to disease progression (NCT02547831).

Hamada and colleagues[24] showed that all patients harboring a *CTNNB1* S45F mutation treated with meloxicam had progressive disease (P = .017), whereas other mutations had no impact on response to treatment. Recently, it has been reported that specific mutations also correlate with response to imatinib in a phase II clinical trial.[25] The progression arrest rate at 6 months was 70%, 81%, and 43% for T41A, S45F, and WT, respectively. *CTNNB1* S45F mutated DF was in fact overrepresented in this trial, which included only progressing patients according to Response Evaluation Criteria in Solid Tumors (RECIST), underlying the more aggressive behavior of this specific subgroup.

Gene Profiles

The ongoing prospective European trial evaluating a watchful-waiting strategy is also focusing on the possible prognostic role of a gene signature for progression (NCT02547831). A specific signature of 36 genes (including FECH, STOML2, and TRIP6) significantly associated with progression-free survival in a subgroup of patients treated with surgery will be tested in the observed population.[26] Dufresne and colleagues[27] previously reported the capability of a specific molecular signature consisting of 15 miRNAs to stratify time to progression following imatinib treatment.

ETIOLOGY

The etiology of DF remains unclear. DF can occur in previous surgical scars, often after caesarian section, or in the abdomen following surgical procedures, especially in patients with FAP. Although the mesentery is the preferred site for FAP-associated DF, the most common anatomic site of sporadic DF is the abdominal wall in patients with a recent history of pregnancy.

Desmoid-Type Fibromatosis and Hormones

This propensity for DF to occur following pregnancy has been postulated to reflect a degree of hormone sensitivity in the tumor within a predisposing microenvironment. However, a direct correlation between estrogen level and DF has never been demonstrated.[28] The positive expression of the sex steroid receptors (estrogen and progesterone) was not described in all series, largely because of different antibodies used for staining.[29,30] So far, no correlation between hormone receptor expression and response to specific antiestrogenic agents has been demonstrated. Moreover, the correlation between female sex, DF, and hormone therapy has never been tested in randomized controlled trials.

Desmoid-Type Fibromatosis and Scars

The occurrence of DF within or close to surgical scars is thought to reflect altered tissue repair processes, based on evidence that β-catenin plays a role in wound healing. In fact, β-catenin is transiently elevated in fibroblasts during tissue repair and forced β-catenin overexpression results in the formation of hypertrophic scars in mice.[31] This abnormal expression is partly related to the release by platelets of growth factors and cytokines (platelet-derived growth factor [PDGF], transforming growth factor [TGF]) at the site of injury, with subsequent induction of β-catenin signaling in fibroblasts.[32] In contrast, a decrease in β-catenin signaling is observed at late stages of the scarring process.[31] Consistently, PDGF receptor (PDGFR) and TGF-β pathways seemed to be downregulated in DF.[17,33]

In Gardner syndrome, the risk of developing mesenteric DF has been shown to be significantly lower after minimally invasive surgical procedures compared to open surgery.[34]

Progenitor Cell

Despite DF cells morphologically resembling fibroblasts in an abundant collagen matrix, the actual progenitor cell of DF is not known. Aberrantly activated mesenchymal stromal cells (MSCs) are present in DF[31,35] and genes and cell surface markers characteristic of MSCs are expressed in DF, suggesting that MSCs may be the progenitor cells of DF.[36]

PATIENT EVALUATION
Symptoms

DF usually presents as a painless mass in the extremity, abdominal wall or trunk. Patients with intra-abdominal DF may note distension or increased abdominal girth. Rarely, DF may result in complications such as bowel perforation or obstruction (**Fig. 3**). Pain is typically a late event, although it can occur or worsen after biopsy. Occasionally neurologic symptoms including both motor and sensory disturbances can be the direct result of DF, particularly those involving the pelvic or scapular girdle. Severe pain may require further evaluation and treatment. It is imperative to establish a relationship between the patient's pain and the location or progression of the tumor, and to rule out other possible etiologies. Often the pain is not directly related to disease progression, though symptoms are clearly related to DF itself. In these cases, targeted intervention for the DF is not indicated, and multidisciplinary evaluation may be required for adequate pain therapy.

DF usually presents as a single lesion but rarely can be multifocal. Multifocality typically occurs in the extremities and in cases of recurrence after previous surgery.

Radiology

Patients with suspected DF are often first evaluated by ultrasound, although sonographic features are fairly nonspecific and further imaging is mandatory. Contrast-enhanced MRI or computed tomography (CT) is required for adequate imaging of intra-abdominal lesions. On CT, DF is isodense to skeletal muscle with inhomogeneous foci corresponding to collagenous or myxoid areas. Contrast enhancement is variable and often prominent, reflecting a rich vascularity. Contrast-enhanced CT is the preferred modality for intra-abdominal DF, as it allows delineation of the tumor from surrounding fat with less peristaltic artifact than MRI.

MRI is the imaging modality of choice for DF arising in the extremities, pelvis, perineum, pelvic and scapular girdles, superficial trunk, and head and neck region. Specific MRI features of DF have been described and have been correlated to disease status. During disease progression, DF is heterogeneously hyperintense on T2-weighted (T2W) images (corresponding to high cellularity), with avid enhancement after administration of intravenous gadolinium and bands of low signal in all

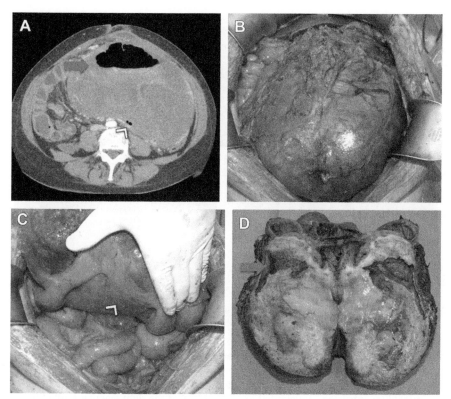

Fig. 3. Intra-abdominal desmoid: Preoperative CT scan (*A*). Intraoperative findings (*B, C*). Surgical specimen (*D*). Disease progression is complicated by bowel perforation in the tumor mass (*arrow*). Arrowheads: radiological and intraoperative evidence of jejunal loop perforated into desmoid mass (*A, C*).

sequences.[37,38] In approximately 90% of cases, the key diagnostic feature of hypointense bands is identifiable on T2W images, which correspond to the dense assemblies of collagen bundles seen histologically. Spontaneous regression and dimensional response to treatment are often predicted by altered characteristics on MRI: increased T2 hypointensity and decreased enhancement (**Figs. 4** and **5**).[37]

RECIST criteria for response to treatment are of little utility in evaluating DF. As these are typically slow-growing lesions, a dimensional response to treatment may not be evident for several months, despite effective therapy. Ongoing investigation into changes in both size and tumor composition on MRI are expected to assist with radiologic surveillance of DF, but at present no formal criteria exist for evaluating response to treatment.

Fluorodeoxyglucose-PET is not currently used in clinical practice, but it has been investigated in the evaluation of DF. Kasper and colleagues[39] demonstrated a 30% decrease in the mean standardized uptake value (SUV) of serial PET scans in patients treated with imatinib. Baseline SUV values are relatively low in DF, compared with high-grade sarcomas. However, the initial mean SUV1 and maximum SUV1 (SUV1max) data suggest that there may be a role for PET in evaluating the response to therapy in DF.[40]

Pathology

DF is composed of proliferations of spindle cells resembling fibroblasts with no malignant features (eg. hyperchromatic nuclei, atypia).[3] These cells are embedded in a

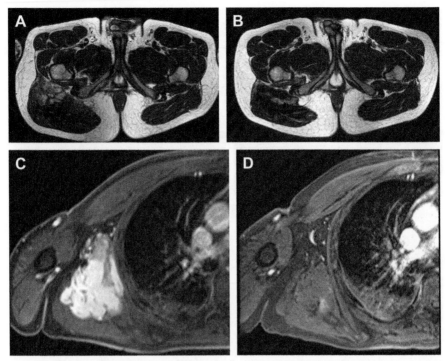

Fig. 4. T2W axial MRI of intramuscular DF of the right buttock (*A*), and spontaneous regression after 4 years of observation, both with reduced tumor size and intensity in T2W sequence (*B*). Gadolinium-enhanced T1-weighted axial MRI of DF of the right scapular girdle (*C*), and near-complete spontaneous regression after 6 years of observation (*D*).

dense collagen matrix with variably prominent blood vessels and tend to have an infiltrative growth pattern. Immunostaining is positive for β-catenin (predominantly nuclear) and vimentin, but it should be noted that nuclear staining for β-catenin is not specific for DF.[41] Other mesenchymal neoplasms, such as solitary fibrous tumor, endometrial stromal sarcoma, and synovial sarcoma can also stain positive for nuclear β-catenin.[42] DF is negative for smooth muscle actin, desmin, h-caldesmon, CD34, c-KIT (CD117), and S-100 and positive for cyclooxygenase 2 (COX-2) and the tyrosine kinase receptor PDGFRb. It is frequently positive for androgen receptor and estrogen receptor beta but not for estrogen receptor alpha.

Given the high incidence of *CTNNB1* mutations in sporadic DF, mutational analysis has become a useful diagnostic tool in challenging cases. For instance, in patients with suspected recurrent DF or patients operated on for different diagnoses (eg. retroperitoneal dedifferentiated liposarcoma) who develop new lesions in the operative field, *CTNNB1* mutational analysis may be essential for diagnosis. Point mutations in exon 3 are pathognomonic of DF among spindle cell lesions. They do not occur among other soft tissue sarcomas, gastrointestinal stromal tumor, or reactive processes (eg. nodular fasciitis, myositis, and scars). However, *CTNNB1* mutations are reported in several epithelial neoplasms.

There are insufficient data at present to use *CTNNB1* mutation status to predict response to treatment, although a correlation has been identified in surgically treated patients.[22,23] Data from the ongoing prospective trial on surveillance of primary DF may eventually add new insight in this area.

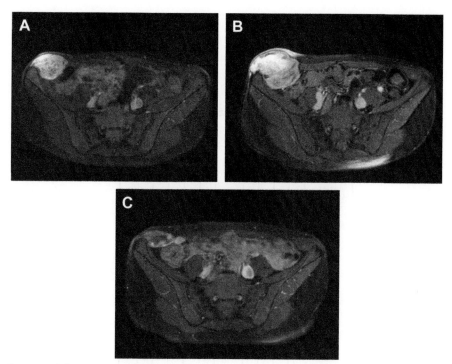

Fig. 5. Gadolinium-enhanced T1-weighted axial MRI of DF of the right abdominal wall (*A*), and dimensional disease progression after 8 months from initial observation (*B*). Partial response to Toremifene 180 daily after 14 months, with both dimensional reduction and attenuation of contrast-enhancement on T1-weighted sequence (*C*).

EVOLVING ROLE OF SURGERY
Surgical Outcomes in Historical Series

Prior to the year 2000, the management of DF mirrored that of soft tissue sarcoma, with surgery as the standard of care. Multiple retrospective single-institution case series have reported local control of DF after complete surgical resection to be approximately 80% at 5 years. Tumor location was found to be a risk factor for recurrence, with extremity DF portending a worse prognosis than abdominal wall and other sites. Recurrent disease was also a risk factor for further recurrence. Surgical margins, however, do not consistently correlate with recurrence (**Table 1**). Of note, microscopically negative surgical margins are more difficult to obtain in DF compared with soft tissue sarcoma because of the infiltrative growth pattern of this disease. This point should be taken into account when considering surgical intervention with the possibility of resultant functional impairment.

Postsurgical Nomogram

A recently published nomogram incorporates tumor site, size, and patient age in estimating risk of local recurrence in patients undergoing surgical resection. As described earlier, abdominal wall DF entails a favorable prognosis, whereas extremity DF portends the worst prognosis. Increased tumor size is associated with continuously increasing risk of local recurrence, and younger patients have the highest risk of recurrent disease.[43]

Table 1
Surgical series

Author, Year	No. of Patients	Primary/Recurrence	Median Follow-up (mo)	5-y DFS (%)		Surgical Margins as Prognostic Factor
				Negative Margins	Positive Margins	
Posner et al,[75] 1989	128	78/53	88	85	50	Yes
Ballo et al,[65] 1999	189	85/104	112	75	50	Yes
Merchant et al,[68] 1999	105	All primary	49	70	78	No
Gronchi et al,[67] 2003	128	Primary	130	82	79	No
	75	Recurrence	153	65	47	No
Huang et al,[76] 2009	151	113/38	102	80	80	Yes
Mullen et al,[77] 2012	177	133/44	40	82	52	Yes
Peng et al,[78] 2012	141	na	26	53	53	Yes
Crago et al,[43] 2013	439	382/113	60	69	69	No
Zeng et al,[79] 2014	233	156/77	54	74	74	Yes
He et al,[80] 2015	114	79/35	73	85	50	Yes

Abbreviations: DFS, disease-free survival; na, not available.

Nonoperative Management

In recent years, evidence of the unpredictable behavior of DF, including long-term disease stabilization and spontaneous regression, has resulted in a paradigm shift toward more conservative treatments.

In 1999, Lewis and colleagues[44] adopted a watchful waiting approach to multiply recurrent DF on the basis that further surgery would result in considerable functional impairment, and demonstrated some long-term disease stabilization without further intervention. Taking into consideration these results along with the local recurrence rate of 20% to 30% (exceedingly high for a benign condition) and the potential morbidity of resection, a nonoperative approach to primary DF was advocated as first-line therapy. This approach initially entailed liberal use of medical and, to a lesser extent, radiation therapy, but eventually a period of observation with no active treatment was systematically offered to most patients with a new diagnosis of primary DF.

In the last 8 years, multiple series of a nonsurgical or observational approach to DF have been published (**Table 2**), with the following major findings:

- Nonoperative management of DF can be safely offered to most patients.
- Disease stabilization is documented for roughly 50% of patients and for a median duration of 14 to 19 months.
- Only a minority of patients require surgical resection after initial observation (16% of abdominal wall DF, 4% of extra-abdominal DF).
- Spontaneous regression is consistently reported in 20% to 28% of cases.
- Disease progression is exceptionally rare after 3 years of initial observation.

At present, the challenge is to find the most suitable treatment for each patient, given the peculiar natural history of the disease and the lack of accepted biological predictive factors.

The recent molecular insights on the possible prognostic role of different *CTNBB1* mutations are mainly based on postsurgical series. Data on primary DF managed with watchful waiting are still pending.

Stepwise Approach

Given the variable and unpredictable behavior of DF and multiplicity of treatment modalities, it is imperative that patients be made aware of the variety of therapeutic strategies and possible disease trajectories at the time of diagnosis.

Two expert consensus statements are now available, one incorporating expertise from a sarcoma patient advocacy group.[45,46] These recommend that a stepwise approach be used for every patient diagnosed with DF, beginning with a period of observation to discriminate active tumors from those that are quiescent or regressing. For progressive and/or symptomatic disease, any available therapeutic option can be considered, beginning with the safest and escalating as necessary (**Fig. 6**).

PHARMACOLOGIC TREATMENT OPTIONS

The period of initial observation should last one to two years. In the case of stabilization or regression, observation should be continued. In the event of progression, alternative treatment options should be discussed. However, progression can be difficult to define. To determine the cutoff for active treatment, different factors have to be taken into account, such as initial tumor size, growth rate, anatomic location, risk to organs/nerves, compression, and worsening of function. In most cases, active treatment is initiated in the context of objective tumor progression in multiple (eg. 3) consecutive imaging studies. Subsequent steps should be tailored according to

Table 2
Wait-and-see policy

Author, Year	Overall Patients	Nonsurgical Approach (No.)	Wait-and-See Approach (No.)	Median Follow-up (mo)	Results of Wait-and-See Approach	Notes
Bonvalot et al,[81] 2008	112	23	11	76	3-y PFS = 68%	—
Nakayama et al,[82] 2008	11	11	11	56	• 10 of 11 growth arrest • 3 of 11 spontaneous regression	—
Fiore et al,[83] 2009	142	142	83	33	• 5-y PFS = 49.9% • Median TTP = 14 mo	—
Barbier et al,[84] 2010	26	26	26	na	Growth arrest after a median of 14 mo	—
Salas et al,[85] 2011	426	56	27	52	• 16 of 27 stable disease • 5 of 27 spontaneous regression • Median TTP = 19 mo	—
Bonvalot et al,[86] 2013	147	106	102	36	• 3-y change to medical therapy = 25% • 3-y change to surgery = 16% • Spontaneous regression in 28%	Abdominal wall DF
Briand et al,[87] 2014	73	55	55	—	• Dropout from wait-and-see policy = 9.6%	Extra-abdominal DF
Colombo et al,[88] 2015	216	122	70	39	• 5-y change to surgery = 3.6% • Median TTP = 18 mo • Spontaneous regression in 20%	Extra-abdominal DF

Abbreviations: PFS, progression-free survival; TTP, time to progression.

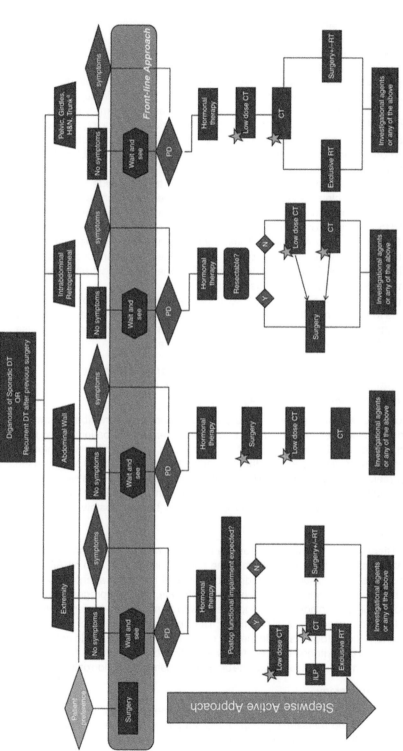

Fig. 6. Consensus algorithm for the treatment of sporadic desmoid-type fibromatosis. First choice in case of rapid progressive disease (PD) (*star*). [a] Abdominal wall excluded. DT, desmoid tumor; H&N, head and neck; ILP, isolated limb perfusion; RT, radiotherapy. (*From* Gronchi A, Colombo C, Le Péchoux C, et al. Sporadic desmoid-type fibromatosis: a stepwise approach to a non-metastatic neoplasm – a position paper from the Italian and the French Sarcoma Group. Ann Oncol 2014;25(3):581; with permission.)

anatomic location, patient age, and comorbidities as depicted in the algorithm in **Fig. 6**.[45,46] In select cases, such as rapidly progressive disease or life-threatening anatomic location, specific treatment may be proposed at the time of diagnosis.

A variety of medical therapies have been found to be effective against DF, including nonsteroidal antiinflammatories (NSAIDs), endocrine therapy, cytotoxic chemotherapy, and targeted therapies such as imatinib.[47–51] The data in support of each of these consist largely of retrospective case series or single-arm cohort studies, with occasional phase II clinical trials. Although clinical trials are ongoing to investigate the efficacy of new agents against DF, there are no randomized controlled trials comparing one pharmacologic treatment strategy versus another (**Tables 3** and **4**). Furthermore, despite our understanding of the disease biology, there are as yet no predictive markers of response to specific therapies to help guide treatment. For example, despite a high prevalence of nuclear estrogen receptor beta positivity in DF, only a small proportion respond to antiestrogen therapy; response to imatinib is not related to expression of c-KIT (KIT staining is generally negative) or to the presence of PDGFR-*alpha* or -*beta* mutations. Thus, the decision of first-line medical therapy must be undertaken by the individual physician and patient after careful consideration of the efficacy and toxicity of available options.[45,46] The use of most pharmacologic agents in the treatment of DF remains off label.[52]

It is important to recognize that because of the slow-growing nature of DF, changes in response to treatment will not be immediately apparent but rather may be appreciated only after serial imaging investigations. In the treatment of progressive disease, growth arrest should be considered a response to therapy.

ESTABLISHED TREATMENTS: NONSTEROIDAL ANTIINFLAMMATORY DRUGS, ANTIESTROGEN AGENTS, CYTOTOXIC CHEMOTHERAPY, IMATINIB
Antiinflammatory and Antiestrogen Agents

The use of NSAIDs against DF was based on the unexpected observation of complete regression of a single recurrent desmoid tumor in the sternum of a patient taking indomethacin for radiation-induced pericarditis.[53] Since then, a variety of antiinflammatory agents, including sulindac, indomethacin, and celecoxib have been widely used. Recently, meloxicam was also found to have some efficacy in DF in a retrospective study.[47] In addition to their antiinflammatory mechanism, the anti–COX-2 activity of these agents may also target downstream events in the β-catenin pathway in DF cells.

Hormone Therapy

Because DF seems to be influenced by the hormonal microenvironment, endocrine manipulation has also been used, both alone and in combination with NSAIDs, with resultant disease stabilization and regression. Several hormonal agents have been studied, including tamoxifen, toremifene, progesterone, medroxyprogesterone acetate, prednisolone, testolactone, and goserelin, with tamoxifen and toremifene being the most frequently used in clinical practice.[52] The mechanism of action of these agents is incompletely understood, as evidenced by the fact that patients who do not respond to tamoxifen can be switched to toremifene with clinical benefit.[54] A role for the TGF-β pathway has been proposed to explain the unique mechanism of action of toremifene.[17]

Cytotoxic Chemotherapy

Chemotherapy has been widely used in DF despite the oncologic dogma that *low-grade tumors with no metastatic potential are not lethal and should not respond to chemotherapy*. DF represents an exception to this rule, especially when associated with FAP.[55] Doxorubicin-based regimens (alone or in combination with dacarbazine)

Table 3
Medical therapy options: established drugs

Authors, Year	Therapy	Potential Target	Study Type	Drug Dose	End Point	Outcome
Nishida et al,[47] 2010	Meloxicam	COX-2	Retrospective study	10 mg daily	NA	95% of SD/PR/CR at 34 mo
Brooks et al,[48] 1992	Toremifene	ER (?)	Retrospective study	200 mg daily	NA	1 CR, 10 PR, 6 SD
Patel et al,[49] 1993	DOX + DTIC	—	Retrospective study	DOX 60–90 mg/m^2; DTIC 750–1000 mg/m^2	ORR	50.00%
Azzarelli et al,[51] 2001	MTX + VBL	—	Retrospective study	MTX 30 mg/m^2/wk VBL 6 mg/m^2/wk	ORR	17.00%
Weiss et al,[50] 1999	MTX + VNR	—	Retrospective study	MTX 50/wk, VNR 20 mg/m^2/wk	ORR	60.00%
Heinrich et al,[56] 2006	Imatinib mesylate	PDGFR-alfa	Phase II clinical trial	800 mg daily	PFS	37% at 1 y
Chugh et al,[57] 2010	Imatinib mesylate	PDGFR-alfa	Phase II clinical trial	200–600 mg daily[a]	PFS	1 y: 66%; 3 y: 58%
Penel et al,[58] 2011	Imatinib mesylate	PDGFR-alfa	Phase II clinical trial	400 mg daily	PFS	1 y: 67%; 2 y: 55%
Kasper et al,[25] ongoing trial	Imatinib mesylate	PDGFR-alfa	Phase II clinical trial	800 mg daily	PFS	65% at 6 mo

Abbreviations: CR, complete response; DOX, doxorubicine; DTIC, dacarbazine; ER, estrogen receptors; MTX, methotrexate; NA, not available; ORR, overall response rate; SD, stable disease; VBL, vinblastine; VNR, vinorelbine.
[a] According to body surface area.

Table 4
Medical treatments: new drugs

Authors, Year or ID Number on clinicaltrial.gov	Drug	Potential Target	Drug Dosage	Study Phase	Primary End Point	Outcome
Jo et al,[59] 2014	Sunitinib	PDGFR, KIT, FLT3, VEGFR inhibitor	37.5 mg/d	Prospective multicenter study	RR	26% PR, 42% SD
NCT01876082	Pazopanib	VEGFR, PDGFR and c-KIT inhibitor	800 mg daily	Phase II clinical trial	PFS	NA
Gounder et al,[61] 2011	Sorafenib[a]	PDGFR and VEGFR inhibitor	400 mg daily	Retrospective study	RR	25% PR, 70% SD, and 4% PD
NCT01981551	PF 03084014	Gamma-secretase inhibitor	150 mg twice a day	Phase II clinical trial	RR	NA
NCT01265030	Sirolimus	mTOR inhibitor	12 mg/m² as loading dose, 4 mg/m²	Phase I/II clinical trial	mTOR pathway activation in preoperative setting	NA

Abbreviations: ID, identification; NA, not available; PD, progressive disease; PFS, progression-free survival; RR, response rate; VEGFR, vascular endothelial growth factor receptor.
[a] NCT02066181 Clinical trial is ongoing.

and methotrexate and vinblastine/vinorelbine have been shown to have activity against DF.[52] Overall response rates to combination chemotherapy in single-arm studies range from 17% to 100%, with a median response rate of 50%. Despite their efficacy, doxorubicin-based regimens have considerable acute and late toxicity (in particular cardiotoxicity); hence, the better-tolerated methotrexate and vinblastine/vinorelbine combination represents a reasonable alternative. Most patients respond slowly, with effects generally observed after months of treatment; but the response is typically durable. Given the toxicity of all chemotherapeutic agents, patients must be carefully selected for this modality.

Imatinib Mesylate

The efficacy of imatinib in patients with DF has been tested in several phase II clinical trials. In a study by Heinrich and colleagues[56] using a dosage of 800 mg daily, the 1-year progression-free survival was 37%, with 16% of partial response (PR). Of 13 cases of stable disease, 3 maintained long-term stability (defined as >18 months). Chugh and colleagues[57] reported 3-year progression-free survival of 58% with 6% regression after a range of 19 to 26 months of treatment, with a clinical benefit (their primary end point) seen in 84% of patients. Penel and colleagues[58] reported 1-year progression-free survival of 67%, including one case of a complete response. Despite the difference in primary end points and the heterogeneity of patients included (not all met RECIST criteria for progressive disease), imatinib was shown to induce disease stability in a proportion of patients. The results of an ongoing trial of imatinib in RECIST progressive patients should provide additional clarity on the subset of patients who derive benefit. Interestingly, in this trial the progression arrest rate seems to be highest among patients harboring a 45F mutation.[25]

NEW FRONTIERS: SUNITINIB, SORAFENIB, PAZOPANIB, GAMMA SECRETASE INHIBITOR, MAMMALIAN TARGET OF RAPAMYCIN INHIBITOR

In light of the efficacy of imatinib in DF, other tyrosine kinase inhibitors have been investigated, including sunitinib, pazopanib, and sorafenib. In a phase II clinical trial involving 19 patients, sunitinib achieved a progression-free survival of 75% at 2 years.[59] Pazopanib, a multi-kinase inhibitor, was reported to be effective in reducing the symptoms of recurrent DF after surgery, with more than 1 year of follow-up.[60] Pazopanib is currently being compared with vinblastine and methotrexate in a phase II clinical trial (NCT01876082). Sorafenib, another PDGFR and VEGF inhibitor, achieved partial response and stable disease rates of 25% and 70%, respectively, after a median of 6 months of treatment in a retrospective study.[61]

Recent studies on the molecular biology of DF have helped identify new potential therapeutic targets, such as the Notch pathway.[62] The expression of Notch1 and Hes1 detected in DF samples suggests a possible correlation between Notch pathway activation and DF. PF-03084014, a gamma-secretase inhibitor in the Notch pathway, is currently being investigated in a phase II trial (NCT0198551) after promising results in phase I.[63]

Another potential therapeutic target is the mammalian target of rapamycin (mTOR) pathway. mTOR activation has been linked to cellular proliferation and tumor growth in transgenic animals harboring *APC* mutations, similar to what is seen in FAP-associated desmoids.[64] Sirolimus, or rapamycin, is an inhibitor of mTOR signaling that is currently being tested in a pilot study aiming to investigate the activation of mTOR and its associated targets in patients with DF (NCT01265030).

NONPHARMACOLOGIC TREATMENT OPTIONS
Radiotherapy

The role of radiotherapy (RT) in DF is limited. Some studies have reported improved local control with adjuvant RT following surgery,[65,66] whereas others have found no benefit.[67–69] The potential sequelae of RT (pathologic fracture, fibrosis, edema, radio-induced malignancy, and neuropathy) must be carefully considered in the decision to use this modality in the treatment of a benign disease. Current consensus guidelines propose the use of RT only after multiple failed lines of treatment. These guidelines also suggest that definitive RT may be considered for tumors in critical anatomic locations (eg. head and neck) where surgery would involve prohibitive risk or functional impairment. Radiation doses should be limited to 50 to 56 Gy, based on results of a recent prospective trial.[70]

Cryoablation

Percutaneous cryoablation is a novel local treatment for small extra-abdominal DF. Small retrospective case series have shown clinical benefit in terms of pain relief and radiologic response, including the possibility of complete response.[71,72] The procedure can be repeated as shown by Cornelis and colleagues[73] in a patient with FAP and multiple extra-abdominal DF. Cryoablation is not appropriate for large tumors or those located close to vital structures. Prospective studies are needed to confirm the safety and efficacy of this procedure.

Isolated Limb Perfusion

Historically, isolated limb perfusion (ILP) has been used in DF as limb-salvage treatment in patients with progressive disease. In a multicenter retrospective series of 28 patients treated with ILP using tumor necrosis factor (TNF) and melphalan, significant antitumor activity was demonstrated. Among 25 patients who received 28 ILP treatments, a complete response was achieved after 2 ILP treatments and a partial response after 17 treatments in 16 patients. Stable disease was reported after 8 treatments in 7 patients. Prolonged disease stabilization has also been documented.[74]

In contrast to the practice in soft tissue sarcoma, surgery for residual disease after ILP is not mandatory and is actually avoided in most patients. Instead, repeat ILP has been described after disease reprogression. ILP represents a valuable therapeutic option for patients with distal (hand/wrist or foot/ankle) or multifocal DF who have failed systemic treatment or for patients who refuse chemotherapy (**Fig. 7**).

SURVEILLANCE RECOMMENDATIONS

In the future, the authors anticipate that an increasing proportion of patients with new diagnoses of DF will undergo active surveillance rather than up-front active treatment. Issues related to frequency, imaging modality, and overall duration of surveillance remain unresolved. Initially, short-interval imaging may be prudent, for example, every 3 to 4 months. The authors recommend using contrast-enhanced MRI for the first 2 years of surveillance. In the case of stable disease or regression, longer time intervals can be adopted as well as sonographic surveillance instead of MRI.

Special consideration should be given to female patients of childbearing age. The complex and incompletely understood relationship between DF and pregnancy warrants a comprehensive discussion to assist patients with family planning and educate them regarding the possible eventualities. Available data do not suggest the need to avoid or interrupt a pregnancy in patients with a history of DF. On the contrary, DF may

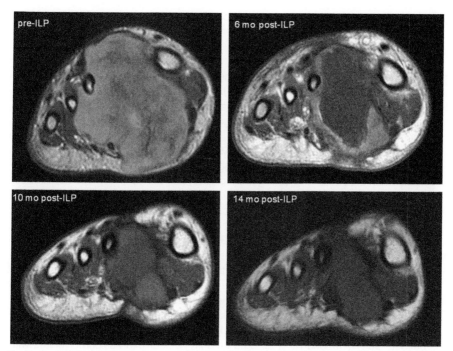

Fig. 7. Gadolinium-enhanced T1-weighted axial MRI of multi-recurrent desmoid of the right foot treated with ILP (TNF + melphalan [Alkeran]), with long-lasting partial response and objective clinical benefit.

be safely managed in the event of progression during or after pregnancy. Obstetric complications are rarely encountered.[28]

ACKNOWLEDGMENTS

The authors thank the Desmoid Tumor Research Foundation for their continued and generous support of their work in this field.

REFERENCES

1. Li M, Cordon-Cardo C, Gerald WL, et al. Desmoid fibromatosis is a clonal process. Hum Pathol 1996;27(9):939–43.
2. Alman BA, Pajerski ME, Diaz-Cano S, et al. Aggressive fibromatosis (desmoid tumor) is a monoclonal disorder. Diagn Mol Pathol 1997;6(2):98–101.
3. Desmoid-type fibromatoses. In: Fletcher JA, Bridge JA, Hogendoorn PCW, editors. WHO Classification of Tumours of Soft Tissue and Bone. Fourth Edition. Lyon (France): IARC; 2013. p. 72–3.
4. Groen EJ, Roos A, Muntinghe FL, et al. Extra-intestinal manifestations of familial adenomatous polyposis. Ann Surg Oncol 2008;15(9):2439–50.
5. Goss KH, Groden J. Biology of the adenomatous polyposis coli tumor suppressor. J Clin Oncol 2000;18(9):1967–79.
6. Barker N. The canonical Wnt/beta-catenin signaling pathway. Methods Mol Biol 2008;468:5–15.
7. Kotiligam D, Lazar AJ, Pollock RE, et al. Desmoid tumor: a disease opportune for molecular insights. Histol Histopathol 2008;23(1):117–26.

8. Lazar AJ, Tuvin D, Hajibashi S, et al. Specific mutations in the beta-catenin gene (CTNNB1) correlate with local recurrence in sporadic desmoid tumors. Am J Pathol 2008;173(5):1518–27.

9. Domont J, Salas S, Lacroix L, et al. High frequency of beta-catenin heterozygous mutations in extra-abdominal fibromatosis: a potential molecular tool for disease management. Br J Cancer 2010;102(6):1032–6.

10. Tejpar S, Nollet F, Li C, et al. Predominance of beta-catenin mutations and beta-catenin dysregulation in sporadic aggressive fibromatosis (desmoid tumor). Oncogene 1999;18(47):6615–20.

11. Crago AM, Chmielecki J, Rosenberg M, et al. Near universal detection of alterations in CTNNB1 and Wnt pathway regulators in desmoid-type fibromatosis by whole-exome sequencing and genomic analysis. Genes Chromosomes Cancer 2015;54(10):606–15.

12. Alman BA, Naber SP, Terek RM, et al. Platelet-derived growth factor in fibrous musculoskeletal disorders: a study of pathologic tissue sections and in vitro primary cell cultures. J Orthop Res 1995;13(1):67–77.

13. Denys H, Jadidizadeh A, Amini Nik S, et al. Identification of IGFBP-6 as a significantly downregulated gene by beta-catenin in desmoid tumors. Oncogene 2004; 23(3):654–64.

14. Locci P, Bellocchio S, Lilli C, et al. Synthesis and secretion of transforming growth factor-beta1 by human desmoid fibroblast cell line and its modulation by toremifene. J Interferon Cytokine Res 2001;21(11):961–70.

15. Saito T, Oda Y, Tanaka K, et al. beta-catenin nuclear expression correlates with cyclin D1 overexpression in sporadic desmoid tumours. J Pathol 2001;195(2): 222–8.

16. Tolg C, Poon R, Fodde R, et al. Genetic deletion of receptor for hyaluronan-mediated motility (Rhamm) attenuates the formation of aggressive fibromatosis (desmoid tumor). Oncogene 2003;22(44):6873–82.

17. Amini Nik S, Ebrahim RP, Van Dam K, et al. TGF-beta modulates beta-Catenin stability and signaling in mesenchymal proliferations. Exp Cell Res 2007; 313(13):2887–95.

18. Fen Li C, Kandel C, Baliko F, et al. Plasminogen activator inhibitor-1 (PAI-1) modifies the formation of aggressive fibromatosis (desmoid tumor). Oncogene 2005; 24(9):1615–24.

19. Colombo C, Creighton CJ, Ghadimi MP, et al. Increased midkine expression correlates with desmoid tumour recurrence: a potential biomarker and therapeutic target. J Pathol 2011;225(4):574–82.

20. Willert K, Nusse R. Beta-catenin: a key mediator of Wnt signaling. Curr Opin Genet Dev 1998;8(1):95–102.

21. Clevers H. Wnt/beta-catenin signaling in development and disease. Cell 2006; 127(3):469–80.

22. Colombo C, Miceli R, Lazar AJ, et al. CTNNB1 45F mutation is a molecular prognosticator of increased postoperative primary desmoid tumor recurrence: an independent, multicenter validation study. Cancer 2013;119(20):3696–702.

23. van Broekhoven DL, Verhoef C, Grunhagen DJ, et al. Prognostic value of CTNNB1 gene mutation in primary sporadic aggressive fibromatosis. Ann Surg Oncol 2015;22(5):1464–70.

24. Hamada S, Futamura N, Ikuta K, et al. CTNNB1 S45F mutation predicts poor efficacy of meloxicam treatment for desmoid tumors: a pilot study. PLoS One 2014;9(5):e96391.

25. Kasper B, Gruenwald V, Reichardt P, et al. Correlation of CTNNB1 mutation status with progression arrest rate in RECIST progressive desmoid tumors treated with imatinib - translational research results from a phase II study of the German Interdisciplinary Sarcoma Group (GISG-01). CTOS Annual Meeting. Salt Lake City, November 4-7, 2015; Paper 045.

26. Salas S, Brulard C, Terrier P, et al. Gene expression profiling of desmoid tumors by cDNA microarrays and correlation with progression-free survival. Clin Cancer Res 2015;21(18):4194–200.

27. Dufresne A, Paturel M, Alberti L, et al. Prediction of desmoid tumor progression using miRNA expression profiling. Cancer Sci 2015;106(5):650–5.

28. Fiore M, Coppola S, Cannell AJ, et al. Desmoid-type fibromatosis and pregnancy: a multi-institutional analysis of recurrence and obstetric risk. Ann Surg 2014; 259(5):973–8.

29. Leithner A, Gapp M, Radl R, et al. Immunohistochemical analysis of desmoid tumours. J Clin Pathol 2005;58(11):1152–6.

30. Deyrup AT, Tretiakova M, Montag AG. Estrogen receptor-beta expression in extra-abdominal fibromatoses: an analysis of 40 cases. Cancer 2006;106(1):208–13.

31. Cheon SS, Cheah AY, Turley S, et al. Beta-catenin stabilization dysregulates mesenchymal cell proliferation, motility, and invasiveness and causes aggressive fibromatosis and hyperplastic cutaneous wounds. Proc Natl Acad Sci U S A 2002;99(10):6973–8.

32. Poon R, Smits R, Li C, et al. Cyclooxygenase-two (COX-2) modulates proliferation in aggressive fibromatosis (desmoid tumor). Oncogene 2001;20(4):451–60.

33. Signoroni S, Frattini M, Negri T, et al. Cyclooxygenase-2 and platelet-derived growth factor receptors as potential targets in treating aggressive fibromatosis. Clin Cancer Res 2007;13(17):5034–40.

34. Vitellaro M, Sala P, Signoroni S, et al. Risk of desmoid tumours after open and laparoscopic colectomy in patients with familial adenomatous polyposis. Br J Surg 2014;101(5):558–65.

35. Carothers AM, Rizvi H, Hasson RM, et al. Mesenchymal stromal cell mutations and wound healing contribute to the etiology of desmoid tumors. Cancer Res 2012;72(1):346–55.

36. Wu C, Amini-Nik S, Nadesan P, et al. Aggressive fibromatosis (desmoid tumor) is derived from mesenchymal progenitor cells. Cancer Res 2010;70(19):7690–8.

37. Otero S, Moskovic EC, Strauss DC, et al. Desmoid-type fibromatosis. Clin Radiol 2015;70(9):1038–45.

38. Kamali F, Wang WL, Guadagnolo BA, et al. MRI may be used as a prognostic indicator in patients with extra-abdominal desmoid tumours. Br J Radiol 2016; 89(1058):20150308.

39. Kasper B, Dimitrakopoulou-Strauss A, Pilz LR, et al. Positron emission tomography as a surrogate marker for evaluation of treatment response in patients with desmoid tumors under therapy with imatinib. Biomed Res Int 2013;2013:389672.

40. Xu H, Koo HJ, Lim S, et al. Desmoid-type fibromatosis of the thorax: CT, MRI, and FDG PET characteristics in a large series from a tertiary referral center. Medicine (Baltimore) 2015;94(38):e1547.

41. Bhattacharya B, Dilworth HP, Iacobuzio-Donahue C, et al. Nuclear beta-catenin expression distinguishes deep fibromatosis from other benign and malignant fibroblastic and myofibroblastic lesions. Am J Surg Pathol 2005;29(5):653–9.

42. Ng TL, Gown AM, Barry TS, et al. Nuclear beta-catenin in mesenchymal tumors. Mod Pathol 2005;18(1):68–74.

43. Crago AM, Denton B, Salas S, et al. A prognostic nomogram for prediction of recurrence in desmoid fibromatosis. Ann Surg 2013;258(2):347–53.
44. Lewis JJ, Boland PJ, Leung DH, et al. The enigma of desmoid tumors. Ann Surg 1999;229(6):866–72 [discussion: 872–3].
45. Gronchi A, Colombo C, Le Pechoux C, et al. Sporadic desmoid-type fibromatosis: a stepwise approach to a non-metastasising neoplasm–a position paper from the Italian and the French Sarcoma Group. Ann Oncol 2014;25(3):578–83.
46. Kasper B, Baumgarten C, Bonvalot S, et al. Management of sporadic desmoid-type fibromatosis: a European consensus approach based on patients' and professionals' expertise - a sarcoma patients EuroNet and European Organisation for Research and Treatment of Cancer/Soft Tissue and Bone Sarcoma Group initiative. Eur J Cancer 2015;51(2):127–36.
47. Nishida Y, Tsukushi S, Shido Y, et al. Successful treatment with meloxicam, a cyclooxygenase-2 inhibitor, of patients with extra-abdominal desmoid tumors: a pilot study. J Clin Oncol 2010;28(6):e107–9.
48. Brooks MD, Ebbs SR, Colletta AA, et al. Desmoid tumours treated with triphenyl-ethylenes. Eur J Cancer 1992;28A(6–7):1014–8.
49. Patel SR, Evans HL, Benjamin RS. Combination chemotherapy in adult desmoid tumors. Cancer 1993;72(11):3244–7.
50. Weiss AJ, Horowitz S, Lackman RD. Therapy of desmoid tumors and fibromatosis using vinorelbine. Am J Clin Oncol 1999;22(2):193–5.
51. Azzarelli A, Gronchi A, Bertulli R, et al. Low-dose chemotherapy with methotrexate and vinblastine for patients with advanced aggressive fibromatosis. Cancer 2001;92(5):1259–64.
52. Janinis J, Patriki M, Vini L, et al. The pharmacological treatment of aggressive fibromatosis: a systematic review. Ann Oncol 2003;14(2):181–90.
53. Waddell WR, Gerner RE. Indomethacin and ascorbate inhibit desmoid tumors. J Surg Oncol 1980;15(1):85–90.
54. Fiore M, Colombo C, Radaelli S, et al. Hormonal manipulation with toremifene in sporadic desmoid-type fibromatosis. Eur J Cancer 2015;51(18):2800–7.
55. Patel SR, Benjamin RS. Desmoid tumors respond to chemotherapy: defying the dogma in oncology. J Clin Oncol 2006;24(1):11–2.
56. Heinrich MC, McArthur GA, Demetri GD, et al. Clinical and molecular studies of the effect of imatinib on advanced aggressive fibromatosis (desmoid tumor). J Clin Oncol 2006;24(7):1195–203.
57. Chugh R, Wathen JK, Patel SR, et al. Efficacy of imatinib in aggressive fibromatosis: results of a phase II multicenter Sarcoma Alliance for Research through Collaboration (SARC) trial. Clin Cancer Res 2010;16(19):4884–91.
58. Penel N, Le Cesne A, Bui BN, et al. Imatinib for progressive and recurrent aggressive fibromatosis (desmoid tumors): an FNCLCC/French Sarcoma Group phase II trial with a long-term follow-up. Ann Oncol 2011;22(2):452–7.
59. Jo JC, Hong YS, Kim KP, et al. A prospective multicenter phase II study of sunitinib in patients with advanced aggressive fibromatosis. Invest New Drugs 2014; 32(2):369–76.
60. Martin-Liberal J, Benson C, McCarty H, et al. Pazopanib is an active treatment in desmoid tumour/aggressive fibromatosis. Clin Sarcoma Res 2013;3(1):13.
61. Gounder MM, Lefkowitz RA, Keohan ML, et al. Activity of Sorafenib against desmoid tumor/deep fibromatosis. Clin Cancer Res 2011;17(12):4082–90.
62. Shang H, Braggio D, Lee YJ, et al. Targeting the Notch pathway: a potential therapeutic approach for desmoid tumors. Cancer 2015;121(22):4088–96.

63. Messersmith WA, Shapiro GI, Cleary JM, et al. A phase I, dose-finding study in patients with advanced solid malignancies of the oral gamma-secretase inhibitor PF-03084014. Clin Cancer Res 2015;21(1):60–7.
64. Fujishita T, Aoki K, Lane HA, et al. Inhibition of the mTORC1 pathway suppresses intestinal polyp formation and reduces mortality in ApcDelta716 mice. Proc Natl Acad Sci U S A 2008;105(36):13544–9.
65. Ballo MT, Zagars GK, Pollack A, et al. Desmoid tumor: prognostic factors and outcome after surgery, radiation therapy, or combined surgery and radiation therapy. J Clin Oncol 1999;17(1):158–67.
66. Spear MA, Jennings LC, Mankin HJ, et al. Individualizing management of aggressive fibromatoses. Int J Radiat Oncol Biol Phys 1998;40(3):637–45.
67. Gronchi A, Casali PG, Mariani L, et al. Quality of surgery and outcome in extra-abdominal aggressive fibromatosis: a series of patients surgically treated at a single institution. J Clin Oncol 2003;21(7):1390–7.
68. Merchant NB, Lewis JJ, Woodruff JM, et al. Extremity and trunk desmoid tumors: a multifactorial analysis of outcome. Cancer 1999;86(10):2045–52.
69. Lev D, Kotilingam D, Wei C, et al. Optimizing treatment of desmoid tumors. J Clin Oncol 2007;25(13):1785–91.
70. Keus RB, Nout RA, Blay JY, et al. Results of a phase II pilot study of moderate dose radiotherapy for inoperable desmoid-type fibromatosis–an EORTC STBSG and ROG study (EORTC 62991-22998). Ann Oncol 2013;24(10):2672–6.
71. Havez M, Lippa N, Al-Ammari S, et al. Percutaneous image-guided cryoablation in inoperable extra-abdominal desmoid tumors: a study of tolerability and efficacy. Cardiovasc Intervent Radiol 2014;37(6):1500–6.
72. Kujak JL, Liu PT, Johnson GB, et al. Early experience with percutaneous cryoablation of extra-abdominal desmoid tumors. Skeletal Radiol 2010;39(2):175–82.
73. Cornelis F, Italiano A, Al-Ammari S, et al. Successful iterative percutaneous cryoablation of multiple extra-abdominal desmoid tumors in a patient with Gardner syndrome. J Vasc Interv Radiol 2012;23(8):1101–3.
74. van Broekhoven DL, Deroose JP, Bonvalot S, et al. Isolated limb perfusion using tumour necrosis factor alpha and melphalan in patients with advanced aggressive fibromatosis. Br J Surg 2014;101(13):1674–80.
75. Posner MC, Shiu MH, Newsome JL, et al. The desmoid tumor. Not a benign disease. Arch Surg 1989;124(2):191–6.
76. Huang K, Fu H, Shi Y, et al. Prognostic factors for extra-abdominal and abdominal wall desmoids: a 20-year experience at a single institution. J Surg Oncol 2009; 100(7):563–9.
77. Mullen JT, Delaney TF, Kobayashi WK, et al. Desmoid tumor: analysis of prognostic factors and outcomes in a surgical series. Ann Surg Oncol 2012;19(13): 4028–35.
78. Peng PD, Hyder O, Mavros MN, et al. Management and recurrence patterns of desmoids tumors: a multi-institutional analysis of 211 patients. Ann Surg Oncol 2012;19(13):4036–42.
79. Zeng WG, Zhou ZX, Liang JW, et al. Prognostic factors for desmoid tumor: a surgical series of 233 patients at a single institution. Tumour Biol 2014;35(8): 7513–21.
80. He XD, Zhang YB, Wang L, et al. Prognostic factors for the recurrence of sporadic desmoid-type fibromatosis after macroscopically complete resection: analysis of 114 patients at a single institution. Eur J Surg Oncol 2015;41(8):1013–9.

81. Bonvalot S, Eldweny H, Haddad V, et al. Extra-abdominal primary fibromatosis: aggressive management could be avoided in a subgroup of patients. Eur J Surg Oncol 2008;34(4):462–8.

82. Nakayama T, Tsuboyama T, Toguchida J, et al. Natural course of desmoid-type fibromatosis. J Orthop Sci 2008;13(1):51–5.

83. Fiore M, Rimareix F, Mariani L, et al. Desmoid-type fibromatosis: a front-line conservative approach to select patients for surgical treatment. Ann Surg Oncol 2009;16(9):2587–93.

84. Barbier O, Anract P, Pluot E, et al. Primary or recurring extra-abdominal desmoid fibromatosis: assessment of treatment by observation only. Orthop Traumatol Surg Res 2010;96(8):884–9.

85. Salas S, Dufresne A, Bui B, et al. Prognostic factors influencing progression-free survival determined from a series of sporadic desmoid tumors: a wait-and-see policy according to tumor presentation. J Clin Oncol 2011;29(26):3553–8.

86. Bonvalot S, Ternes N, Fiore M, et al. Spontaneous regression of primary abdominal wall desmoid tumors: more common than previously thought. Ann Surg Oncol 2013;20(13):4096–102.

87. Briand S, Barbier O, Biau D, et al. Wait-and-see policy as a first-line management for extra-abdominal desmoid tumors. J Bone Joint Surg Am 2014;96(8):631–8.

88. Colombo C, Miceli R, Le Pechoux C, et al. Sporadic extra abdominal wall desmoid-type fibromatosis: surgical resection can be safely limited to a minority of patients. Eur J Cancer 2015;51(2):186–92.

Dermatofibrosarcoma Protuberans

Wide Local Excision Versus Mohs Micrographic Surgery

John T. Mullen, MD

KEYWORDS

- Dermatofibrosarcoma protuberans • Mohs surgery • Wide local excision
- Recurrence • Cutaneous sarcoma

KEY POINTS

- Dermatofibrosarcoma protuberans (DFSP) is a rare dermal soft tissue sarcoma characterized by a typically indolent clinical course.
- Complete surgical resection is the mainstay of treatment, and this is accomplished with either a standard wide local excision (WLE) or with Mohs micrographic surgery (MMS), as long as a comprehensive pathologic examination of the margins is completed before reconstruction of the defect.
- MMS is the ideal surgical approach for relatively small DFSPs in cosmetically sensitive areas (ie, face, scalp, or neck), where tissue preservation is critical to achieve optimal cosmetic and functional outcomes.
- WLE with a 1.0- to 1.5-cm margin width is the ideal approach for most DFSPs on the trunk or extremities, because it is likely to achieve complete tumor clearance with excellent cosmetic and functional outcomes in a single stage.

INTRODUCTION

Dermatofibrosarcoma protuberans (DFSP) is a rare dermal soft tissue sarcoma characterized by a typically indolent clinical course. Although transformation to a high-grade fibrosarcoma is possible, particularly in the case of recurrent DFSP, by far the greatest clinical challenge in the management of DFSP is achieving local control. Because DFSP arises in the dermis and invades radially through preexisting collagen bundles and deeply along connective tissue septae,[1] its extent of invasion is often difficult to clinically appreciate, and thus determining the appropriate width

The author has nothing to disclose.
Division of Surgical Oncology, Massachusetts General Hospital, Harvard Medical School, 55 Fruit Street, Yawkey 7B, Boston, MA 02114, USA
E-mail address: jmullen@mgh.harvard.edu

Surg Oncol Clin N Am 25 (2016) 827–839
http://dx.doi.org/10.1016/j.soc.2016.05.011
1055-3207/16/$ – see front matter © 2016 Elsevier Inc. All rights reserved.
surgonc.theclinics.com

of the margins of resection is challenging. There has been vigorous debate in the literature as to the optimal surgical approach to these tumors, with some groups advocating for radical resection with defined margins of excision, and others advocating for Mohs micrographic surgery (MMS).

Ultimately, there is no "one size fits all" surgical technique for the treatment of DFSP. Indeed, the choice between wide local excision (WLE) and MMS for DFSP should be governed by the attainment of the following three goals: (1) to completely excise the tumor with negative margins, which is tantamount to cure, because these tumors very rarely metastasize; (2) to preserve function, optimize cosmesis, and minimize the morbidity of resection; and (3) to minimize the cost and inconvenience to the patient and the health care system at large. Both WLE and MMS are capable of achieving the first goal, such that the choice of surgical approach may be driven more by individual patient and tumor factors that make the attainment of the second and third goals important.

EPIDEMIOLOGY

DFSP is a rare sarcoma, accounting for less than 0.1% of all malignancies and between 2% and 6% of all soft tissue sarcomas,[2] although it is the most common sarcoma of the skin. Rouhani and colleagues,[2] in an analysis of the Surveillance, Epidemiology, and End Results database from 1992 to 2004, reported that the incidence of DFSP was 4.5 cases per million person-years and that DFSP comprised 18.4% of all cutaneous sarcomas during that time period. It typically occurs in the third and fourth decades of life, has an equal gender distribution, and has a higher incidence among black persons than seen for other cutaneous sarcomas.

CLINICAL PRESENTATION AND NATURAL HISTORY

DFSP most commonly presents as a slow-growing, asymptomatic nodular or plaque-like lesion that may have a violaceous or reddish brown appearance. The tumor has a hard consistency and is fixed to the dermis but is usually freely movable over the underlying fascia and muscle. Over time, which can vary from months to years, DFSP may grow radially to generate a larger plaque and vertically to generate multiple nodules within the plaque, from which its name "protuberans" is derived. The average tumor diameter is on the order of a few centimeters, although neglected tumors can grow to much larger sizes. DFSP can occur anywhere on the body, although the most common locations are the extremities, trunk, and head and neck. Diagnostic delays are common with these tumors, which are often mistaken as dermatofibromas, sebaceous cysts, lipomas, and scars.

Despite the frequent, long delays in diagnosis, distant metastasis is exceedingly rare, with a reported rate of 2% to 4%.[2,3] The main site of distant recurrence is the lung, via hematogenous tumor spread, and in nearly all cases metastases are preceded by multiple local recurrences or in the context of transformation to a higher-grade fibrosarcoma.[3] As with most other soft tissue sarcomas, DFSP rarely metastasizes to the regional lymph nodes, having been reported to occur in 1% or fewer cases.[4]

PATHOLOGY

Grossly, DFSP appears as a solitary, poorly circumscribed, gray-white mass that infiltrates the dermis and subcutaneous tissue (**Fig. 1**). Histologically, the tumor is composed of a dense, uniform array of cells with spindle-shaped nuclei embedded within collagen and may demonstrate a cartwheel or storiform pattern. Tumor cells

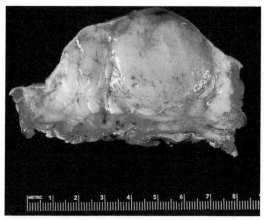

Fig. 1. Gross image of a classic DFSP, which appears as a solitary, poorly circumscribed, gray-white mass that infiltrates the dermis and subcutaneous tissue. (*Courtesy of* Massachusetts General Hospital Pathology Department, Boston, MA.)

have large nuclei with low pleomorphism and rare mitotic figures. A defining characteristic of DFSP is its capacity to invade the surrounding tissues to a considerable distance, with tumor cells forming tentacle-like projections along the fibrous septae and into fat lobules in a distinctive honeycomb pattern (**Fig. 2**).[5] Notably, this infiltration is often eccentric, with long, narrow tumor extensions in one direction but not in another, making it difficult to determine the true extent of the lesion.[1]

There are several histologic subtypes of DFSP, including pigmented (Bednar tumor), myxoid, sclerosing, granular cell, atrophic, and giant cell fibroblastoma variants. Approximately 80% to 90% of DFSPs are low-grade lesions, whereas the remaining 10% to 20% of DFSPs contain a high-grade fibrosarcomatous (DFSP-FS) component classically showing a "herringbone" pattern with hypercellularity, atypical cells, and an increased mitotic rate (**Fig. 3**).[6] This histologic variant is associated with a more

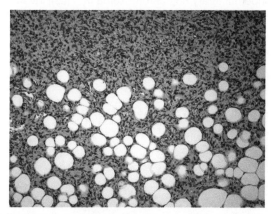

Fig. 2. Histologically, DFSP is composed of a dense, uniform array of cells with spindle-shaped nuclei embedded within collagen and may demonstrate a cartwheel or storiform pattern. A defining characteristic of DFSP is its capacity to invade the surrounding tissues, as this DFSP demonstrates with invasion of the adjacent fat lobules in a distinctive honeycomb pattern (H&E, 100×).

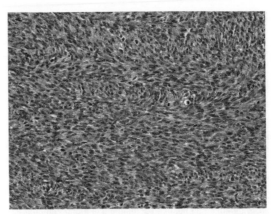

Fig. 3. DFSP with a high-grade fibrosarcomatous component, which classically demonstrates a "herringbone" pattern with hypercellularity, atypical cells, and an increased mitotic rate (H&E, 200×).

aggressive clinical behavior, with a higher rate of local recurrence after resection and an increased risk of distant metastasis.[7]

Immunohistochemical expression of the CD34 antigen is the most helpful diagnostic marker of DFSP (**Fig. 4**), and immunostaining for CD34 and factor XIIIa may be necessary to distinguish a DFSP from a benign dermatofibroma, respectively.[8] However, CD34 expression is by no means specific for DFSP and may be absent in a significant percentage of these tumors, including in DFSP-FS.[9]

MOLECULAR BIOLOGY AND PATHOGENESIS

Advances in understanding the molecular pathogenesis of DFSP have enabled the diagnosis of most of these tumors using modern molecular pathologic techniques. Genetically, DFSP is characterized by either a reciprocal translocation [t(17;22)] or, more often, by a supernumerary ring chromosome [r(17;22)] involving chromosomes 17 and 22.[10] These chromosomal rearrangements lead to a fusion of the collagen

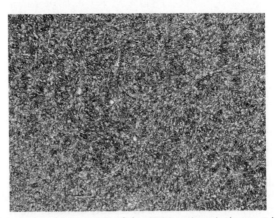

Fig. 4. Immunohistochemical expression of the CD34 antigen is the most helpful diagnostic marker of DFSP (immunostain, 200×).

type Iα1 (*COL1A1*) gene on chromosome 17 and the platelet-derived growth factor β (*PDGFB*) gene on chromosome 22, which leads to constitutive activation of the PDGFB receptor and its tyrosine kinases that results in cell growth and proliferation. The chromosomal translocation is detected by fluorescence in situ hybridization, and although this study is not absolutely necessary for the routine pathologic diagnosis of DFSP, identification of the *COL1A1/PDGFB* rearrangement is mandatory in cases where standard pathologic studies are inconclusive.

MANAGEMENT OF DERMATOFIBROSARCOMA PROTUBERANS: OVERVIEW

The diagnostic work-up of DFSP entails a complete history and physical examination. Radiographic imaging of the primary tumor is generally not necessary, especially in the case of small tumors. However, for larger tumors in difficult locations, MRI may be helpful.[11] Because the risk of metastasis is very low, staging scans of the chest or other sites are generally not indicated unless there are worrisome findings on the history and physical examination or high-risk features on pathology. Patients with larger tumors and/or tumors in cosmetically sensitive areas may benefit from a multidisciplinary approach to optimize the clinical and reconstructive outcomes.[3]

Complete surgical resection is the mainstay of treatment, and this is accomplished with either a standard WLE or with MMS, as long as a comprehensive pathologic examination of the margins is completed before reconstruction of the defect. In the occasional circumstance when a surgical margin is positive or very narrow and further surgical resection is not possible, adjuvant radiation therapy may be considered.[12,13] In the case of locally advanced or recurrent DFSP, neoadjuvant imatinib mesylate (Gleevec) therapy has been shown to reduce the preoperative tumor size and to lessen surgical morbidity associated with the resection of residual DFSP.[14–16] Indeed, because the pathogenesis of DFSP is caused by activation of the PDGFRB receptor, which has tyrosine kinase activity, it makes perfect sense that tyrosine kinase inhibitors, such as imatinib, would have activity in DFSP. Conventional chemotherapy, however, is generally considered ineffective in the treatment of DFSP.

SURGICAL TREATMENT: WIDE LOCAL EXCISION

WLE down to and including the underlying fascia has long been the standard surgical approach to DFSP, and in most cases this is all that is required.[17] However, the optimal width of excision around the primary tumor has never been defined in prospective studies. Older retrospective studies describing 1- to 3-cm margins of excision report local recurrence rates of 50% or more.[17–22] Such high recurrence rates are thought to be caused by the extensive and eccentric pattern of local invasion of DFSP, which is difficult to appreciate at the time of resection, making it difficult to do a margin-negative excision.[21] Thus, even lesions that have been said to have been excised with "negative" margins exhibit high rates of local recurrence.[23] More recent large series evaluating WLE for DFSP have advocated for margin widths ranging from 1 cm to greater than or equal to 3 cm, with positive margin rates and local recurrence rates ranging from 3% to 32% and 0% to 50%, respectively (**Table 1**).

Bowne and colleagues[7] reported outcomes from Memorial Sloan-Kettering Cancer Center in 159 patients with primary (n = 111) or locally recurrent (n = 48) DFSP. Most tumors were low-grade (n = 134), and the remainder was the higher grade DFSP-FS variant. All patients underwent WLE, and on final pathologic review, only 58% of the patients had confirmed negative microscopic margins, whereas 32% had positive margins and 10% had "close" (<1 mm) margins. Not unexpectedly, 34 of the 159 patients (21%) developed a local recurrence at a median of 32 months, and 29 of these

Table 1
Recent studies evaluating the risk of local recurrence after wide local excision of dermatofibrosarcoma protuberans

Authors/Year	Patient (N)	Margin Width (cm)	Negative Margins (%)	Positive Margins (%)	Local Recurrence (%)
Bowne et al,[7] 2000	159	NA	58	32	21
Chang et al,[26] 2004	60	≥3.0	NA	NA	16
DuBay et al,[3] 2004	43	1–2	95	5	0
Khatri et al,[29] 2003	24	2.5–3.3	100	0	0
Fiore et al,[34] 2005	136 primary	NA	88	12	4
	82 recurrent	NA	85	15	5
Monnier et al,[24] 2006	4	<0.9	NA	NA	50
	31	1–2.9	NA	NA	46
	31	≥3.0	NA	NA	7
Kimmel et al,[32] 2007	98	2.0	NA	NA	41
	—	2.5	NA	NA	24
	—	3.0	NA	NA	11–20
Popov et al,[30] 2007	40	1.5–6.0	100	0	0
Yu et al,[25] 2008	25	3.0	NA	NA	0
Paradisi et al,[28] 2008	38	2–5	NA	NA	13
Meguerditchian et al,[31] 2010	28	2.0	79	21	3.6
Heuvel et al,[27] 2010	38	2–3	95	5	7
Farma et al,[35] 2010	206	2 (median)	97	3	1
Cai et al,[45] 2012	81	1.5–2.5	NA	NA	13.6
	141	≥3.0	—	—	5.7
Woo et al,[36] 2016	21	<3.0	95	5	0
	28	≥3.0	96	4	0
Kim et al,[37] 2015	90	1–5	100	0	5.5

Abbreviation: NA, not available.

34 patients (85%) had either positive or "close" margins. Even for patients with low-grade DFSP with reportedly negative margins, the 5-year local recurrence rate was 7%. On multivariate analysis, "close" or positive microscopic margins and DFSP-FS variant proved to be independent prognostic factors for local recurrence.

In 2006, Monnier and colleagues[24] conducted a retrospective review of DFSP using a population-based cancer registry in France. In 66 patients followed for a median of 9.6 years, they found a significant difference in recurrence rates based on margin width, with a 47% local recurrence rate for margins less than 3 cm versus 7% for margins from 3 to 5 cm. Yu and colleagues[25] reported no recurrences in 25 patients treated with either a 3-cm WLE, a modified WLE incorporating careful pathologic processing of the specimens, Mohs surgery, or some combination of these techniques. In 60 patients with DFSP treated with WLE with margins greater than or equal to 3 cm, Chang and colleagues[26] noted a local recurrence rate of 16%. Heuvel and colleagues[27] from the Netherlands reported margin-negative and local recurrence rates of 95% and 7%, respectively, in 38 patients treated with WLE with 2- to 3-cm margins. The local control rate was 100% for patients in whom negative microscopic margins were achieved. Paradisi and colleagues[28] compared the local recurrence rates with WLE versus MMS in 79 patients with DFSP. The margins of excision in those undergoing WLE ranged from 2 to 5 cm, and the local recurrence rate was 13% in the 38 patients treated with WLE compared with 0% in the 41 patients treated with MMS.

Khatri and colleagues[29] reported a 100% local recurrence-free survival after WLE with gross margins of 2.5 to 3.3 cm in 24 patients with either primary (n = 11) or recurrent (n = 13) DFSPs. Popov and colleagues[30] from Helsinki treated 40 patients with DFSP with WLE alone to an average gross margin of 3.1 cm and an average microscopic margin of 1.6 cm and found no recurrences at a mean follow-up of 40 months. Most of the patients were operated on in one stage, but 58% (n = 23) of the patients required reconstructive procedures, including split-thickness skin grafts (n = 11) and local flaps (n = 7). Meguerditchian and colleagues[31] performed a retrospective review of 48 patients with primary DFSP undergoing either WLE with a median margin width of 2 cm (n = 28) or MMS (n = 20) at Roswell Park Cancer Center. The rates of positive margins and local recurrence were 21% and 0% and 3.6% and 0% for the WLE and MMS patients, respectively.

In 2007 Kimmel and colleagues[32] reported a meta-analysis of DFSP case reports identified from a Medline search from 1994 to 2004 and among 98 patients with DFSP found local recurrence rates of 41% for a 2-cm WLE margin width, 24% for a 2.5-cm width, and 11% to 20% for a 3-cm width. These authors concluded that 4-cm margins of excision would be necessary to clear 95% of DFSPs, although this conclusion was deemed to be misleading and unsubstantiated by Zager and colleagues[33] in their letter to the editor.

Fiore and colleagues[34] reported one of the largest series of WLE of DFSP in the literature in 2005, including 218 patients, of whom 136 had primary disease and 82 had recurrent disease. The margin width was not defined in this study, but negative margins were achieved in 87% of patients. These authors used a liberal policy of re-excision after inadequate prior surgery and identified residual disease in 62% of cases. The crude cumulative incidence of local failure was 4% at 10 years, and the rate of distant metastasis at 10 years was only 2%. Reconstructive surgery, including flaps and skin grafts, was needed in 30% of the patients, particularly those with recurrent tumors and head and neck tumors.

Two particularly significant publications demonstrate that remarkably low rates of local recurrence can be achieved with WLE provided that there is meticulous pathologic evaluation of the margins. DuBay and coworkers[3] espoused a multidisciplinary approach to the treatment of DFSPs at the University of Michigan, and 43 of 63 DFSPs included in this study were approached initially with WLE with 1- to 2-cm margins of excision. Ninety-five percent of these lesions were cleared histologically, and two (5%) patients received postoperative radiation therapy for positive margins after undergoing maximal excision. At a median follow-up of 4 years, there were no local recurrences. Farma and colleagues[35] combined this experience from the University of Michigan with that from the Moffitt Cancer Center in a retrospective study spanning 1991 to 2008. They reported a local recurrence rate of only 1% at a median follow-up of greater than 5 years for 206 low-grade DFSPs in 204 patients. The median width of excision was 2 cm (range, 0.5–3 cm), and the median number of excisions to achieve negative margins was 1 (range, 1–4). Primary wound closure was achieved in 69% of patients, whereas 25% of patients required a skin graft and 4% a tissue flap. Importantly, in both of these series, the tissue from all of the peripheral margins underwent meticulous pathologic analysis of en face 2-mm tangential sections using routine hematoxylin and eosin staining. Immunohistochemistry using anti-CD34 antibody staining was performed as deemed necessary by the pathologist.

Two of the most recent studies examining long-term outcomes after WLE of DFSP were published from South Korea. Woo and colleagues[36] examined the outcomes of 63 patients who underwent WLE of primary DFSPs at Samsung Medical Center from 1999 to 2011, and they reported no local recurrences in patients undergoing a margin-negative resection of any width, although they recommended WLE with gross margins of 1.5 to 2 cm along with frozen section pathologic analysis before wound closure. Kim and colleagues[37] examined the outcomes of 90 patients who underwent WLE with gross margins of 1 to 5 cm of DFSPs at Seoul National University from 1992 to 2015. They found a local recurrence rate of 5.5% at a mean follow-up of 43 months, and there were no significant risk factors for local recurrence on multivariate analysis.

SURGICAL TREATMENT: MOHS MICROGRAPHIC SURGERY

MMS is an alternative to WLE that uses en face tangential sectioning of the radial margins and horizontal sectioning of the base of the DFSP, which thereby enables the clinician to microscopically examine almost 100% of the deep and peripheral margins of the tumor. This precise mapping and orienting of the tumor specimen using MMS allows the surgeon to trace out the tentacle-like projections of DFSP and to develop a map to guide residual tumor resection. The process is repeated, typically the same day, until the surgical margin is clear. This meticulous margin assessment with MMS is in stark contrast to the conventional histologic examination with vertical sectioning of a permanently fixed, paraffin-embedded WLE specimen, in which perhaps only 1% to 5% of the tumor margin is assessed. It is argued that the comprehensive margin assessment with MMS accounts for the extremely low rates of local recurrence with this technique, with multiple studies reporting a median local recurrence rate of less than 1%.[1,3,28,31,38–43]

Ratner and colleagues[1] published one of the largest series of MMS for the treatment of DFSP in 1997. This study included 58 patients with primary and recurrent DFSP treated with MMS at one of three institutions from 1981 to 1994. They reported a local recurrence rate of only 1.7% (0% for primary tumors and 4.8% for recurrent tumors), the sole recurrence developing in a patient with a twice-recurrent DFSP. These authors also calculated, based on the Mohs surgical determination of microscopic tumor extent, the minimum excision width that would have been required to eradicate all tumors with a standard WLE. Standard WLE with a width of 1 cm around the primary tumor would have left residual microscopic tumor in more than 70% of patients; a width of 2 cm, 40%; 3 cm, 15.5%; and 5 cm, 5%. Indeed, Ratner and colleagues concluded that even a WLE with a width of 10 cm around the primary tumor would not have cleared some DFSPs despite resecting a huge excess of normal tissue. Despite the excellent results with MMS for DFSP in this series, the authors did not conclude that all cases of DFSP should be treated by MMS. Rather, they stated that MMS is the treatment of choice for DFSPs at sites where the maximum conservation of normal tissue is required, such as on the face, scalp, or neck, whereas WLE with standard margins is a very reasonable approach for well-defined tumors on the trunk or extremities because it is likely to achieve complete tumor clearance with excellent cosmetic and functional outcomes.

Loghdey and colleagues[42] reviewed the outcomes of 76 patients with DFSP treated with MMS at Queens Medical Centre in Nottingham, United Kingdom from 1996 to 2013. At a mean follow-up of 50 months, the local recurrence rate was 1.5%, and complete tumor clearance was achieved in 80% of cases with a margin less than or equal to 2 cm and in 91% of cases with a margin less than or equal to 3 cm. Twenty-seven percent of patients required plastic surgical reconstruction of the defect with either a skin graft or a local flap the following day, whereas 73% of patients had their wounds primarily closed by the Mohs surgeon on the same day as the resection. These authors concluded that MMS is the optimal treatment choice for DFSPs arising anywhere on the body.

There have been no randomized clinical trials comparing the outcomes of MMS with WLE for DFSP, but there have been several nonrandomized comparative trials to date.[3,28,31,38] Gloster and colleagues[38] from the Mayo Clinic identified one local recurrence in 15 patients (6.6%) undergoing MMS for DFSP compared with four local recurrences in 39 patients (10%) undergoing WLE. Paradisi and colleagues[28] examined the outcomes of 79 patients with DFSP who underwent either WLE with gross margins of 2 to 5 cm (n = 38) or MMS (n = 41) at one of three institutions in Italy and Germany. They reported five (13.2%) local recurrences in the WLE group compared with zero local recurrences in the MMS group at a mean follow-up of approximately 5 years. Furthermore, in the study referenced previously by DuBay and coworkers[3] 13 patients with DFSP underwent attempted MMS, and complete tumor extirpation was achieved by MMS in 11 patients, including seven with head and neck tumors and four with trunk or extremity tumors. DFSPs excised by MMS were smaller than those treated by WLE (n = 44), and the average number of Mohs stages performed was 2.4. A subsequent surgical procedure was performed to reconstruct 5 of the 11 defects with either a skin graft or a local flap. There were no local recurrences in the MMS group at a median follow-up of 5.2 years, but note that there were also no local recurrences in the WLE group in this study, because these patients had meticulous pathologic margin assessment. Lastly, Meguerditchian and colleagues[31] published a 3.6% rate of local recurrence in 28 patients undergoing WLE for DFSP compared with a 0% local recurrence rate in 20 patients treated with MMS for DFSP at Roswell Park Cancer Institute, although WLE was faster (median operative time of 77 minutes vs 257 minutes) and resulted in a defect that was less likely to require advanced closure techniques (18% vs 65%).

WIDE LOCAL EXCISION OR MOHS MICROGRAPHIC SURGERY FOR DERMATOFIBROSARCOMA PROTUBERANS?

Based on the data presented on the outcomes of patients with DFSP treated with either WLE or MMS, what is one to conclude about the optimal surgical treatment of this indolent tumor? Because MMS offers the advantage of precise and complete evaluation of the surgical margins and, as a result, very low rates of local recurrence, why not choose this technique over WLE for all patients with DFSP? The answer lies in the significant drawbacks of MMS. First, MMS is a highly specialized procedure, which requires considerable training and a specialized ancillary team, thus limiting its widespread application. Second, MMS is very labor intensive, requiring the creation and review of multiple histologic tumor sections while the patient waits. For many patients, a staged surgical procedure ("slow Mohs") requiring many hours over several days is necessary, followed by plastic surgical reconstruction on yet another day for many of these patients. These facts make MMS both costly and inconvenient for the patient. Lastly, MMS is generally performed under local anesthesia, thus limiting its application to bigger, bulkier tumors. Thus, most experts in this field agree that MMS is an ideal surgical approach for relatively small DFSPs in cosmetically sensitive areas where tissue preservation is critical to achieve optimal cosmetic and functional outcomes.

For patients with larger DFSPs, or for those with tumors harboring a higher-grade, fibrosarcomatous element, few would argue that aggressive WLE under general anesthesia is appropriate. The real question is what to do about the relatively small DFSP on the trunk or the extremity. Does one accept the higher rate of local recurrence for the cost savings and speed of a standard WLE? Based on the work published by DuBay, Farma, and Sondak, who have reported near-zero local recurrence rates with WLE if coupled with comprehensive margin assessment, this tradeoff does not have to be made.[3,35,44] Although this technique is more labor intensive for the dermatopathologist, the local recurrence rates are as low as those reported with MMS, and most truncal and extremity DFSPs are simply excised in one stage with primary wound closure, with an excellent cosmetic and functional outcome at minimal cost and inconvenience to the patient. An important caveat to this approach is that primary wound closure should be accomplished with minimal, if any, undermining such that as few tissue planes as possible are subjected to possible tumor implantation in the event that a re-excision is necessary for positive margins on final pathology.

That then leaves one remaining controversial question. What margin width should be chosen for the WLE? Obviously, there are no randomized data to help answer this question. In our experience, most DFSPs can be completely excised with a 1.0- to 1.5-cm gross margin, and so we start with this and check multiple frozen section margins with our dedicated soft tissue pathology team while the patient is under anesthesia. If the margins are negative (as they usually are), we primarily close the wound. If there is a focally positive margin, we excise additional tissue along that margin and again perform frozen sections, closing the wound once assured that the margin is microscopically negative. Note that it is important to raise the possibility of the need to perform a very wide excision, with or without the need for complex wound reconstruction (eg, a skin graft), with the patient during the preoperative consultation and informed consent process, because these DFSPs can be quite infiltrative. Lastly, if one or more margins are positive after the initial conservative (1.0- to 1.5-cm gross margin) resection such that primary wound closure seems unlikely, and if we have not had a preoperative discussion with the patient about the possibility of local flap and/or skin graft reconstruction of the defect (which is rare), we would stop the procedure and place a temporary dressing (eg, vacuum-assisted closure device) on the wound and plan to return a subsequent day for wider resection and plastic surgical reconstruction.

SUMMARY

Most patients with DFSP are successfully and efficiently treated with standard WLE when combined with careful pathologic analysis of the entire surgical margin. MMS is the ideal surgical approach for relatively small DFSPs in cosmetically sensitive areas where tissue preservation is critical to achieve optimal cosmetic and functional outcomes. Radiation therapy is rarely necessary but is effective for patients with multiply recurrent lesions or for those in whom a negative margin cannot be achieved despite aggressive resection. The small but definite risk of transformation to a higher grade fibrosarcoma justifies an aggressive surgical approach to DFSP.

REFERENCES

1. Ratner D, Thomas CO, Johnson TM, et al. Mohs micrographic surgery for the treatment of dermatofibrosarcoma protuberans. Results of a multiinstitutional series with an analysis of the extent of microscopic spread. J Am Acad Dermatol 1997;37:600–13.
2. Rouhani P, Fletcher CD, Devesa SS, et al. Cutaneous soft tissue sarcoma incidence patterns in the U.S.: an analysis of 12,114 cases. Cancer 2008;113: 616–27.
3. DuBay D, Cimmino V, Lowe L, et al. Low recurrence rate after surgery for dermatofibrosarcoma protuberans: a multidisciplinary approach from a single institution. Cancer 2004;100:1008–16.
4. Rutgers EJ, Kroon BB, Albus-Lutter CE, et al. Dermatofibrosarcoma protuberans: treatment and prognosis. Eur J Surg Oncol 1992;18:241–8.
5. Llombart B, Monteagudo C, Sanmartin O, et al. Dermatofibrosarcoma protuberans: a clinicopathological, immunohistochemical, genetic (COL1A1-PDGFB), and therapeutic study of low-grade versus high-grade (fibrosarcomatous) tumors. J Am Acad Dermatol 2011;65:564–75.
6. Mentzel T, Beham A, Katenkamp D, et al. Fibrosarcomatous ("high-grade") dermatofibrosarcoma protuberans: clinicopathologic and immunohistochemical study of a series of 41 cases with emphasis on prognostic significance. Am J Surg Pathol 1998;22:576–87.
7. Bowne WB, Antonescu CR, Leung DH, et al. Dermatofibrosarcoma protuberans: a clinicopathologic analysis of patients treated and followed at a single institution. Cancer 2000;88:2711–20.
8. Abenoza P, Lillemoe T. CD34 and factor XIIIa in the differential diagnosis of dermatofibroma and dermatofibrosarcoma protuberans. Am J Dermatopathol 1993;15:429–34.
9. Goldblum JR. CD34 positivity in fibrosarcomas which arise in dermatofibrosarcoma protuberans. Arch Pathol Lab Med 1995;119:238–41.
10. Pedeutour F, Simon MP, Minoletti F, et al. Translocation, t(17;22)(q22;q13), in dermatofibrosarcoma protuberans: a new tumor-associated chromosome rearrangement. Cytogenet Cell Genet 1996;72:171–4.
11. Serra-Guillen C, Sanmartin O, Llombart B, et al. Correlation between preoperative magnetic resonance imaging and surgical margins with modified Mohs for dermatofibrosarcoma protuberans. Dermatol Surg 2011;37:1638–45.
12. Ballo MT, Zagars GK, Pisters P, et al. The role of radiation therapy in the management of dermatofibrosarcoma protuberans. Int J Radiat Oncol Biol Phys 1998;40: 823–7.
13. Suit H, Spiro I, Mankin HJ, et al. Radiation in management of patients with dermatofibrosarcoma protuberans. J Clin Oncol 1996;14:2365–9.
14. Johnson-Jahangir H, Sherman W, Ratner D. Using imatinib as neoadjuvant therapy in dermatofibrosarcoma protuberans: potential pluses and minuses. J Natl Compr Canc Netw 2010;8:881–5.

15. McArthur GA, Demetri GD, van Oosterom A, et al. Molecular and clinical analysis of locally advanced dermatofibrosarcoma protuberans treated with imatinib: imatinib target exploration consortium study B2225. J Clin Oncol 2005;23:866–73.
16. Ugurel S, Mentzel T, Utikal J, et al. Neoadjuvant imatinib in advanced primary or locally recurrent dermatofibrosarcoma protuberans: a multicenter phase II DeCOG trial with long-term follow-up. Clin Cancer Res 2014;20:499–510.
17. Roses DF, Valensi Q, LaTrenta G, et al. Surgical treatment of dermatofibrosarcoma protuberans. Surg Gynecol Obstet 1986;162:449–52.
18. Burkhardt BR, Soule EH, Winkelmann RK, et al. Dermatofibrosarcoma protuberans. Study of fifty-six cases. Am J Surg 1966;111:638–44.
19. McPeak CJ, Cruz T, Nicastri AD. Dermatofibrosarcoma protuberans: an analysis of 86 cases–five with metastasis. Ann Surg 1967;166:803–16.
20. Pack GT, Tabah EJ. Dermato-fibrosarcoma protuberans. A report of 39 cases. AMA Arch Surg 1951;62:391–411.
21. Rowsell AR, Poole MD, Godfrey AM. Dermatofibrosarcoma protuberans: the problems of surgical management. Br J Plast Surg 1986;39:262–4.
22. Taylor HB, Helwig EB. Dermatofibrosarcoma protuberans. A study of 115 cases. Cancer 1962;15:717–25.
23. Parker TL, Zitelli JA. Surgical margins for excision of dermatofibrosarcoma protuberans. J Am Acad Dermatol 1995;32:233–6.
24. Monnier D, Vidal C, Martin L, et al. Dermatofibrosarcoma protuberans: a population-based cancer registry descriptive study of 66 consecutive cases diagnosed between 1982 and 2002. J Eur Acad Dermatol Venereol 2006;20: 1237–42.
25. Yu W, Tsoukas MM, Chapman SM, et al. Surgical treatment for dermatofibrosarcoma protuberans: the Dartmouth experience and literature review. Ann Plast Surg 2008;60:288–93.
26. Chang CK, Jacobs IA, Salti GI. Outcomes of surgery for dermatofibrosarcoma protuberans. Eur J Surg Oncol 2004;30:341–5.
27. Heuvel ST, Suurmeijer A, Pras E, et al. Dermatofibrosarcoma protuberans: recurrence is related to the adequacy of surgical margins. Eur J Surg Oncol 2010;36: 89–94.
28. Paradisi A, Abeni D, Rusciani A, et al. Dermatofibrosarcoma protuberans: wide local excision vs. Mohs micrographic surgery. Cancer Treat Rev 2008;34:728–36.
29. Khatri VP, Galante JM, Bold RJ, et al. Dermatofibrosarcoma protuberans: reappraisal of wide local excision and impact of inadequate initial treatment. Ann Surg Oncol 2003;10:1118–22.
30. Popov P, Bohling T, Asko-Seljavaara S, et al. Microscopic margins and results of surgery for dermatofibrosarcoma protuberans. Plast Reconstr Surg 2007;119: 1779–84.
31. Meguerditchian AN, Wang J, Lema B, et al. Wide excision or Mohs micrographic surgery for the treatment of primary dermatofibrosarcoma protuberans. Am J Clin Oncol 2010;33:300–3.
32. Kimmel Z, Ratner D, Kim JY, et al. Peripheral excision margins for dermatofibrosarcoma protuberans: a meta-analysis of spatial data. Ann Surg Oncol 2007;14: 2113–20.
33. Zager JS, Bui MM, Farma JM, et al. Proper margins of excision in dermatofibrosarcoma protuberans: wide or narrow? Ann Surg Oncol 2008;15:2614–6.
34. Fiore M, Miceli R, Mussi C, et al. Dermatofibrosarcoma protuberans treated at a single institution: a surgical disease with a high cure rate. J Clin Oncol 2005;23: 7669–75.

35. Farma JM, Ammori JB, Zager JS, et al. Dermatofibrosarcoma protuberans: how wide should we resect? Ann Surg Oncol 2010;17:2112–8.
36. Woo KJ, Bang SI, Mun GH, et al. Long-term outcomes of surgical treatment for dermatofibrosarcoma protuberans according to width of gross resection margin. J Plast Reconstr Aesthet Surg 2016;69(3):395.
37. Kim BJ, Kim H, Jin US, et al. Wide local excision for dermatofibrosarcoma protuberans: a single-center series of 90 patients. Biomed Res Int 2015;2015:642549.
38. Gloster HM Jr, Harris KR, Roenigk RK. A comparison between Mohs micrographic surgery and wide surgical excision for the treatment of dermatofibrosarcoma protuberans. J Am Acad Dermatol 1996;35:82–7.
39. Hafner HM, Moehrle M, Eder S, et al. 3D-Histological evaluation of surgery in dermatofibrosarcoma protuberans and malignant fibrous histiocytoma: differences in growth patterns and outcome. Eur J Surg Oncol 2008;34:680–6.
40. Lemm D, Mugge LO, Mentzel T, et al. Current treatment options in dermatofibrosarcoma protuberans. J Cancer Res Clin Oncol 2009;135:653–65.
41. Llombart B, Serra-Guillen C, Monteagudo C, et al. Dermatofibrosarcoma protuberans: a comprehensive review and update on diagnosis and management. Semin Diagn Pathol 2013;30:13–28.
42. Loghdey MS, Varma S, Rajpara SM, et al. Mohs micrographic surgery for dermatofibrosarcoma protuberans (DFSP): a single-centre series of 76 patients treated by frozen-section Mohs micrographic surgery with a review of the literature. J Plast Reconstr Aesthet Surg 2014;67:1315–21.
43. Snow SN, Gordon EM, Larson PO, et al. Dermatofibrosarcoma protuberans: a report on 29 patients treated by Mohs micrographic surgery with long-term follow-up and review of the literature. Cancer 2004;101:28–38.
44. Sondak VK, Cimmino VM, Lowe LM, et al. Dermatofibrosarcoma protuberans: what is the best surgical approach? Surg Oncol 1999;8:183–9.
45. Cai H, Wang Y, Wu J, et al. Dermatofibrosarcoma protuberans: clinical diagnoses and treatment results of 260 cases in China. J Surg Oncol 2012;105:142–8.

Radiation Therapy for Soft Tissue Sarcoma

Indications and Controversies for Neoadjuvant Therapy, Adjuvant Therapy, Intraoperative Radiation Therapy, and Brachytherapy

Nicole A. Larrier, MD, MSc[a], Brian G. Czito, MD[a],
David G. Kirsch, MD, PhD[a,b,*]

KEYWORDS

- Radiation therapy • Brachytherapy • Intraoperative radiation therapy • Sarcoma

KEY POINTS

- Radiotherapy is an effective treatment of soft tissue sarcomas.
- Randomized trials show that radiation therapy in combination with surgery increases local control compared with surgery alone; no statistically significant differences in survival were observed in these small studies.
- In large national cancer databases, treatment of high-grade soft tissue sarcomas with adjuvant radiation therapy is associated with a 10% improvement in survival.
- Preoperative radiotherapy doubles the risk of a wound complication, whereas postoperative radiotherapy increases the risk of late effects, such as fibrosis, edema, and joint stiffness.

INTRODUCTION

For more than 100 years, radiation therapy has been a mainstay of cancer therapy because of the exquisite ability of ionizing radiation to kill cancer cells.[1] Historically, even though James Ewing used short-term tumor response to radiation therapy to

Disclosure: Dr D.G. Kirsch is on the scientific advisory board and owns stock in Lumicell Inc; is a founder of and own stock in XRad Therapeutics; has received research funding from Lumicell Inc, GlaxoSmithKline, and Janssen; and serves as the Chair of the Developmental Therapeutics Committee for the Sarcoma Alliance for Research through Collaboration (SARC). Dr N.A. Larrier and Dr B.G. Czito have nothing to disclose.
[a] Department of Radiation Oncology, Duke University Medical Center, 450 Research Drive, Durham, NC 27708, USA; [b] Department of Pharmacology & Cancer Biology, Duke University Medical Center, 450 Research Drive, Durham, NC 27708, USA
* Corresponding author. Department of Radiation Oncology, Duke University Medical Center, 450 Research Drive, Durham, NC 27708.
E-mail address: david.kirsch@duke.edu

help differentiate Ewing sarcoma from osteosarcoma, short-term changes in the size of a tumor following radiotherapy do not accurately quantify its efficacy. For some cancers (including soft tissue sarcoma), if they do not dramatically shrink following radiation therapy, clinicians may surmise that they are radiation resistant. However, this misconception is not consistent with clinical trials of radiation therapy in which the end point is local control. As discussed in this article, randomized clinical trials show that radiation therapy improves local control after surgery to a similar extent as surgery for breast cancer or rectal cancer. Therefore, radiation therapy is an effective modality for treating patients with soft tissue sarcoma.

PATIENT EVALUATION OVERVIEW

Because radiation therapy is an effective therapy for soft tissue sarcoma and can be integrated with surgical resection before, during, or after surgery, it is critical that a radiation oncologist experienced in treating sarcomas evaluates patients at the time of initial diagnosis. The 2015 National Comprehensive Cancer Network (NCCN) guidelines for the management of soft tissue sarcomas state that, "prior to the initiation of therapy, all patients should be evaluated and managed by a multidisciplinary team with expertise and experience in sarcoma."[2] Except for the rare clinical scenario in which a soft tissue sarcoma is causing progressive neurologic deficits or life-threatening bleeding, there is almost always sufficient time for evaluation by a radiation oncologist, facilitating a multidisciplinary consensus treatment plan before definitive surgical resection.

The 2015 NCCN guidelines for soft tissue sarcoma state that, before the initiation of therapy, all patients should be evaluated and managed by a multidisciplinary team with expertise and experience in sarcoma.

SURGERY ALONE

For extremity soft tissue sarcomas, the goals of local therapy include maximizing local control and function. Therefore, most patients with extremity soft tissue sarcomas undergo limb-sparing surgical resection. Limb-sparing surgery by surgeons experienced in soft tissue sarcoma resection achieves local control in approximately two-thirds of patients.[3] In a setting in which limb-sparing surgery would not lead to a functional extremity, amputation without radiation therapy is an established treatment option. When limb-sparing surgery can lead to a functional extremity, surgery alone may still be the optimal local therapy, particularly in the clinical setting in which local recurrence is unlikely to lead to the development of metastases or loss of limb function. Soft tissue sarcomas in this category include small (<5 cm), low-grade tumors, particularly those superficial to the fascia. If a tumor with these clinical features recurs after surgery alone, salvage therapy including radiotherapy and surgery is likely to lead to a functional limb. Data supporting this· approach come from a retrospective series from the Dana Farber Cancer Institute, concerning 74 patients with soft tissue sarcoma of the extremity or trunk with a median tumor size of 4 cm, of which 54% were low grade. These patients were treated with function-sparing surgery alone (ie, no radiotherapy) and the 10-year actuarial rate of local control was 93%.[4] All of the sarcomas with a histologic resection margin of at least 1 cm achieved local control with surgery alone.

Intermediate-grade and high-grade, large (>5 cm) sarcomas have a higher risk of developing metastases. Sarcomas deep to the fascia generally require a more extensive resection of normal muscle so surgery for a recurrence may substantially increase morbidity and decrease limb function. Because there are currently no reliable methods to detect residual microscopic sarcoma at the time of surgery, large sarcomas that are deep to the fascia are frequently treated with radiation therapy, particularly if they are intermediate or high grade. Several investigators are developing different approaches to imaging microscopic residual cancer during surgery.[5,6] If these intraoperative imaging techniques can better identify patients at high risk of residual cancer, then this may enable more patients to be managed with surgery alone.

Limb-sparing surgery alone (without radiotherapy) may be adequate local therapy for extremity soft tissue sarcomas that are small (<5 cm), low grade, and superficial to the fascia.

RADIATION THERAPY OPTIONS
Definitive Radiation Therapy Without Surgery

Although surgery is usually the cornerstone of local therapy for soft tissue sarcomas, there are certain clinical settings in which surgical resection may not be possible. For example, a soft tissue sarcoma may be located in the head and neck in a location that cannot be removed without sacrificing major blood vessels and/or nerves. Similarly, patients may refuse an amputation that may be recommended to achieve an en bloc resection and optimize local control. In these settings, definitive radiation therapy, with or without concurrent chemotherapy, is an alternative treatment option. Kepka and colleagues[7] reported the Massachusetts General Hospital institutional experience treating 112 patients with soft tissue sarcoma with definitive radiation therapy for gross disease. Locations included the extremities (43%), retroperitoneum (24%), head and neck (24%), and truncal wall (7%). The median size was 8 cm and 89% were intermediate or high grade. Median radiation dose was 64 Gy and 20% of patients received chemotherapy. With a median follow-up of 139 months, the 5-year actuarial local control, disease-free survival, and overall survival rates were 45%, 24%, and 35% respectively. Tumor size was a critical factor in 5-year local control: 51% for sarcomas less than 5 cm, 45% for sarcomas 5 to 10 cm, and 9% for sarcomas greater than 10 cm. Radiation dose also influenced outcome. Patients receiving less than 63 Gy achieved 5-year local control and overall survival rates of 22% and 14% respectively. Patients receiving 63 Gy or more achieved 5-year local control and overall survival rates of 60% and 52% respectively. Thus, for sarcomas less than 10 cm to which a radiation dose of 63 Gy or more can safely be delivered, definitive radiation therapy is a useful treatment option when surgery is not feasible or is declined by the patient.

For soft tissue sarcomas less than 10 cm, definitive radiation therapy (≥63 Gy) without surgery can achieve local control in approximately 50% of patients.

Radiation Therapy Plus Surgery

External beam radiotherapy as adjuvant therapy for extremity sarcomas
The use of adjuvant external beam radiotherapy (EBRT) with limb-sparing surgery for extremity sarcomas was initially implemented as an alternative approach to amputation in adult extremity soft tissue sarcomas.[8] This approach was prospectively

evaluated in 2 randomized studies conducted by the US National Cancer Institute (NCI) in the United States from the 1970s to 1990s. Rosenberg and colleagues[9] compared amputation with a limb salvage approach in extremity sarcomas, consisting of resection of the involved limb compartment and adjuvant EBRT. All patients (n = 43) received chemotherapy (doxorubicin, cyclophosphamide, methotrexate). Postoperative radiotherapy was administered (60–70 Gy) to 27 patients. A local recurrence rate of 15% was seen in the limb salvage group versus 0% in the amputation group (P = .06). However, overall survival was similar.

This result prompted the investigators at the NCI to ask whether radiotherapy was necessary in addition to limb-sparing surgery.[10] This second NCI study compared limb salvage (surgery and postoperative EBRT) with surgery alone. Surgery consisted of resection of gross tumor with a 1-cm to 2-cm margin where feasible. After surgical healing, patients with high-grade tumors (n = 91) were randomized to chemotherapy alone (doxorubicin, cyclophosphamide) versus chemotherapy and radiotherapy (63 Gy). Patients with low-grade (n = 50) tumors did not receive chemotherapy, but were randomized to observation versus radiotherapy. With a median follow-up of 9.6 years, patients treated with limb-sparing surgery alone showed increased local recurrence (24.3% vs 1.4%). Of note, overall survival was not statistically different. This randomized clinical trial established that EBRT in addition to limb-sparing surgery increases local control.

Even in this early study, there was a prospective evaluation of quality of life. Patients receiving adjuvant radiotherapy experienced decreased limb strength, increased edema, and worse range of motion of joints. However, these late effects did not seem to affect global quality of life or activities of daily living. Remarkably, follow-up for this study was recently extended for a median of 17.9 years and 54 patients completed a telephone interview.[11] During this extended follow-up, 1 of 24 patients in the surgery-alone group developed a local recurrence, but none of 30 patients in the radiotherapy group recurred locally. Twenty-year overall survival with surgery alone was 64% and 71% for patients who received EBRT. The 7% increase in overall survival for patients receiving adjuvant radiation therapy was not statistically significant, but the trial included low-grade and high-grade soft tissue sarcomas and was not powered to detect a 7% survival difference. The investigators appropriately concluded that EBRT following limb-sparing surgery provides excellent local control with acceptable toxicity with long-term follow-up, but no statistically significant improvement in overall survival.

A randomized clinical trial at the NCI showed that adjuvant radiation therapy after limb-sparing surgery significantly increases local control (24.3% vs 1.4%), with an improved overall survival of 7% (which was not statistically significant) in this small group of patients.

It is conceivable that, with a much larger sample size of patients with high-grade sarcoma, adjuvant radiation therapy would improve overall survival for some patients with soft tissue sarcoma. A retrospective study from the Surveillance, Epidemiology, and End Results (SEER) database with 6960 patients with soft tissue sarcoma of the extremities treated from 1998 through 2005 found that, for patients with high-grade sarcomas, 3-year overall survival was increased for patients receiving adjuvant radiation therapy: 73% versus 63% (P<.001).[12] No difference in 3-year overall survival was observed in patients with low-grade sarcomas. Similarly, a retrospective analysis of 10,290 patients from the National Cancer Database from 1998 through 2006 also found improved survival for patients with intermediate-grade and high-grade soft tissue sarcoma of the extremity treated with adjuvant radiation therapy.[13] To create 2 similar groups of patients treated with or without adjuvant radiation therapy, propensity matching was performed to match age, sex, tumor size, tumor grade, histology, margin type, tumor location (upper vs lower extremity), and extent of resection. Overall survival was compared for 2584 patients treated with adjuvant radiation therapy and 2582 patients without radiation therapy. Overall survival was increased by approximately 10% for patients receiving adjuvant radiation therapy ($P<.001$). In summary, retrospective studies from large databases show that adjuvant radiation therapy is associated with improved survival by up to 10% for patients with high-grade extremity sarcomas, although randomized trials of EBRT powered to detect a 10% survival difference have not been performed.

Retrospective studies from large databases (SEER, National Cancer Data Base) suggest that adjuvant radiation therapy may improve survival for patients with high-grade extremity sarcomas by as much as 10%.

Following the randomized trial of limb-sparing surgery with or without adjuvant radiotherapy at the NCI, limb salvage (surgery and EBRT) became the standard of care for eligible patients. Discussion then ensued regarding the timing of surgery and radiotherapy. Some clinicians proposed preoperative radiotherapy using a lower radiation dose and smaller treatment fields, as used in the treatment of other malignancies. One advantage of this approach is that the radiation oncologist can image and define the location of the tumor and more easily identify the adjacent area at risk of microscopic disease at the time of treatment planning. In contrast, if the radiation therapy is delivered after gross tumor resection, it is more challenging to define the treatment target. In addition, sarcoma cells can seed the surgical wound during surgery. Thus, the postoperative radiation field typically encompasses the entire operative bed, which can increase the size of the radiation field. Thus, a lower radiation dose delivered to a smaller treatment volume in a preoperative approach might decrease long-term complications. However, surgical oncologists expressed concern regarding the risk of wound complications associated with preoperative radiotherapy.

The National Cancer Institute Canada (NCIC) SR2 study addressed the question of preoperative versus postoperative radiotherapy in a seminal randomized trial published in 2002.[14] To date, this is the largest randomized study addressing the role of radiotherapy in extremity sarcoma. Nearly 200 patients were randomized to preoperative (50 Gy) versus postoperative (66 Gy) radiotherapy. The primary end point was wound complications at 120 days. Wound complications were defined as the need for a second surgery, or wound interventions requiring readmission, deep packing, or an invasive procedure. Secondary end points included local control and overall survival. At 120 days the wound complication rate was 17% in the postoperative radiotherapy group compared with 35% in the preoperative radiotherapy group. The rate of wound complication varied by anatomic site in multivariate analysis. In the upper extremity, in the absence of preoperative radiotherapy the rate of wound complications was 0% (0 of 19), which increased to 5.6% (1 of 18) after preoperative radiotherapy. In contrast, in the lower extremity the risk of a wound complication in the absence of preoperative radiotherapy was 21.3% (16 of 75), which increased to 42.9% (30 of 70) after preoperative radiotherapy. Therefore, a dose of radiation (50 Gy) does not seem to cause wound complications equally in all anatomic sites. Instead, it seems to double the risk of the baseline wound complication rate, which is much higher for lower extremity sarcomas. Local control (approximately 90%) and overall survival were similar between the groups.

Late effects on functional outcomes in the NCIC SR2 trial were also analyzed 2 years after therapy using the Musculoskeletal Tumor Rating Scale and the Toronto Extremity Salvage Score.[15] There was a trend toward increased grade 2 or greater fibrosis in the postoperative radiotherapy group (48.2% vs 31.5%), which at that time point was not statistically significant ($P = .07$). Although not statistically significant, extremity edema (23.2% vs 15.5%) and joint stiffness (23.2% vs 17.8%) were also more frequent in the postoperative arm. Radiation field size was predictive for greater fibrosis and joint stiffness, which correlated with lower functional scores. These data provide the basis for counseling patients with extremity sarcomas who are eligible for limb-sparing surgery about the risks and benefits of preoperative versus postoperative radiotherapy. Based on individual patient's particular risk profiles for wound complications and goals regarding functionality after treatment of sarcoma, surgical or orthopedic oncologists and radiation oncologists can make recommendations regarding the timing of radiotherapy. In general, for younger patients, who may better tolerate a temporary wound complication, the authors usually offer preoperative radiation therapy to limit the risk of late effects, which might be permanent. For older patients with comorbidities, including diabetes and significant heart disease, in whom a wound complication could cause more serious morbidity and even increase the risk of mortality, the authors often recommend postoperative radiation therapy, particularly in patients in whom late effects from radiation may be less of a concern.

A randomized clinical trial from the NCIC showed that preoperative and postoperative radiotherapy achieved similar rates of local control and overall survival. Preoperative radiotherapy doubled the risk for a surgical wound complication, but used a lower radiation dose and a smaller treatment field, which resulted in fewer long-term side effects.

Practical aspects of EBRT treatment planning for extremity sarcomas include:

1. Before any therapy, review all available data and consult with a multidisciplinary team. Specifically, the radiation oncologist should review the diagnostic MRI with a musculoskeletal radiologist and ensure that the pathology has been reviewed by a pathologist with experience interpreting soft tissue sarcomas.
2. Discuss the planned (or completed) surgery with the surgeon. This discussion alerts the radiation oncologist to any special concerns regarding scars, ecchymoses, or drain sites to be treated, including a margin that may be particularly close at the time of surgery and may therefore benefit from higher doses of radiation therapy, and unusual patterns of spread related to specific histologic subtypes.
3. After signing informed consent for radiotherapy, the patient undergoes a computed tomography (CT) simulation in the treatment position. Reproducibility is key to ensuring that treatment is delivered precisely to the target on a daily basis. Positioning of the involved extremity should take into consideration potential radiation beam arrangements. The position of the contralateral extremity and other critical structures such as the genitalia needs to be considered. Therefore, at the time of simulation a patient-specific immobilization device[16] is used to ensure patient comfort and maximize reproducibility of the position of the extremity. Once the patient is in a satisfactory position and the immobilization is built, then a CT scan is acquired. Intravenous contrast can be used to show the tumor more clearly. This CT scan is used by the radiation oncologist to contour the tumor target and the normal tissue avoidance structures. If possible, MRI can be obtained in the

treatment position, but the narrow bore of many MRI scanners may preclude imaging the extremity after it has been immobilized. The diagnostic MRI may be merged with the treatment planning CT. The contrasted T1 and T2 series are often the most useful. The tumor is outlined on the CT and MRI as the gross tumor volume (GTV), which is shown in red in **Fig. 1**. This volume is expanded to include regions at risk for microscopic spread. The MRI T2 peritumoral edema is usually included

A

B

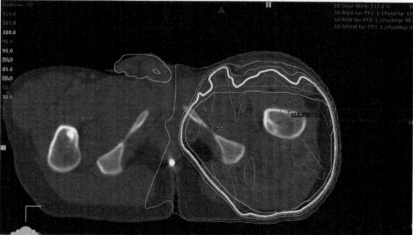

Fig. 1. (*A*) Contours of radiation target volumes on a CT simulation for radiation therapy planning. The gross tumor volume (GTV) is contoured in red. The clinical target volume (CTV) provides an additional margin for microscopic spread of the tumor and is contoured in green. A planning target volume (PTV) includes additional margin for setup error and is contoured in pink. The radiation dose is routinely prescribed to the PTV. The genitalia are contoured in yellow as a radiation avoidance structure. (*B*) The treatment plan shows the radiation dose distribution compared with the contoured volumes in (*A*). Each color within the dose distribution represents a relative percentage of the prescription dose with the key in the upper left.

because of the risk of harboring microscopic extension of tumor. Typically, this clinical target volume (CTV) is an expansion of the GTV by 3 cm in the longitudinal direction and 1.5 cm radially.[17] The CTV, which is outlined in green in **Fig. 1**, is routinely customized to exclude regions that would not be characteristic of tumor spread, such as entering another compartment or invasion into the bone. The final expansion to the planning target volume (PTV), which is outlined in pink in **Fig. 1**, accounts for setup error and is usually 0.5 cm when daily image-guided radiation therapy (IGRT) is used.[17] Normal tissues are also contoured. These tissues include bone, genitalia, joints, and a normal strip of tissue on the opposite side of the extremity, which can be used as an avoidance structure.

4. Volumetric-based treatment planning is then performed using three-dimensional planning or inverse planning for intensity-modulated radiation therapy (IMRT). Care is taken to avoid treating the entire circumference of the extremity by limiting radiation dose to a normal strip of tissue (to decrease risk of edema), to avoid treating an entire joint (to decrease risk of joint stiffness), and to minimize dose to weight-bearing bones (to minimize risk of fracture). For example, the risk of fracture after treatment in one series was decreased if the mean radiation dose to the bone was less than 37 Gy and the volume of the bone receiving 40 Gy was less than 64%.[18]

5. At the time of treatment, the patient is repositioned within the immobilization device in the identical position as at the time of CT simulation. Verification images with kilovoltage radiographs are taken at the center of the radiation plan as well as the treatment fields for quality assurance. Some treatment machines have the capability of performing a cone beam CT scan to aid in verification of soft tissues to further confirm an accurate setup. These types of images may be taken daily before treatment if IGRT is needed to minimize the daily setup error.

The clinical trials described earlier used conventional radiotherapy approaches. More recently, advances in physics, imaging, and computing have enabled more sophisticated methods of radiation delivery, such as IMRT and IGRT. IGRT was recently studied prospectively in extremity sarcoma in a multi-institutional setting in radiation therapy oncology group (RTOG) 0630.[17] The rationale for IGRT is that the setup of the patient on the treatment table can vary from day to day and introduce error into treatment delivery. To minimize the risk of missing the target, the radiation field size can be increased, but this results in additional normal tissue irradiation, which may further increase side effects. To limit the expansion of the radiation field because of setup uncertainty, patient positioning can be verified by imaging the treatment area just before delivering radiotherapy. IGRT uses pretreatment imaging so that shifts (often measured in millimeters) can be made before delivering the daily treatment. Pretreatment imaging may consist of kilovoltage orthogonal radiographs or cone beam CT. By aligning the patient's position with the treatment plan before delivery (**Fig. 2**), the daily setup error can be decreased, which may allow the radiation field size to be safely reduced. In RTOG 0630, 86 patients were treated preoperatively to 50 Gy with daily IGRT using tailored radiotherapy fields with a PTV margin of 0.5 cm. Late toxicities at 2 years were compared with those in the preoperative arm of the NCIC SR2 cohort. In the IGRT group, 10% of patients had late toxicity compared with 37% in the NCIC group ($P<.001$). Note that the wound complication rate and local control were similar in both studies. In a secondary analysis of the daily shifts made from the pretreatment imaging with IGRT in RTOG 0630, a PTV expansion of 1.5 cm in all directions would have been required to cover the CTV and account for the setup variations in the absence of daily pretreatment imaging.[19] Patients with optimal

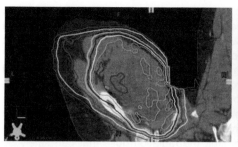 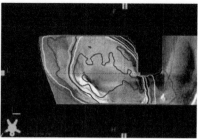

Fig. 2. Image-guided radiation therapy. A treatment plan was generated for a proximal thigh sarcoma (*left*). Just before treatment, a cone beam CT scan was acquired on the treatment couch. The treatment couch can then be moved to align the patient position to match the pretreatment simulation before delivering the daily radiation treatment (*right*).

immobilization may not need daily IGRT if the shifts following initial pretreatment images require shifts to correct patient position that are less than the PTV expansion.

IMRT uses radiation fields with nonuniform fluence so that the high-dose radiation can be distributed to better conform to the treatment target and avoid adjacent normal tissue. IMRT was used with IGRT in 75% of patients enrolled on RTOG 0630. Image guidance combined with IMRT also was used by the sarcoma group in Toronto in a prospective clinical trial of 70 patients with extremity sarcoma, attempting to reduce the risk of acute wound complications associated with preoperative radiotherapy.[20] At the time of radiation treatment planning, the surgeon was asked to outline the structures on the planning CT scan deemed at high risk for a wound healing complication. In particular, the site of the future scar and surgical flaps were contoured. The radiation physics planning team then used IMRT techniques to minimize the radiation dose to these regions. A standard preoperative radiotherapy dose of 50 Gy was used. Furthermore, at the time of surgery, the radiotherapy planning data were transferred to the operating suite to assist in recreating the planned surgical incisions. Results showed that the need for tissue transfer was reduced (6.8% vs 28.6%; $P = .002$). The overall wound complication rate was reduced (30.5% vs 43%) compared with the preoperative arm of the NCIC SR2 trial, but this did not reach statistical significance ($P = .2$). A retrospective review of 319 patients with extremity sarcomas treated at Memorial Sloan Kettering Cancer Center compared outcomes treated with conventional EBRT (n = 154) and IMRT (n = 165).[21] On multivariate analysis, treatment with IMRT was an independent predictor for reduced local recurrence (hazard ratio = 0.46; 95% confidence interval, 0.24–0.89; $P = .02$). Thus, when IMRT may provide a significant advantage by sparing normal tissues from a high radiation dose, then it is a reasonable treatment option.

External beam radiotherapy as adjuvant therapy for retroperitoneal sarcomas

In contrast with extremity soft tissue sarcomas, in which local control can be achieved in approximately 90% of patients with the combination of limb-sparing surgery and radiation therapy, the management of patients with retroperitoneal soft tissue sarcoma poses a greater therapeutic challenge. Even in the setting of an en bloc resection, the natural history of retroperitoneal sarcoma is characterized by high rates of local recurrence. In contemporary series, macroscopically complete resection rates range from 64% to 95%,[22] but, even in the setting of gross total resection, margins for retroperitoneal sarcomas are likely to be close if not microscopically involved secondary to anatomic constraints. Surgery-alone series have shown that local recurrence is the primary mode of failure for many patients with retroperitoneal sarcoma, occurring in 41% to 82% of patients undergoing gross total resection, with higher rates seen with long-term follow-up.[23,24] Local failure may result in uncontrolled local disease and lead to morbidity, including bowel obstruction/perforation/fistula, pain, ureteral obstruction, renal failure, gastrointestinal bleeding, biliary obstruction, failure to thrive, and neuropathy. Unlike other sarcoma sites, uncontrolled local disease remains a major source of mortality. Therefore, if radiation therapy increased the local control of retroperitoneal sarcomas, then it might decrease morbidity and improve survival. The large size of retroperitoneal sarcomas and the proximity of adjacent normal structures limit the radiation dose that can safely be delivered. Therefore, standard EBRT techniques are limited to delivering 45 to 55 Gy using daily fractions of 1.8 to 2 Gy, which may be insufficient to reliably control local regional disease. After surgery, normal bowel often falls into the tumor bed, making postoperative radiotherapy particularly challenging for this anatomic site. Technical details for the treatment of retroperitoneal sarcomas with radiotherapy have recently been summarized by an international consensus[25] and are outside of the scope of this article. However, it is worth noting that the kidneys are radiosensitive organs. If the tumor is close to one kidney, a renal scan should be performed to verify the function of the contralateral kidney before initiating treatment that may render the ipsilateral kidney nonfunctional.

The value of preoperative radiotherapy for retroperitoneal sarcomas remains ill-defined. ACOSOG (American College of Surgeons Oncology Group) Z9031 was a clinical trial in the United States that randomized patients with retroperitoneal sarcomas to preoperative radiotherapy versus no radiation therapy. However, this trial closed early because of poor accrual. The phase III EORTC (European Organisation for Research and Treatment of Cancer) 62092-22092 STRASS trial (NCT01344018) is currently randomizing patients with retroperitoneal sarcomas to preoperative radiotherapy (50.4 Gy) versus no radiation therapy. Until the results of this randomized trial are available, clinicians must look to retrospective analyses to assess the potential impact of adjuvant radiation therapy. For example, one recent study examined patients with retroperitoneal sarcoma treated at 2 institutions from 2003 to 2011. At Memorial Sloan Kettering Cancer Center, 172 patients were treated with surgery alone. At Massachusetts General Hospital, 32 patients were treated with neoadjuvant or adjuvant EBRT with or without intraoperative radiation therapy (IORT). EBRT was delivered by IMRT using photons or with proton beam radiation therapy. Proton beam radiation therapy is a charged particle treatment that does not have any exit radiation dose beyond the treatment target, and therefore decreases the amount of radiation to some normal tissues. After a median follow-up of 39 months, 5-year local relapse-free survival was 91% in the radiotherapy group and 65% in the surgery-alone group ($P = .02$).[26] In the absence of randomized data, patients with retroperitoneal sarcoma should be evaluated by a multidisciplinary team that includes a radiation oncologist with experience treating these tumors to consider whether radiation therapy is indicated. The authors routinely recommend preoperative radiation therapy (45–50.4 Gy) for intermediate and high-grade retroperitoneal sarcomas. Because of the high rate of recurrence, the authors often consider including IORT at the time of surgery.

Intraoperative radiation therapy for retroperitoneal sarcomas

IORT is the delivery of radiation therapy during surgery. The underlying rationale for IORT is that increasing doses of radiation therapy during surgery, beyond what is safe to deliver with EBRT alone, may enhance local tumor control. During surgery and IORT, radiation dose–limiting structures adjacent to the tumor, such as the bowel, can be displaced away from the tumor bed and shielded. Thus, IORT has the potential to improve local control and the therapeutic ratio by (1) excluding part or all of the dose-limiting normal structures from the irradiated field by operative mobilization or direct shielding, (2) delivering high-dose radiation to the tumor bed, and (3) reducing the volume of the high radiation boost dose by direct tumor/tumor bed visualization and treatment to that site. IORT was first used almost 100 years ago. Presently, there more than 160 centers in at least 29 countries worldwide with active IORT programs (Don Goer, personal communication, 2016).

IORT is frequently used in combination with fractionated neoadjuvant or adjuvant EBRT and resection. The rationale for combining IORT with EBRT is that EBRT fields encompass not only the primary tumor but also adjacent surrounding tissues that potentially harbor microscopic disease. In contrast with a large single fraction of radiation during surgery, EBRT is typically given in small (1.8 to 2 Gy) daily fractions, which takes advantage of radiobiological features, such as cell cycle redistribution and tumor reoxygenation, which promotes tumor control while minimizing late normal tissue injury. The biological effectiveness of single-dose IORT in tumor relative to equivalent total dose of fractionated EBRT has been estimated to be 1.5 to 2.5 times the IORT dose delivered. When combined with EBRT and resection, IORT at doses ranging from 10 to 20 Gy may provide local control for sarcomas, particularly in the setting of microscopic residual disease.

Practical aspects of treatment planning for IORT for retroperitoneal sarcomas include:

1. The authors' preferred treatment strategy in most patients with intermediate-grade to high-grade retroperitoneal sarcomas is to obtain tissue diagnosis by core-needle biopsy. Before initiating treatment of a retroperitoneal sarcoma, the patient should be evaluated by a multidisciplinary team that includes a radiation oncologist to determine whether EBRT and/or IORT are indicated.
2. For intermediate-grade and high-grade retroperitoneal sarcomas, the authors typically deliver preoperative EBRT (45–55 Gy using fractions of 1.8–2 Gy) using highly conformal techniques. Because the tumor frequently displaces normal tissue away from what will become the tumor bed margin, this approach offers theoretic and clinical advantages compared with resection with IORT followed by postoperative EBRT. Preoperative EBRT seems to be well tolerated and is associated with less acute and chronic toxicity compared with postoperative approaches that use a higher radiation dose.[14]
3. Maximal resection usually occurs 4 to 6 weeks after completing EBRT.
4. Criteria that the authors use to select patients for IORT include:
   a. Surgery is likely to be incomplete and leave behind microscopic or gross residual disease, which will lead to a high probability of subsequent failure within the tumor bed.
   b. There is no evidence of distant metastases. Possible exceptions include patients with resectable oligometastatic or single-organ metastasis and a high probability of symptomatic local failure.
   c. EBRT doses required for a high probability of local control following subtotal or no resection exceed normal tissue tolerance. In retroperitoneal sarcoma, total doses required for a high likelihood of eradication of microscopic disease exceed 60 to 70 Gy, and for eradication of gross disease the required dose is even higher.
   d. Surgical displacement or shielding of dose-limiting structures or organs can be accomplished during IORT administration, allowing for acceptable risks of immediate toxicity and late effects.

5. IORT may be administered with either electrons (IOERT) or high-dose-rate (HDR) photon afterloading techniques. IOERT uses a linear accelerator in the operating room to generate electrons of different energies that are shaped by a cone to match the geometric target of the tumor bed. Electron energies can range from 6 MeV to 20 MeV, which allows treatment of shallow targets with low energy (1–2 cm) or gross disease with high energy. For HDR afterloading, an applicator such as the Harrison-Anderson-Mick (HAM) applicator is placed directly onto the surface of the tumor bed (**Fig. 3**). The applicator contains catheters that are separated in 1-cm intervals. The catheters are then attached to the HDR unit, which remotely delivers a radioactive isotope, such as ^{192}iridium, through each catheter. The isotope stops at different dwell positions within the catheters for various lengths of time according to a computer-generated treatment plan in order to deliver the prescribed dose to a specified area.

6. For patients with completely resected tumors and negative margins, an IORT dose of 10 to 12 Gy is usually selected, whereas a grossly resected tumor bed with positive microscopic margins usually receives 12.5 to 15 Gy (depending on volume treated). For gross residual disease, doses range from 15 to 20 Gy depending on the extent of residual tumor, the volume treated, and normal tissue within the IORT field.

The sole randomized study evaluating EBRT with or without IOERT for retroperitoneal sarcomas was performed at the NCI.[27] This small study of 35 patients undergoing gross total resection randomized patients to receive IOERT to a dose of 20 Gy followed by reduced-dose EBRT (35–40 Gy) or postoperative EBRT alone to doses of 50 to 55 Gy. Patients receiving IOERT also received misonidazole as a radiosensitizer. Mature results of this study showed a significant reduction in local failure with the use of IOERT (20% in-field local recurrence vs 80% in-field local recurrence; $P<.001$), although median survival was similar between both groups. Multiple single and collective institutional experiences evaluating the role of IORT in retroperitoneal sarcomas suggest that IORT reduces local failure rates compared with historical controls treated with surgery alone or surgery with EBRT, particularly in patients undergoing gross total resection.[28]

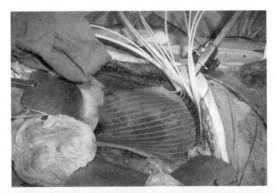

Fig. 3. HAM applicator for IORT in a patient with a retroperitoneal sarcoma. The bowel has been moved away from the tumor bed. The HAM applicator is placed directly on the tumor bed. After moving the patient into a shielded area of the operating room, an iridium source travels through each catheter to deliver IORT to the tumor bed.

Simultaneous integrated boost radiation for retroperitoneal sarcomas

An alternative approach to delivering high-dose radiation therapy to the resection margin of a retroperitoneal sarcoma during surgery with IORT is to simultaneously deliver an additional dose to the anticipated resection margin during preoperative EBRT. This approach uses IMRT with a technique called a simultaneous integrated boost. In most patients with retroperitoneal sarcoma, the anterior margin can be widely resected and, if it is invading an organ, such as the colon, then this portion of the organ can be resected. In contrast, the posterior margin, such as the psoas muscle, is more difficult to resect and frequently harbors microscopic residual cancer. Because the tumor displaces the normal tissues anteriorly and away from this posterior margin, it is possible to simultaneously escalate the radiation dose to this anticipated positive margin while retaining a standard dose to the anterior margin of the tumor to avoid exceeding normal tissue radiation dose constraints. A group at the University of Alabama at Birmingham treated 16 patients with retroperitoneal sarcoma with preoperative radiation therapy with 45 Gy in 25 fractions to the tumor and a simultaneous integrated boost of 57.5 Gy in 25 fractions to the posterior volume predicted to be at high risk for positive surgical margins.[29] With a median follow-up of 28 months, there were 2 local recurrences.[29] Toxicity seemed to be similar to that of standard preoperative EBRT. There is now an ongoing phase I/II clinical trial (NCT01659203) for retroperitoneal sarcomas at several institutions in the United States using IGRT with IMRT or proton radiation therapy to escalate the simultaneous integrated dose to the posterior margin to 63 Gy in 28 fractions while the rest of the tumor is treated to 50.4 Gy in 28 fractions.

A simultaneous integrated boost approach for preoperative radiation therapy is also being combined with IORT for retroperitoneal sarcomas in a phase I/II clinical trial in Heidelberg, Germany (NCT01566123). Interim analysis of this prospective, single-center trial of 27 patients with primary/recurrent retroperitoneal sarcomas (>5 cm, M0, at least marginally resectable) was recently reported.[30] Neoadjuvant IMRT using an integrated boost with doses of up to 56 Gy to the boost volume in 25 fractions was used, followed by surgery and IOERT (10–12 Gy). Gross total resection was feasible in all but 1 patient. Final margin status was R0 in 6 (22%) and R1 in 20 patients (74%). IOERT was performed in 23 patients (85%) with a median dose of 12 Gy (10–20 Gy). Three-year and 5-year local control rates were 72%, with 2 recurrences located outside of the EBRT area. The investigators concluded that the combination of neoadjuvant IMRT with simultaneous integrated boost to the margin at high risk, surgery, and IOERT is feasible with acceptable toxicity and yields good results in terms of local control and overall survival in patients with high-risk retroperitoneal sarcomas.

Brachytherapy as adjuvant therapy for sarcomas

Brachytherapy, which refers to therapy over a short distance, describes techniques that deliver radiation from radioactive sources that are located in or next to the target. In contrast with EBRT (teletherapy), which is delivered noninvasively from a linear accelerator, brachytherapy requires interstitial placement of radioactive seeds directly into a tumor or into catheters that have been placed into the tumor bed during surgical resection. Investigators at Memorial Sloan Kettering Cancer Center tested the efficacy of brachytherapy for extremity soft tissue sarcoma in a prospective randomized clinical trial.[3] During surgery for soft tissue sarcomas of the extremity or superficial trunk, 164 patients were randomized to no additional therapy or to brachytherapy, in which case catheters were placed into the tumor bed intraoperatively. Approximately 5 days later, the catheters were loaded with low-dose-rate (LDR) [192]iridium for 4 to 6 days to deliver 42 to 45 Gy. With a median follow-up of 76 months, the 5-year actuarial rate of local control for patients with high-grade sarcomas treated with surgery alone was 66%, whereas local control with brachytherapy was 89% ($P = .0025$). However, these patients did not have improved overall survival. Surprisingly, patients with low-grade sarcomas failed to benefit from LDR brachytherapy in this study.

A randomized clinical trial showed that brachytherapy in addition to limb-sparing surgery significantly improved local control, but did not change overall survival.

Although this study established that LDR brachytherapy significantly improves local control for high-grade soft tissue sarcomas, most institutions use EBRT rather than LDR brachytherapy for several reasons. First, the dose distribution with LDR brachytherapy depends on the placement of the catheters in the tumor bed, which is typically at 1-cm intervals and covers 2 cm above and below the location of the tumor. If catheters are too far apart, then an area at risk may be underdosed. If catheters are too close together, then an area may be overdosed. Thus, the success of brachytherapy depends on accurate catheter placement. The impact of suboptimal catheter placement can be ameliorated to a degree with HDR brachytherapy, in which dwell times for the radioactive source can be increased or decreased depending on the distance to adjacent sources. HDR brachytherapy is usually delivered twice a day for a total of 8 to 10 treatments. However, even when HDR brachytherapy is used, for most sarcoma implants the catheters are placed in a single plane. This single plane may not adequately cover the three-dimensional tissue at risk of harboring microscopic residual sarcoma, which can be more easily treated with EBRT. Thus, the authors generally prefer EBRT to brachytherapy for the management of extremity sarcomas. However, we do consider brachytherapy in cases in which the geometry of the sarcoma and normal anatomy enable a single-plane implant to provide excellent coverage of the area at risk and for certain clinical scenarios. For example, we would consider brachytherapy for a patient who is not available for a 5-week to 6-week course of EBRT and therefore requests a compressed radiotherapy course. We also consider brachytherapy for patients with a locally recurrent sarcoma after prior EBRT and limb-sparing surgery, recognizing that this approach to managing previously irradiated tissue has an increased risk for complications.[31]

Brachytherapy was also studied in a prospective trial in Toronto in patients with retroperitoneal sarcomas.[32] Forty patients were treated with preoperative EBRT (45–50 Gy) and 19 patients also received brachytherapy (20–25 Gy) to the tumor bed. At 10 years, relapse-free survival and overall survival were similar between the two groups. Brachytherapy in the upper abdomen was associated with substantial acute postoperative toxicity (≥grade 3) and death in 2 patients.[33] Therefore, postoperative brachytherapy is not routinely used to treat patients with retroperitoneal sarcomas.

Radiation Therapy and Chemotherapy

Radiation therapy can also be used concurrently with chemotherapy. The rationale of combined modality therapy is that chemotherapy may sensitize the sarcoma to radiotherapy and early use of chemotherapy (ie, before surgery) may have maximal benefit against microscopic metastatic disease. For more information on the use of chemotherapy for sarcomas please see Robert J. Canter: Chemotherapy: Does Neoadjuvant or Adjuvant Therapy Improve Outcomes, in this issue.

In the context of radiotherapy, note that some institutions prefer to treat patients with soft tissue sarcomas at high risk of metastases with combined radiation therapy and chemotherapy. For example, at Massachusetts General Hospital, patients with large ($\geq$8 cm) intermediate-grade and high-grade sarcomas were treated with 3 cycles of neoadjuvant chemotherapy (mesna, Adriamycin, ifosfamide, dacarbazine [MAID]) interdigitated between two 22-Gy (11 fractions) courses (total 44 Gy) of preoperative radiotherapy.[34] Up to 3 cycles of MAID chemotherapy were delivered after surgery. With a median follow-up of 46 months, a cohort of 66 patients had a local control rate of 91%, a 5-year distant recurrence-free survival rate of 64%, and a 5-year overall survival rate of 86%.[35] The RTOG tested a similar approach in a multi-institutional prospective phase II study in RTOG 9514. Sixty-six patients with high-grade, large ($\geq$8 cm) soft tissue sarcomas of the extremity and body wall were treated with interdigitated MAID chemotherapy and 44-Gy preoperative radiotherapy.[36] Three cycles of MAID were offered after surgery. Ninety-seven percent of patients experienced grade 3 or higher toxicity, including 3 deaths. With a median follow-up of 7.7 years, 5-year distant disease-free survival and overall survival rates were 64.1% and 71.2%, respectively. Other institutions have used other combinations of concurrent chemotherapy and radiotherapy for soft tissue sarcomas. For example, at the University of California, Los Angeles, reduced-dose radiotherapy (28 Gy) has been combined with various chemotherapy regimens, including (1) intra-arterial Adriamycin; (2) intravenous ifosfamide; and (3) intravenous cisplatin, Adriamycin, and ifosfamide.[37] In this study of 496 patients with intermediate-grade and high-grade extremity soft tissue sarcoma, at least 95% necrosis after neoadjuvant therapy correlated with decreased local recurrence and improved overall survival. At MD Anderson, a phase I trial in 36 patients with high-risk extremity and trunk sarcoma tested escalating doses of gemcitabine with 50 Gy concurrent preoperative radiation therapy.[38] In addition, the authors have used concurrent ifosfamide chemotherapy and radiotherapy in selected patients treated with definitive radiotherapy or in the setting in which surgery may not achieve a negative margin, such as a pulmonary sarcoma adjacent to the aorta.[39] Despite the rationale for combination chemoradiotherapy for high-risk extremity sarcoma, there are limited prospective randomized data supporting this approach.

An ongoing phase II clinical trial in Europe is testing the combination of the tyrosine kinase inhibitor pazopanib with preoperative radiotherapy (NCT02575066). In the United States, the impact of adding pazopanib to preoperative radiotherapy (with or without chemotherapy) is being tested in a randomized phase II/III trial through the adult NRG Oncology and Children's Oncology Group (NCT02180867). Given the promising results of immunotherapy for other cancers, clinical trials testing immunotherapy with preoperative radiation therapy are also being planned. It is hoped that combining radiation therapy with these or other novel agents will improve overall survival for patients with high-risk soft tissue sarcoma.

RADIATION THERAPY COMPLICATIONS

Like all forms of cancer therapy, radiation therapy is associated with risks of short-term toxicity and long-term side effects. Short-term radiation toxicity includes fatigue, skin erythema and desquamation, as well as site-specific toxicity. For example, patients treated with radiotherapy for retroperitoneal sarcoma may experience nausea and diarrhea, which would not occur in patients receiving radiation therapy for extremity sarcoma. Similarly, patients treated for head and neck sarcoma may uniquely experience oral mucositis and xerostomia. As described earlier, the NCIC SR2 randomized trial of preoperative versus postoperative radiation therapy for extremity soft tissue sarcomas showed that preoperative radiotherapy doubles the risk of a wound complication after surgery.[14] Although these wound complications can require a return trip to the operating room to debride the wound, these complications can generally be managed without adversely affecting the long-term function of the extremity.

In contrast, postoperative radiation therapy, which delivers a 20% to 30% higher radiation dose to a significantly larger volume of normal tissue, increases late effects, such as extremity edema, fibrosis, and joint stiffness.[15] Because the risk of fracture after radiotherapy also correlates with radiation dose and volume of the weight-bearing bone exceeding certain levels, postoperative radiotherapy can also increase the risk of subsequent fracture.[18] Although radiation oncologists routinely consider the risk of toxicity in terms of the percentage of the normal organ or tissue irradiated to specific radiation dose thresholds (ie, using dose-volume histograms), these risks are superimposed on comorbidities specific to each patient. For example, patients with osteoporosis may develop fractures after a lower dose of radiation compared with patients with good bone health. Similarly, the same 50 Gy of preoperative radiotherapy that substantially increases the risk of a lower extremity wound complication (from 21% to 43%) is unlikely to cause a wound complication in the upper extremity, where surgery alone has a very low baseline risk of wound complications.[14] An important area for future clinical research is to identify patient-specific and anatomy-specific risks for radiotherapy complications so that they can be integrated into radiation dose–volume complication probability models.

This concept can also be extended to the rare, but potentially life-threatening, late effect of radiation-associated cancer. Relative to the potency of killing cancer cells, radiation is a weak carcinogen.[40] Studies that attempt to define the risk of radiation-induced cancer frequently compare second cancers with a normal, noncancer control group. However, this overestimates the risk of radiation for causing cancer because cancer survivors have a higher rate of developing a second cancer than the normal population. For example, randomized clinical trials in Europe that included 2554 adults with rectal cancer or endometrial cancer compared second cancers after surgery alone versus surgery and pelvic radiotherapy.[41] With a median follow-up of 13 years, compared with healthy controls, the risk of a second cancer was approximately 3-fold higher. However, the risk was similar for patients who received surgery alone and surgery with pelvic radiotherapy. It is also worth considering the results of the 20-year follow-up of the randomized clinical trial of EBRT for extremity sarcoma at the NCI.[11] Although patients treated with postoperative EBRT tended to have more wound complications, clinically significant edema, and functional limb deficits, they did not have a large number of second cancers and tended to have an increased overall survival ($P = .22$). However, just as a low risk of wound complications from preoperative EBRT in the upper extremity does not correlate with the risk of wound complications in the lower extremity, the same radiotherapy that does not significantly increase rates of second cancer in one population may substantially increase second cancers in susceptible patients. Because the risk of radiation-associated cancer varies by organ, developmental stage, and radiation dose, it is difficult to estimate a general risk factor. Nevertheless, patients with an inherited (ie, germline) susceptibility to cancer may be at particular risk for radiation-induced cancer because every cell in the body already has 1 cancer-causing mutation. Although family history of cancer in a patient who has cancer can predict for the presence of a germline mutation, whole-genome sequencing of pediatric patients with cancer identified germline mutations in cancer-predisposing genes in only 8.5% of patients, and family history did not predict the presence of an underlying cancer predisposition syndrome in most patients.[42] Thus, pediatric and young adult patients with sarcoma may be at particular risk for carrying a germline mutation and at higher risk for developing a treatment-associated malignancy.

The risk of developing these late effects is not only a function of radiation dose and volume treated but also radiation technique. For example, avoiding circumferential limb irradiation or minimizing the amount of a joint within a radiation field can decrease the risk of late effects. Therefore, patients with sarcoma should be encouraged to seek care from radiation oncologists with expertise in sarcoma not only to maximize the likelihood for local control but also to minimize the risk of long-term side effects. Moreover, when considering risks of radiation therapy based on prior studies, it is important to recognize that radiotherapy techniques and target volumes evolve over time. For example, the recent prospective phase II trials of preoperative IGRT for extremity sarcoma from the RTOG 0630[17] and the Toronto sarcoma group[20] show reduced risk for late effects compared with conventional radiotherapy.

SUMMARY

Soft tissue sarcomas are rare cancers that can be challenging to treat. Optimal management requires coordinating multidisciplinary treatment from a team of physicians with experience caring for patients with sarcoma. Once a diagnosis is established, a consultation with a radiation oncologist is indicated so that the risks and benefits of preoperative, intraoperative, and postoperative radiotherapy can be discussed. Randomized controlled trials have established that radiation therapy increases local control for extremity sarcomas compared with limb-sparing surgery alone. Although surgery alone can be optimal therapy for certain patients, for patients with large intermediate and high-grade sarcomas, radiotherapy should be delivered in addition to surgery in order to maximize local control. For patents with high-grade sarcomas, retrospective studies from cancer registries have shown that adjuvant radiotherapy results in an approximately 10% improvement in survival. However, prospective randomized trials of radiation therapy were not powered to detect such a survival difference. Therefore, improving local control as part of a limb-preserving strategy is the primary rationale for including radiation therapy as a key component in the multidisciplinary management of these challenging patients.

REFERENCES

1. Coleman CN, Lawrence TS, Kirsch DG. Enhancing the efficacy of radiation therapy: premises, promises, and practicality. J Clin Oncol 2014;32(26):2832–5.
2. Von Mehren M, Randall RL, Benjamin RS, et al. Soft tissue sarcoma. J Natl Compr Canc Netw 2014;12(4):473–83.
3. Pisters PW, Harrison LB, Leung DH, et al. Long-term results of a prospective randomized trial of adjuvant brachytherapy in soft tissue sarcoma. J Clin Oncol 1996;14(3):859–68.
4. Baldini EH, Goldberg J, Jenner C, et al. Long-term outcomes after function-sparing surgery without radiotherapy for soft tissue sarcoma of the extremities and trunk. J Clin Oncol 1999;17(10):3252–9.
5. Whitley MJ, Weissleder R, Kirsch DG. Tailoring adjuvant radiation therapy by intraoperative imaging to detect residual cancer. Semin Radiat Oncol 2015;25(4): 313–21.
6. Whitley MJ, Cardona DM, Lazarides AL, et al. A mouse-human phase 1 co-clinical trial of a protease-activated fluorescent probe for imaging cancer. Sci Transl Med 2016;8(320):320ra324.
7. Kepka L, DeLaney TF, Suit HD, et al. Results of radiation therapy for unresected soft-tissue sarcomas. Int J Radiat Oncol Biol Phys 2005;63(3):852–9.

8. Suit HD, Russell WO, Martin RG. Management of patients with sarcoma of soft tissue in an extremity. Cancer 1973;31(5):1247–55.

9. Rosenberg SA, Tepper J, Glatstein E, et al. The treatment of soft-tissue sarcomas of the extremities: prospective randomized evaluations of (1) limb-sparing surgery plus radiation therapy compared with amputation and (2) the role of adjuvant chemotherapy. Ann Surg 1982;196(3):305–15.

10. Yang JC, Chang AE, Baker AR, et al. Randomized prospective study of the benefit of adjuvant radiation therapy in the treatment of soft tissue sarcomas of the extremity. J Clin Oncol 1998;16(1):197–203.

11. Beane JD, Yang JC, White D, et al. Efficacy of adjuvant radiation therapy in the treatment of soft tissue sarcoma of the extremity: 20-year follow-up of a randomized prospective trial. Ann Surg Oncol 2014;21(8):2484–9.

12. Koshy M, Rich SE, Mohiuddin MM. Improved survival with radiation therapy in high-grade soft tissue sarcomas of the extremities: a SEER analysis. Int J Radiat Oncol Biol Phys 2010;77(1):203–9.

13. Hou CH, Lazarides AL, Speicher PJ, et al. The use of radiation therapy in localized high-grade soft tissue sarcoma and potential impact on survival. Ann Surg Oncol 2015;22(9):2831–8.

14. O'Sullivan B, Davis AM, Turcotte R, et al. Preoperative versus postoperative radiotherapy in soft-tissue sarcoma of the limbs: a randomised trial. Lancet 2002;359(9325):2235–41.

15. Davis AM, O'Sullivan B, Turcotte R, et al. Canadian Sarcoma Group, NCI Canada Clinical Trial Group Randomized Trial. Late radiation morbidity following randomization to preoperative versus postoperative radiotherapy in extremity soft tissue sarcoma. Radiother Oncol 2005;75(1):48–53.

16. Dickie CI, Parent A, Griffin A, et al. A device and procedure for immobilization of patients receiving limb-preserving radiotherapy for soft tissue sarcoma. Med Dosim 2009;34(3):243–9.

17. Wang D, Zhang Q, Eisenberg BL, et al. Significant reduction of late toxicities in patients with extremity sarcoma treated with image-guided radiation therapy to a reduced target volume: results of Radiation Therapy Oncology Group RTOG-0630 Trial. J Clin Oncol 2015;33(20):2231–8.

18. Dickie CI, Parent AL, Griffin AM, et al. Bone fractures following external beam radiotherapy and limb-preservation surgery for lower extremity soft tissue sarcoma: relationship to irradiated bone length, volume, tumor location and dose. Int J Radiat Oncol Biol Phys 2009;75(4):1119–24.

19. Li XA, Chen X, Zhang Q, et al. Margin reduction from image guided radiation therapy for soft tissue sarcoma: Secondary analysis of Radiation Therapy Oncology Group 0630 results. Pract Radiat Oncol 2015. [Epub ahead of print].

20. O'Sullivan B, Griffin AM, Dickie CI, et al. Phase 2 study of preoperative image-guided intensity-modulated radiation therapy to reduce wound and combined modality morbidities in lower extremity soft tissue sarcoma. Cancer 2013; 119(10):1878–84.

21. Folkert MR, Singer S, Brennan MF, et al. Comparison of local recurrence with conventional and intensity-modulated radiation therapy for primary soft-tissue sarcomas of the extremity. J Clin Oncol 2014;32(29):3236–41.

22. Schwarzbach MH, Hohenberger P. Current concepts in the management of retroperitoneal soft tissue sarcoma. [Fortschritte der Krebsforschung. Progres dans les recherches sur le cancer]. Recent Results Cancer Res 2009;179:301–19.

23. Hu KS, Harrison LC. Adjuvant radiation therapy of retroperitoneal sarcoma: the role of intraoperative radiotherapy (IORT). Sarcoma 2000;4(1–2):11–6.

24. Pierie JPEN, Betensky RA, Choudry U, et al. Outcomes in a series of 103 retroperitoneal sarcomas. Eur J Surg Oncol 2006;32(10):1235–41.
25. Baldini EH, Wang D, Haas RL, et al. Treatment guidelines for preoperative radiation therapy for retroperitoneal sarcoma: preliminary consensus of an international expert panel. Int J Radiat Oncol Biol Phys 2015;92(3):602–12.
26. Kelly KJ, Yoon SS, Kuk D, et al. Comparison of perioperative radiation therapy and surgery versus surgery alone in 204 patients with primary retroperitoneal sarcoma: a retrospective 2-institution study. Ann Surg 2015;262(1):156–62.
27. Sindelar WF, Kinsella TJ, Chen PW, et al. Intraoperative radiotherapy in retroperitoneal sarcomas. Final results of a prospective, randomized, clinical trial. Arch Surg 1993;128(4):402–10.
28. Czito BG, Willett CG. Intraoperative irradiation. In: Gunderson LL, Tepper JE, editors. Clinical radiation oncology. 3rd edition. Philadelphia: Elsevier; 2011. p. 317–30.
29. Tzeng CW, Fiveash JB, Popple RA, et al. Preoperative radiation therapy with selective dose escalation to the margin at risk for retroperitoneal sarcoma. Cancer 2006;107(2):371–9.
30. Roeder F, Ulrich A, Habl G, et al. Clinical phase I/II trial to investigate preoperative dose-escalated intensity-modulated radiation therapy (IMRT) and intraoperative radiation therapy (IORT) in patients with retroperitoneal soft tissue sarcoma: interim analysis. BMC Cancer 2014;14:617.
31. Torres MA, Ballo MT, Butler CE, et al. Management of locally recurrent soft-tissue sarcoma after prior surgery and radiation therapy. Int J Radiat Oncol Biol Phys 2007;67(4):1124–9.
32. Smith MJ, Ridgway PF, Catton CN, et al. Combined management of retroperitoneal sarcoma with dose intensification radiotherapy and resection: long-term results of a prospective trial. Radiother Oncol 2014;110(1):165–71.
33. Jones JJ, Catton CN, O'Sullivan B, et al. Initial results of a trial of preoperative external-beam radiation therapy and postoperative brachytherapy for retroperitoneal sarcoma. Ann Surg Oncol 2002;9(4):346–54.
34. DeLaney TF, Spiro IJ, Suit HD, et al. Neoadjuvant chemotherapy and radiotherapy for large extremity soft-tissue sarcomas. Int J Radiat Oncol Biol Phys 2003;56(4):1117–27.
35. Look Hong NJ, Hornicek FJ, Harmon DC, et al. Neoadjuvant chemoradiotherapy for patients with high-risk extremity and truncal sarcomas: a 10-year single institution retrospective study. Eur J Cancer 2013;49(4):875–83.
36. Kraybill WG, Harris J, Spiro IJ, et al. Long-term results of a phase 2 study of neoadjuvant chemotherapy and radiotherapy in the management of high-risk, high-grade, soft tissue sarcomas of the extremities and body wall: Radiation Therapy Oncology Group Trial 9514. Cancer 2010;116(19):4613–21.
37. Eilber FC, Rosen G, Eckardt J, et al. Treatment-induced pathologic necrosis: a predictor of local recurrence and survival in patients receiving neoadjuvant therapy for high-grade extremity soft tissue sarcomas. J Clin Oncol 2001;19(13): 3203–9.
38. Tseng WW, Zhou S, To CA, et al. Phase 1 adaptive dose-finding study of neoadjuvant gemcitabine combined with radiation therapy for patients with high-risk extremity and trunk soft tissue sarcoma. Cancer 2015;121(20):3659–67.
39. Cuneo KC, Riedel RF, Dodd LG, et al. Pathologic complete response of a malignant peripheral nerve sheath tumor in the lung treated with neoadjuvant ifosfamide and radiation therapy. J Clin Oncol 2012;30(28):e291–3.

40. Suit H, Goldberg S, Niemierko A, et al. Secondary carcinogenesis in patients treated with radiation: a review of data on radiation-induced cancers in human, non-human primate, canine and rodent subjects. Radiat Res 2007;167(1): 12–42.
41. Wiltink LM, Nout RA, Fiocco M, et al. No increased risk of second cancer after radiotherapy in patients treated for rectal or endometrial cancer in the randomized TME, PORTEC-1, and PORTEC-2 trials. J Clin Oncol 2015; 33(15):1640–6.
42. Zhang J, Walsh MF, Wu G, et al. Germline mutations in predisposition genes in pediatric cancer. N Engl J Med 2015;373(24):2336–46.

Chemotherapy

Does Neoadjuvant or Adjuvant Therapy Improve Outcomes?

Robert J. Canter, MD, MAS

KEYWORDS

- Soft tissue sarcoma • Surgery • Chemotherapy • Multimodality therapy
- Limb salvage • Survival

KEY POINTS

- More effective systemic therapy is a critical unmet need in the combined modality therapy of locally advanced soft tissue sarcoma.
- Meta-analyses of adjuvant/neoadjuvant clinical trials of chemotherapy for soft tissue sarcoma show a modest, but statistically significant, improvement in oncologic outcome favoring chemotherapy.
- Adjuvant/neoadjuvant chemotherapy for soft tissue sarcoma has not been widely adopted in large part because of the modest benefits and substantial risk of toxicity from intensive anthracycline-based regimens.
- Outcomes with adjuvant/neoadjuvant chemotherapy in soft tissue sarcoma vary by histologic subtype, and approaches based on tumor histology and individual patient and tumor factors are indicated.

INTRODUCTION

Soft tissue sarcomas (STS) are an uncommon and diverse group of tumors with mesenchymal differentiation, accounting for approximately 1% of US cancer diagnoses annually.[1,2] As such, clinical behavior of these tumors can vary greatly, and robust prospectively obtained outcomes data are difficult to achieve. The rarity of incidence and diversity of disease biology also make consensus on treatment guidelines challenging, especially for key clinical questions in which the benefit/risk ratio for therapy may be narrow. As a general rule, the primary treatment modality for nonmetastatic STS in all locations and for most histologic types remains wide en bloc surgical resection, frequently in combination with radiotherapy (RT). Although distant disease control

The author has nothing to disclose.

Division of Surgical Oncology, Department of Surgery, UC Davis Comprehensive Cancer Center, Davis School of Medicine, University of California, Suite 3010, 4501 X Street, Sacramento, CA 95817, USA

E-mail address: rjcanter@ucdavis.edu

Surg Oncol Clin N Am 25 (2016) 861–872
http://dx.doi.org/10.1016/j.soc.2016.05.013
1055-3207/16/$ – see front matter © 2016 Elsevier Inc. All rights reserved.

and effective systemic therapy remain critical unmet needs in the multimodality management of STS, the role of systemic therapy in the management of primary, nonmetastatic disease remains an area of significant debate.[2,3]

Overall, local therapy, particularly for extremity and body wall/truncal STS, has proven highly effective. For the past 30 years, function-preserving/limb-sparing surgery combined with RT has successfully replaced amputation and other radical extirpative procedures in 90% to 95% of patients with STS.[1–3] Long-term local control rates with these combined modality approaches exceed 85% to 90%. However, distant control and overall survival (OS) remain a challenge, particularly for patients with more aggressive disease (typically characterized by tumors larger than 10 cm, high-grade histology, and/or histologic subtypes with high risk of metastasis, such as synovial sarcoma, myxoid/round liposarcoma, and undifferentiated pleomorphic sarcoma).[4] In fact, patients with high-grade tumors (typically American Joint Committee on Cancer [AJCC] stage III) have a risk of distant recurrence and death as high as 50% within 5 years of diagnosis.[4,5] For these patients, neoadjuvant/adjuvant chemotherapy has frequently been advocated to improve metastasis-free survival and OS. However, the role of chemotherapy in the treatment of patients with STS amenable to complete surgical resection remains a controversial subject. The handful of prospective studies showing survival, local-recurrence, or distant-recurrence benefits to adjuvant/neoadjuvant chemotherapy in localized STS are mitigated by other studies demonstrating no benefit.[2]

In this article, we focus on the role of chemotherapy in the definitive management of STS amenable to surgical resection with curative intent. Although current data are equivocal and the approach to adjuvant/neoadjuvant chemotherapy varies by institution, by specialty, and even by practitioner, there is increasing recognition that outcomes with adjuvant/neoadjuvant chemotherapy in STS vary by histologic subtype and that multimodality treatment approaches based on tumor histology and individual patient and tumor factors are indicated.[5,6]

TREATMENT APPROACHES

Current National Comprehensive Cancer Network (NCCN) guidelines for the multimodality management of STS, particularly for locally advanced disease amenable to resection with curative intent, clearly endorse management by sarcoma specialists in a tertiary referral center.[2] However, the specific recommendations regarding treatment sequencing and specific modalities (such as chemotherapy and RT) used in a combined modality approach are equivocal. Wide, but function-preserving, surgery in combination with RT remain the backbone of therapy in all possible treatment scenarios in which curative treatment is the goal. Moreover, NCCN guidelines acknowledge that it is acceptable to either include or omit chemotherapy from combined modality treatment, even in cases of locally advanced/stage III disease (http://www.nccn.org/professionals/physician_gls/PDF/sarcoma.pdf) despite the substantial risk of distant disease progression and death.

As a result, there is wide variation in the utilization of adjuvant/neoadjuvant chemotherapy in the management of primary STS. For example, an analysis by Wasif and colleagues[7] showed that orthopedic oncologists and physicians with more than 75% of their clinical practice devoted to patients with sarcoma had the greatest preference for chemotherapy in the adjuvant/neoadjuvant management of STS. In contrast, surgical oncologists reported a statistically significant lower predilection for incorporating chemotherapy into the treatment plan for patients with locally advanced STS. Overall, the results of this survey study reinforced the impression that there is no clear consensus to the multimodality approach for localized STS, especially regarding the indications and implementation of adjuvant/neoadjuvant chemotherapy.

In a related analysis, Sherman and colleagues[8] evaluated national practice patterns in the United States using the hospital-based National Cancer Database (NCDB), which has detailed demographic, pathologic, and treatment-related information on cancer-related diagnoses and outcomes. The investigators found that for the time period 2000 to 2009, neoadjuvant therapy with both RT and chemotherapy was increasing, whereas trimodality therapy was decreasing. Factors predictive of receipt of chemotherapy included younger age, synovial histology, high-grade histology, and positive surgical margins. Overall, however, chemotherapy was administered to only 31% of patients with stage III STS and 13.5% of patients with stage II STS. Taken together, these studies underscore the impression that the use of adjuvant/neoadjuvant chemotherapy has failed to gain widespread adoption in the United States in the primary management of nonmetastatic STS.

BIOLOGICAL QUESTIONS IN SARCOMA CHEMOTHERAPY

It is important to remember that the routine use of adjuvant/neoadjuvant chemotherapy has been unequivocally accepted into the combined modality therapy for certain types of sarcoma. For example, in pediatric bone and STSs, there is clearly an established role for adjuvant/neoadjuvant chemotherapy, and this approach has been shown to improve outcomes.[9] In the early 1980s, the standard treatment of osteosarcoma was wide surgical resection, including amputation. However, more than 80% of patients with osteosarcoma developed metastatic disease, typically within 6 months of surgical intervention, in the setting of surgical monotherapy.[10] The short disease-free interval routinely observed in these patients suggested that occult micrometastasis was present at diagnosis, and the introduction of adjuvant/neoadjuvant chemotherapy for patients with osteosarcoma improved outcomes dramatically.

In fact, over the past 30 years, the 5-year survival of patients with malignant bone sarcoma has improved from approximately 16% without chemotherapy to approximately 70% with multiagent chemotherapy.[10] These dramatic (and clearly unequivocal) results have provided proof-in-principle that chemotherapy can be effective for primary bone sarcomas, reinforcing the concept that subclinical metastatic disease is present at diagnosis, which can be effectively eradicated by systemic cytotoxic chemotherapy. Similarly, multiagent chemotherapy is a routine component of primary therapy for small round blue sarcomas, such as rhabdomyosarcoma and Ewing sarcoma.[2] In fact, some practitioners consider chemotherapy to be primary therapy in these chemosensitive subtypes with surgical resection/local therapy serving as adjuvant therapy. Irrespective of these considerations, it is clear that chemotherapy has been established as a critical component of combined modality therapy in these histologies, and the role of chemotherapy has been endorsed by major oncology organizations, such as the NCCN and European Society for Medical Oncology.

However, it has also been observed that survival outcomes are significantly worse when adult patients (using variable age cutoffs between 18 and 40) are diagnosed with sarcoma histologies typically diagnosed in pediatric patients. For example, using surveillance, epidemiology, and end results (SEER) data, Mirabello and colleagues[11] observed that 5-year OS rates for patients with osteosarcoma were 62% for patients younger than 24 years, 59% for patients 25 to 59 years, and 24% for patients 60 years and older. Similarly, a single-institution analysis by Koohbanani and colleagues[12] demonstrated significant differences in survival of patients with Ewing sarcoma by age. Patients younger than 18 experienced a 5-year OS of 61%, whereas the 5-year OS for patients older than 40 was 38%. Several hypotheses have been offered to explain these age-related differences with chemotherapy in typically chemosensitive sarcomas. Some have hypothesized that these differences in oncologic outcome among pediatric and adult patients with similar bone and STS histologies are related to intrinsic differences in tumor biology between pediatric and adult patients with similar sarcoma histologies. On the other hand, others have attributed these differences in outcome between pediatric and adult patients to their respective ability to tolerate maximal cytotoxic chemotherapy, with greater dose intensity of chemotherapy in younger patients correlating with better outcomes.

Collins and colleagues[13] performed a pooled analysis of individual data from multiple prospective neoadjuvant chemotherapy trials involving nearly 5000 patients with osteosarcoma. Consistent with prior studies assessing the impact of age on outcome, the investigators observed that younger patients had significantly better OS than older patients, including adults. However, using a landmark analysis analytical technique that incorporated chemotherapy-induced tumor necrosis into the model (an established biomarker of survival in patients with osteosarcoma receiving neoadjuvant chemotherapy), the investigators found that age was no longer a statistically significant predictor of OS. The investigators therefore concluded that the receipt of high-dose chemotherapy and the manner of its metabolism by the host was the key driver of outcome rather than differences in tumor biology among young and older patients. Despite these results, it is important to remember that STS subtypes in adult patients are different from those diagnosed in children, and although chemotherapy may be critical to outcomes in osteosarcoma and Ewing sarcoma, it may not be in adult STS histologies, such as liposarcoma, leiomyosarcoma, and high-grade undifferentiated pleomorphic sarcoma, in which tumor biology and intrinsic chemosensitivity may be different.

CLINICAL TRIALS EVALUATING OUTCOMES

Based on the results of chemotherapy in osteosarcoma and other pediatric sarcoma treatment paradigms, proponents of chemotherapy have advocated for a similar treatment approach in adult STS given the risk of distant metastasis and poor survival in the subgroup of patients with locally advanced disease. The risk of poor OS is particularly relevant for patients with high-grade primary STS larger than 5 cm in maximal dimension (AJCC stage IIb and III). These patients carry a risk of distant recurrence and death that approaches 50% at 5 years.[4,14,15] This cohort of patients has traditionally been the subject of much controversy regarding the risks and benefits of adjuvant/neoadjuvant chemotherapy.

Approximately 20 randomized trials and 2 meta-analyses have been performed to evaluate the role of chemotherapy in patients undergoing surgery and RT with curative intent, and there are data both for and against the routine use of perioperative chemotherapy for patients with STS. Ultimately, despite the importance of this research question in the STS community, there remain fundamental unresolved questions regarding the role of chemotherapy in the management of primary disease, primarily because the rarity and diversity of these tumors, as well as differences in chemotherapy regimens and dosing, hinder an adequate patient accrual for definitive randomized trials.

Doxorubicin Monotherapy Trials

Studies analyzing the utility of adjuvant chemotherapy for adult STS were first performed in 1970s. In fact, from the 1970s to the 1990s, 14 randomized trials were performed comparing surgical resection (±RT) to surgical resection (±RT) plus chemotherapy.[16] These studies primarily used doxorubicin as monotherapy in the adjuvant setting. Ultimately, these studies set the stage for subsequent decades of controversy, as there was a minority of studies showing survival, local-recurrence, and distant-recurrence benefits to adjuvant chemotherapy that were offset by other studies demonstrating no benefit. Further confounding the results of these studies were methodological and other flaws that left question marks over the validity of these data. For example, the use of doxorubicin monotherapy is considered a limitation by chemotherapy proponents, especially in the United States, as the combination of doxorubicin-ifosfamide is associated with greater response rates and is widely considered a more active regimen.[6] In addition, these studies were confounded by a lack of standardization of surgical and RT techniques at the time, a lack of widespread adoption of cross-sectional imaging for accurate staging assessment, and a lack of uniform pathologic diagnostic criteria, among others. All of these issues raise legitimate questions regarding the generalizability and external validity of the study results.

Given these concerns, the role of adjuvant chemotherapy in STS was considered an important clinical problem that warranted further evaluation in a meta-analysis. Previous published results were equivocal, but these clinical trials were small and therefore potentially underpowered to detect moderate, but clinical meaningful, treatment effects. This equipoise lead to the Sarcoma Meta-Analysis Collaboration (SMAC), which was the first meta-analysis of pooled data involving 1568 patients with localized, resectable STS.[17] Overall, the investigators of this meta-analysis observed statistically significant reductions in local recurrence-free survival (LRFS), distant recurrence-free survival (DRFS), and recurrence-free survival (RFS). These results corresponded to an absolute benefit at 10 years of 6% in LRFS, 10% in DRFS, and 10% in RFS. There was a 4% absolute benefit in OS with chemotherapy, but importantly, this result was not statistically significant (hazard ratio [HR] 0.89, 95% confidence interval [CI] 0.76–1.03). Skeptics of chemotherapy frequently point to this overall negative result for the primary endpoint of OS as the essential finding. Conversely, advocates of chemotherapy emphasize that a significant improvement in OS was observed in patients with extremity and truncal STS with a 7% absolute benefit at 10 years ($P = .029$).

Despite the 10% improvement in RFS at 10 years with chemotherapy in this much cited meta-analysis, the lack of clear statistically significant improvements in OS undermined any conclusions that adjuvant chemotherapy was routinely indicated in STS, especially given the potential toxicity of doxorubicin-based regimens. Moreover, the statistical power of this meta-analysis was weakened by important methodological flaws, such as missing patient data, absence of central pathologic review of cases, and heterogeneity of the study population, including 5% low-grade tumors, 18% with tumor size smaller than 5 cm, and nonsarcoma diagnoses in approximately 10% of cases. These factors are cited as evidence undermining the case for adjuvant/neoadjuvant chemotherapy in primary STS. Finally, and significantly, a 2011 study of meta-analyses by Roseman and colleagues[18] observed that possible conflicts of interest, including industry/pharmaceutical sponsor funding, were rarely disclosed in the research methods of meta-analyses. In their analysis, Roseman and colleagues[18] provided evidence that these conflicts of interest are significant factors impacting the inclusion of studies, synthesis methods, and investigator assumptions about patient status and censoring strategies that affect the results of meta-analyses. In the SMAC meta-analysis, the authors of the meta-analysis were many of the same investigators from the individual randomized clinical trials evaluating chemotherapy for STS. In addition, the SMAC meta-analysis did not evaluate for the risk of bias across individual studies (as recommended by the PRISMA criteria) nor did they disclose any external sources of funding.[17]

Combination Doxorubicin-Ifosfamide Trials

Following the adoption of ifosfamide for the treatment of sarcoma in the 1990s, subsequent studies of adjuvant and neoadjuvant therapy of primary STS focused on the combination of ifosfamide and an anthracycline. These have included both prospective, randomized trials and retrospective cohort analyses with more complete data and more homogeneity of the study groups. Although these studies have shown improved outcomes for patients with specific sarcoma histologies receiving chemotherapy, the results with doxorubicin/ifosfamide combination regimens have also been equivocal, and the risk/benefit ratio of adjuvant/neoadjuvant chemotherapy in these patients remains an unresolved question.

Studies have generally shown that regimens using doxorubicin and ifosfamide result in the greatest response rates ($\sim$25%).[19] Frustaci and colleagues[20] assessed high-dose epirubicin and ifosfamide in a randomized phase II trial of 104 patients with STS undergoing radical surgery with or without RT. The investigators focused on extremity and truncal primary sites (given the SMAC results). Patients with both primary and locally recurrent disease were included, but patients with metastatic disease were excluded. The trial was further complicated by a stratification schema based on both primary versus locally recurrent disease as well as tumor size larger or smaller than 10 cm in maximal tumor dimension. Eight tumor histologies were included, but they were all high grade.

In this study, it was notable that a large majority of patients (42/46 or 91%) were able to complete all 5 cycles of chemotherapy, but aggressive supportive therapy, including hydration, mesna, and granulocyte colony-stimulating factor, was administered and most patients were younger than 55 (with no patients >65). Importantly, the rate of distant recurrence was markedly better in the chemotherapy arm at 2 years (28% recurrence with chemotherapy vs 45% with observation, $P = .04$). Similarly, OS at 4 years was improved in the chemotherapy group (69% chemotherapy vs 50% observation, $P = .03$). Although these results suggested important benefits to combination chemotherapy in the adjuvant setting, the patient stratification process in a small cohort created imbalances in the treatment groups, which may have contributed to differences in patient outcome. Furthermore, the results were also likely contingent on careful patient selection, which may not translate to other treatment scenarios.

A subsequent analysis of the same patient population with longer follow-up demonstrated that the benefits of adjuvant chemotherapy were not durable.[21] With a median follow-up of 90 months, OS remained better in the chemotherapy cohort compared with the observation cohort (59% vs 43%), but this difference was no longer statistically significant ($P = .07$). Although this result could be interpreted as type II error from an underpowered trial of a rare disease in which it is difficult to detect moderate but clinically meaningful treatment effects, another valid interpretation of the updated analysis of Frustaci and colleagues[21] is that early benefits from chemotherapy may be lost with longer follow-up because chemotherapy given at the time of recurrence may be as beneficial to patient outcome as chemotherapy given in the adjuvant setting. This ongoing reservation regarding the benefits of early versus late chemotherapy was articulated in a retrospective analysis of the MD Anderson Cancer Center and Memorial Sloan Kettering Cancer Center combined experience with anthracycline-based perioperative chemotherapy for patients with large, deep, and high-grade extremity STS.[22] This study demonstrated a time-varying effect associated with chemotherapy. During the first year, the HR of disease-specific death for patients treated with chemotherapy compared with those who were not was 0.37. However, following the first year, the HR of disease-specific death was 1.36, favoring the patients treated without chemotherapy. Although the findings in this study are potentially confounded by the effects of selection bias, an important implication of this article is that studies showing benefit to chemotherapy in patients with primary STS should be interpreted with caution because early benefits may be counteracted by later detrimental effects.

In a subsequent randomized trial, Petrioli and colleagues[23] evaluated 88 patients with STS, of whom 45 were randomized to surgical resection plus chemotherapy (58% epirubicin alone and 42% epirubicin/ifosfamide) compared with 43 patients who were randomized to surgical resection alone. Despite the locally advanced disease present in this patient population, only 50% received RT. This trial was open from 1985 until 1996, but closed prematurely because of poor patient accrual. An analysis of the accrued patients revealed that OS was significantly improved in the chemotherapy group (5-year OS 72% with chemotherapy vs 47% with observation). However, despite the 25% absolute improvement in OS in the chemotherapy group, this difference approached, but did not reach, statistical significance ($P = .06$) because of the sample size. As with the studies by Frustaci and colleagues,[20,21] the results of the study by Petrioli and colleagues[23] provided evidence both for and against adjuvant/neoadjuvant chemotherapy depending on one's interpretation of the data.

Updated Meta-Analysis

After the publication of the 1997 SMAC meta-analysis, adjuvant chemotherapy was not routinely adopted. In addition, new systemic agents, specifically ifosfamide, were in use. Finally, the results of additional randomized controlled trials were available for analysis. Given this background, investigators at the University of Waterloo conducted an updated meta-analysis of the impact of adjuvant/neoadjuvant chemotherapy on outcomes in STS.[24]

Overall, the results were similar to the prior meta-analysis. Statistically significant improvements in LRFS, DRFS, and RFS were observed in the chemotherapy group, corresponding to an absolute benefit at 10 years of 5% in LRFS, 9% in DRFS, and 10% in RFS. In this analysis, there was a 6% absolute benefit in OS with chemotherapy, which was statistically significant (HR 0.77, 95% CI 0.64–0.93). Although this updated meta-analysis confirmed the modest efficacy of adjuvant/neoadjuvant chemotherapy for STS and demonstrated incrementally superior effects with the addition of ifosfamide, the study was criticized for failing to include an important European Organisation for the Research and Treatment of Cancer (EORTC) trial of adjuvant chemotherapy that demonstrated no benefit in the chemotherapy arm.[25]

Neoadjuvant Treatment

Although historically adjuvant chemotherapy has received greater evaluation in clinical trials and therefore has greater evidence on which to base treatment decisions, the results of survey studies demonstrate that neoadjuvant chemotherapy is typically favored in the management of locally advanced STS, perhaps because clinical response and downstaging can be followed prospectively and patients with rapidly progressive disease can be spared operation.[7,26]

The only randomized trial of neoadjuvant chemotherapy for STS was conducted by the EORTC.[27] This study enrolled 150 patients (analyzing 134) in a phase II trial, comparing 3 cycles of neoadjuvant doxorubicin (50 mg/m^2 per cycle) plus ifosfamide

(5 g/m^2 per cycle) with surgical monotherapy. With more than 7 years of follow-up, 5-year OS was 65% with chemotherapy compared with 64% without chemotherapy ($P = .22$). Although the phase II design of this study may be viewed as a sign of inadequate statistical power, many consider the results of this study to provide additional evidence against the routine use of adjuvant/neoadjuvant chemotherapy for STS. However, it is also important to acknowledge another frequent criticism of this study, namely that the doses of chemotherapy were low and considered suboptimal to provide a benefit, at least according to US standards.

SUBTYPE-SPECIFIC ANALYSES

Another recurring theme of the clinical trials evaluating the efficacy of adjuvant/neoadjuvant chemotherapy in STS is that they have all included multiple histologies.[2] In fact, there are no clinical trials testing the hypothesis that the benefits of adjuvant/neoadjuvant chemotherapy are subtype-specific. Increasing evidence highlights the impact of tumor histology on survival and response to therapy in patients with STS, and efforts to study the natural history and biology of individual histologic subtypes are increasing.[5]

Synovial Sarcoma

Based on early reports of significant response of synovial sarcoma to chemotherapy, especially ifosfamide-containing regimens in the metastatic setting,[28] STS experts have tended to consider synovial sarcoma a chemosensitive histology for which chemotherapy in the adjuvant/neoadjuvant setting is indicated. Although there are no adequately powered randomized trials evaluating adjuvant/neoadjuvant chemotherapy for synovial sarcoma, there is evidence from high-volume sarcoma centers in the United States and Europe to suggest that perioperative chemotherapy may improve outcomes.

For example, a pooled analysis from 2 US institutions of 101 patients with locally advanced extremity synovial sarcoma demonstrated a 21% absolute improvement in 4-year disease-specific survival (DSS) with chemotherapy (88% vs 67%, $P = .01$).[29] An analysis by Ferrari and colleagues[30] of 271 patients with synovial sarcoma demonstrated a 12% absolute improvement in DRFS (60% with chemotherapy vs 48% without chemotherapy, $P<.05$) among the 61 patients (24%) who received chemotherapy following complete tumor resection. Canter and colleagues[31] constructed a nomogram for DSS using data from 255 patients with synovial sarcoma undergoing resection with curative intent. The investigators then calculated the observed to expected DSS for patients receiving doxorubicin/ifosfamide chemotherapy. Based on the nomogram, patients treated with chemotherapy had a statistically superior 3-year DSS, although these improvements dissipated over time. Despite these positive results, it is important to remember the limitations of retrospective analyses. Selection bias, particularly when applied to which patients receive or do not receive chemotherapy, is a key confounding factor, as are secular trends in the evaluation and management of patients, which may evolve considerably over studies encompassing 20 to 30 years of accrual. As a result, despite the widely accepted view that synovial sarcoma is a chemosensitive histology, it is by no means assured that adjuvant/neoadjuvant chemotherapy improves outcomes for synovial sarcoma in the setting of resection with curative intent, and the EORTC study evaluating adjuvant chemotherapy for STS showed no benefit to chemotherapy, including among the subgroup of patients with synovial sarcoma.[25]

A cooperative group randomized trial is currently under way in Europe sponsored by the Italian Sarcoma Group (http://www.italiansarcomagroup.org/studi-clinici/)

evaluating neoadjuvant chemotherapy. The primary endpoint of this trial is disease-free survival (DFS) in adult patients ($\geq$18) with high-risk STS of the extremities and trunk eligible for complete resection. Importantly, the trial will be stratified based on histology and will incorporate a histology-based chemotherapy approach.

Myxoid/Round Cell Liposarcoma

High-grade myxoid liposarcoma (typically defined as >5% round cell component) is characterized by a chromosome 12;16 translocation in more than 95% of cases that results in an FUS-DDIT3 gene fusion. Myxoid/round cell liposarcoma is associated with a poor prognosis with 5-year OS of approximately 50%.[32] However, despite the risk of metastases and death, myxoid/round liposarcoma has also been observed to be responsive to chemotherapy, prompting consideration of chemotherapy in the adjuvant/neoadjuvant setting. Ultimately, data favoring this approach are limited. Eilber and colleagues[33] retrospectively analyzed 129 patients with liposarcoma, including 61 (47%) with myxoid/round cell liposarcoma. The 5-year DSS for patients with myxoid/round cell liposarcoma treated with chemotherapy was 100% compared with 78% for patients with surgical monotherapy ($P = .01$). Similarly, Grobmyer and colleagues[34] analyzed 282 patients, including 56 with locally advanced liposarcoma (pT2bG3). For patients with tumors larger than 10 cm, neoadjuvant chemotherapy improved 3-year DSS from 62% (without chemotherapy) to 83% with chemotherapy ($P = .02$), although specific results among the myxoid/round liposarcoma subgroup were not provided. Given the lack of level I data in support of oncologic benefit for adjuvant/neoadjuvant chemotherapy for myxoid/round cell liposarcoma, it is reasonable to base the decision for neoadjuvant chemotherapy on the anticipated response, which may promote better tumor clearance/less morbidity at the time of operation for these patients.

Undifferentiated Pleomorphic Sarcoma

Undifferentiated pleomorphic sarcoma (UPS) remains a challenging STS histology with a generally poor prognosis. Depending on clinical-pathological factors, 5-year OS ranges from 35% to 60%. Although UPS has classically been considered a chemo-resistant histology, a recent large-scale analysis of the National Cancer Data Base involving 5377 patients with stage III STS demonstrated a statistically significant benefit for adjuvant/neoadjuvant chemotherapy, particularly among patients with UPS in whom median OS improved from 49 months without chemotherapy to 78 months with chemotherapy ($P = .02$).[35] Notwithstanding the large sample size and risk-adjusted analyses, the results of this retrospective study should be interpreted with caution, especially given the diversity of sarcoma subtypes and tumor locations studied, as well as the numerous imbalances in the chemotherapy and no chemotherapy cohorts.

TARGETED THERAPY/NOVEL AGENTS
Antiangiogenic Targeted Therapy

Similar to other malignancies, STS has been shown to overexpress angiogenic factors in both tumor tissue and serum, suggesting that antiangiogenic therapy may prove effective for patients with STS.[36,37] Although data such as these support the hypothesis that angiogenesis inhibition with targeted agents may prove efficacious in the adjuvant/neoadjuvant setting for patients with STS, only phase I studies have been conducted to date, with ambiguous results.[38,39]

Trabedectin and Eribulin

In 2015 and 2016, both trabedectin (for liposarcoma and leiomyosarcoma) and eribulin were approved by the Food and Drug Administration in the United States for patients with metastatic and unresectable STS who had failed prior chemotherapy. However, there are limited data assessing the utility of these novel agents in the adjuvant/neoadjuvant setting. In a phase II study of 23 patients with locally advanced myxoid liposarcoma treated with neoadjuvant trabedectin, 7 had an objective partial response, and at surgery, 3 had a pathologic complete response after 3 to 6 cycles.[40]

SUMMARY

Overall, the evidence suggests that there is a small absolute benefit to adjuvant/neoadjuvant chemotherapy in primary STS amenable to resection with curative intent. However, it is likely that these benefits do not apply equally to all sarcoma subtypes, and limited data suggest that synovial sarcoma and myxoid/round cell liposarcoma are the most chemosensitive histologies. A tailored, personalized approach to adjuvant/neoadjuvant chemotherapy in localized STS should weigh the benefits of increased DFS and OS against the risks of acute morbidity from chemotherapy, including neutropenia and neutropenic sepsis, the risks of chronic morbidity, such as impaired fertility, future cardiomyopathy, and future secondary malignancy, as well as quality of life effects in an individualized, multidisciplinary treatment plan. Moving forward, heightened emphasis and attention should be placed on phase I and II clinical trials and innovative co-clinical trials, such as outbred large animals like canines who carry a large burden of spontaneous sarcomas, to more rigorously link molecular drivers of poor STS outcome with systemic agents able to target those pathways and thereby improve outcomes for patients with STS.

REFERENCES

1. Canter RJ. Surgical approach for soft tissue sarcoma: standard of care and future approaches. Curr Opin Oncol 2015;27(4):343–8.
2. Demetri GD, Antonia S, Benjamin RS, et al. Soft tissue sarcoma. J Natl Compr Canc Netw 2010;8(6):630–74.
3. Gronchi A, Colombo C, Raut CP. Surgical management of localized soft tissue tumors. Cancer 2014;120(17):2638–48.
4. Kattan MW, Leung DH, Brennan MF. Postoperative nomogram for 12-year sarcoma-specific death. J Clin Oncol 2002;20(3):791–6.
5. Canter RJ, Beal S, Borys D, et al. Interaction of histologic subtype and histologic grade in predicting survival for soft-tissue sarcomas. J Am Coll Surg 2010;210(2):191–8.e2.
6. Reynoso D, Subbiah V, Trent JC, et al. Neoadjuvant treatment of soft-tissue sarcoma: a multimodality approach. J Surg Oncol 2010;101(4):327–33.
7. Wasif N, Tamurian RM, Christensen S, et al. Influence of specialty and clinical experience on treatment sequencing in the multimodal management of soft tissue extremity sarcoma. Ann Surg Oncol 2012;19(2):504–10.
8. Sherman KL, Wayne JD, Chung J, et al. Assessment of multimodality therapy use for extremity sarcoma in the United States. J Surg Oncol 2014;109(5):395–404.
9. Biermann JS, Adkins DR, Agulnik M, et al. Bone cancer. J Natl Compr Canc Netw 2013;11(6):688–723.
10. Geller DS, Gorlick R. Osteosarcoma: a review of diagnosis, management, and treatment strategies. Clin Adv Hematol Oncol 2010;8(10):705–18.

11. Mirabello L, Troisi RJ, Savage SA. Osteosarcoma incidence and survival rates from 1973 to 2004: data from the Surveillance, Epidemiology, and End Results Program. Cancer 2009;115(7):1531–43.
12. Koohbanani B, Han G, Reed D, et al. Ethnicity and age disparities in Ewing sarcoma outcome. Fetal Pediatr Pathol 2013;32(4):246–52.
13. Collins M, Wilhelm M, Conyers R, et al. Benefits and adverse events in younger versus older patients receiving neoadjuvant chemotherapy for osteosarcoma: findings from a meta-analysis. J Clin Oncol 2013;31(18):2303–12.
14. Mariani L, Miceli R, Kattan MW, et al. Validation and adaptation of a nomogram for predicting the survival of patients with extremity soft tissue sarcoma using a three-grade system. Cancer 2005;103(2):402–8.
15. Eilber FC, Brennan MF, Eilber FR, et al. Validation of the postoperative nomogram for 12-year sarcoma-specific mortality. Cancer 2004;101(10):2270–5.
16. Patrikidou A, Domont J, Cioffi A, et al. Treating soft tissue sarcomas with adjuvant chemotherapy. Curr Treat Options Oncol 2011;12(1):21–31.
17. Adjuvant chemotherapy for localised resectable soft-tissue sarcoma of adults: meta-analysis of individual data. Sarcoma Meta-analysis Collaboration. Lancet 1997;350(9092):1647–54.
18. Roseman M, Milette K, Bero LA, et al. Reporting of conflicts of interest in meta-analyses of trials of pharmacological treatments. JAMA 2011;305(10):1008–17.
19. Judson I, Verweij J, Gelderblom H, et al. Doxorubicin alone versus intensified doxorubicin plus ifosfamide for first-line treatment of advanced or metastatic soft-tissue sarcoma: a randomised controlled phase 3 trial. Lancet Oncol 2014; 15(4):415–23.
20. Frustaci S, Gherlinzoni F, De Paoli A, et al. Adjuvant chemotherapy for adult soft tissue sarcomas of the extremities and girdles: results of the Italian randomized cooperative trial. J Clin Oncol 2001;19(5):1238–47.
21. Frustaci S, De Paoli A, Bidoli E, et al. Ifosfamide in the adjuvant therapy of soft tissue sarcomas. Oncology 2003;65(Suppl 2):80–4.
22. Cormier JN, Huang X, Xing Y, et al. Cohort analysis of patients with localized, high-risk, extremity soft tissue sarcoma treated at two cancer centers: chemotherapy-associated outcomes. J Clin Oncol 2004;22(22):4567–74.
23. Petrioli R, Coratti A, Correale P, et al. Adjuvant epirubicin with or without ifosfamide for adult soft-tissue sarcoma. Am J Clin Oncol 2002;25(5):468–73.
24. Pervaiz N, Colterjohn N, Farrokhyar F, et al. A systematic meta-analysis of randomized controlled trials of adjuvant chemotherapy for localized resectable soft-tissue sarcoma. Cancer 2008;113(3):573–81.
25. Woll PJ, Reichardt P, Le Cesne A, et al. Adjuvant chemotherapy with doxorubicin, ifosfamide, and lenograstim for resected soft-tissue sarcoma (EORTC 62931): a multicentre randomised controlled trial. Lancet Oncol 2012;13(10):1045–54.
26. Wasif N, Smith CA, Tamurian RM, et al. Influence of physician specialty on treatment recommendations in the multidisciplinary management of soft tissue sarcoma of the extremities. JAMA Surg 2013;148(7):632–9.
27. Gortzak E, Azzarelli A, Buesa J, et al. A randomised phase II study on neoadjuvant chemotherapy for 'high-risk' adult soft-tissue sarcoma. Eur J Cancer 2001;37(9):1096–103.
28. Rosen G, Forscher C, Lowenbraun S, et al. Synovial sarcoma. Uniform response of metastases to high dose ifosfamide. Cancer 1994;73(10):2506–11.
29. Eilber FC, Brennan MF, Eilber FR, et al. Chemotherapy is associated with improved survival in adult patients with primary extremity synovial sarcoma. Ann Surg 2007;246(1):105–13.

30. Ferrari A, De Salvo GL, Brennan B, et al. Synovial sarcoma in children and ado-lescents: the European Pediatric Soft Tissue Sarcoma Study Group prospective trial (EpSSG NRSTS 2005). Ann Oncol 2015;26(3):567–72.

31. Canter RJ, Qin LX, Maki RG, et al. A synovial sarcoma-specific preoperative nomogram supports a survival benefit to ifosfamide-based chemotherapy and improves risk stratification for patients. Clin Cancer Res 2008;14(24):8191–7.

32. Dalal KM, Antonescu CR, Singer S. Diagnosis and management of lipomatous tu-mors. J Surg Oncol 2008;97(4):298–313.

33. Eilber FC, Eilber FR, Eckardt J, et al. The impact of chemotherapy on the survival of patients with high-grade primary extremity liposarcoma. Ann Surg 2004; 240(4):686–95 [discussion: 695–7].

34. Grobmyer SR, Maki RG, Demetri GD, et al. Neo-adjuvant chemotherapy for pri-mary high-grade extremity soft tissue sarcoma. Ann Oncol 2004;15(11):1667–72.

35. Movva S, von Mehren M, Ross EA, et al. Patterns of chemotherapy administration in high-risk soft tissue sarcoma and impact on overall survival. J Natl Compr Canc Netw 2015;13(11):1366–74.

36. Yoon SS, Segal NH, Olshen AB, et al. Circulating angiogenic factor levels corre-late with extent of disease and risk of recurrence in patients with soft tissue sar-coma. Ann Oncol 2004;15(8):1261–6.

37. Yudoh K, Kanamori M, Ohmori K, et al. Concentration of vascular endothelial growth factor in the tumour tissue as a prognostic factor of soft tissue sarcomas. Br J Cancer 2001;84(12):1610–5.

38. Canter RJ, Borys D, Olusanya A, et al. Phase I trial of neoadjuvant conformal radiotherapy plus sorafenib for patients with locally advanced soft tissue sar-coma of the extremity. Ann Surg Oncol 2014;21(5):1616–23.

39. Jakob J, Simeonova A, Kasper B, et al. Combined radiation therapy and sunitinib for preoperative treatment of soft tissue sarcoma. Ann Surg Oncol 2015;22(9): 2839–45.

40. Gronchi A, Bui BN, Bonvalot S, et al. Phase II clinical trial of neoadjuvant trabec-tedin in patients with advanced localized myxoid liposarcoma. Ann Oncol 2012; 23(3):771–6.

UNITED STATES POSTAL SERVICE

Statement of Ownership, Management, and Circulation (All Periodicals Publications Except Requester Publications)

1. Publication Title	2. Publication Number	3. Filing Date
SURGICAL ONCOLOGY CLINICS OF NORTH AMERICA	012 – 565	9/18/2016

4. Issue Frequency	5. Number of Issues Published Annually	6. Annual Subscription Price
JAN, APR, JUL, OCT	4	$290.00

7. Complete Mailing Address of Known Office of Publication (Not printer) (Street, city, county, state, and ZIP+4®)

ELSEVIER INC.
360 PARK AVENUE SOUTH
NEW YORK, NY 10010-1710

Contact Person
STEPHEN R. BUSHING

Telephone (Include area code)
215-239-3688

8. Complete Mailing Address of Headquarters or General Business Office of Publisher (Not printer)

ELSEVIER INC.
360 PARK AVENUE SOUTH
NEW YORK, NY 10010-1710

9. Full Names and Complete Mailing Addresses of Publisher, Editor, and Managing Editor (Do not leave blank)

Publisher (Name and complete mailing address)

LINDA BELFUS, ELSEVIER INC.
1600 JOHN F KENNEDY BLVD. SUITE 1800
PHILADELPHIA, PA 19103-2899

Editor (Name and complete mailing address)

JOHN VASSALLO, ELSEVIER INC.
1600 JOHN F KENNEDY BLVD. SUITE 1800
PHILADELPHIA, PA 19103-2899

Managing Editor (Name and complete mailing address)

ADRIANNE BRIGIDO, ELSEVIER INC.
1600 JOHN F KENNEDY BLVD. SUITE 1800
PHILADELPHIA, PA 19103-2899

10. Owner (Do not leave blank. If the publication is owned by a corporation, give the name and address of the corporation immediately followed by the names and addresses of all stockholders owning or holding 1 percent or more of the total amount of stock. If not owned by a corporation, give the names and addresses of the individual owners. If owned by a partnership or other unincorporated firm, give its name and address as well as those of each individual owner. If the publication is published by a nonprofit organization, give its name and address.)

Full Name	Complete Mailing Address
WHOLLY OWNED SUBSIDIARY OF REED/ELSEVIER, US HOLDINGS	1600 JOHN F KENNEDY BLVD. SUITE 1800 PHILADELPHIA, PA 19103-2899

11. Known Bondholders, Mortgagees, and Other Security Holders Owning or Holding 1 Percent or More of Total Amount of Bonds, Mortgages, or Other Securities. If none, check box ☐ None

Full Name	Complete Mailing Address
N/A	

12. Tax Status (For completion by nonprofit organizations authorized to mail at nonprofit rates) (Check one)
The purpose, function, and nonprofit status of this organization and the exempt status for federal income tax purposes:
☐ Has Not Changed During Preceding 12 Months
☐ Has Changed During Preceding 12 Months (Publisher must submit explanation of change with this statement)

13. Publication Title	14. Issue Date for Circulation Data Below
SURGICAL ONCOLOGY CLINICS OF NORTH AMERICA	JULY 2016

15. Extent and Nature of Circulation		Average No. Copies Each Issue During Preceding 12 Months	No. Copies of Single Issue Published Nearest to Filing Date
a. Total Number of Copies (Net press run)		261	237
b. Paid Circulation (By Mail and Outside the Mail)	(1) Mailed Outside-County Paid Subscriptions Stated on PS Form 3541 (include paid distribution above nominal rate, advertiser's proof copies, and exchange copies)	86	94
	(2) Mailed In-County Paid Subscriptions Stated on PS Form 3541 (include paid distribution above nominal rate, advertiser's proof copies, and exchange copies)	0	0
	(3) Paid Distribution Outside the Mails Including Sales Through Dealers and Carriers, Street Vendors, Counter Sales, and Other Paid Distribution Outside USPS®	45	61
	(4) Paid Distribution by Other Classes of Mail Through the USPS (e.g., First-Class Mail®)	0	0
c. Total Paid Distribution (Sum of 15b (1), (2), (3), and (4))		131	155
d. Free or Nominal Rate Distribution (By Mail and Outside the Mail)	(1) Free or Nominal Rate Outside-County Copies included on PS Form 3541	24	62
	(2) Free or Nominal Rate In-County Copies Included on PS Form 3541	0	0
	(3) Free or Nominal Rate Copies Mailed at Other Classes Through the USPS (e.g., First-Class Mail)	0	0
	(4) Free or Nominal Rate Distribution Outside the Mail (Carriers or other means)	0	0
e. Total Free or Nominal Rate Distribution (Sum of 15d (1), (2), (3) and (4))		24	62
f. Total Distribution (Sum of 15c and 15e)		155	217
g. Copies not Distributed (See Instructions to Publishers #4 (page 83))		106	20
h. Total (Sum of 15f and g)		261	237
i. Percent Paid (15c divided by 15f times 100)		85%	71%

* If you are claiming electronic copies, go to line 16 on page 3. If you are not claiming electronic copies, skip to line 17 on page 3.

16. Electronic Copy Circulation	Average No. Copies Each Issue During Preceding 12 Months	No. Copies of Single Issue Published Nearest to Filing Date
a. Paid Electronic Copies	0	0
b. Total Paid Print Copies (Line 15c) + Paid Electronic Copies (Line 16a)	131	155
c. Total Print Distribution (Line 15f) + Paid Electronic Copies (Line 16a)	155	217
d. Percent Paid (Both Print & Electronic Copies) (16b divided by 16c × 100)	85%	71%

☒ I certify that 50% of all my distributed copies (electronic and print) are paid above a nominal price.

17. Publication of Statement of Ownership

☒ If the publication is a general publication, publication of this statement is required. Will be printed in the OCTOBER 2016 issue of this publication.

☐ Publication not required

18. Signature and Title of Editor, Publisher, Business Manager, or Owner

STEPHEN R. BUSHING - INVENTORY DISTRIBUTION CONTROL MANAGER

Date 9/18/2016

I certify that all information furnished on this form is true and complete. I understand that anyone who furnishes false or misleading information on this form or who omits material or information requested on the form may be subject to criminal sanctions (including fines and imprisonment) and/or civil sanctions (including civil penalties).

PS Form **3526**, July 2014 (Page 3 of 4) PSN: 7530-01-000-9931 PRIVACY NOTICE: See our privacy policy on www.usps.com.

PS Form **3526**, July 2014 (Page 1 of 4 (see instructions page 4)) PSN: 7530-01-000-9931 PRIVACY NOTICE: See our privacy policy on www.usps.com.

Printed and bound by CPI Group (UK) Ltd, Croydon, CR0 4YY

07/10/2024

01040505-0004